Chemical Rejuvenation of the Face

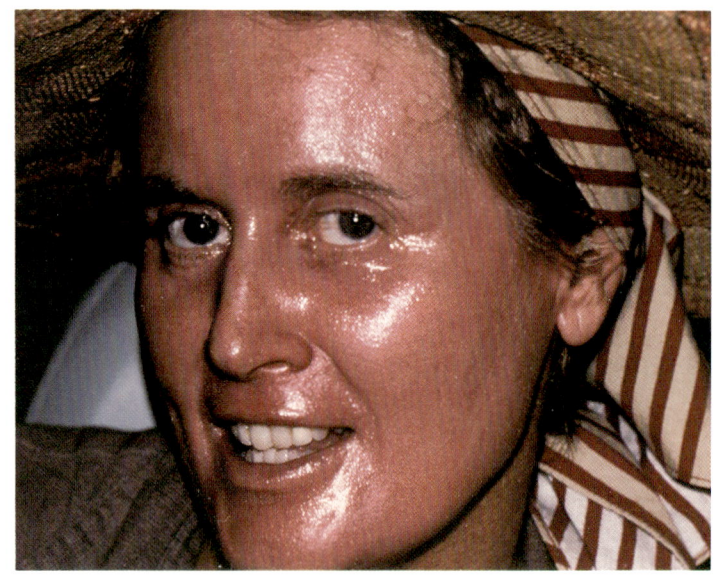

"Sunburn is very becoming—but only when it is even—one must be careful not to look like a mixed grill."

Noel Coward*

*Leonard Safir and William Safire, Good Advice, Times Books 1982

Chemical Rejuvenation
of the Face

ROBERT KOTLER, MD, FACS
Clinical Instructor
Division of Head and Neck Surgery
Department of Surgery
UCLA Center for the Health Sciences
Los Angeles, California

With Contributions by
Willard L. Marmelzat, MD
Richard G. Glogau, MD
Thomas J. Baker, MD

with 301 illustrations, including 296 4-color illustrations

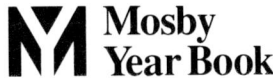

St. Louis Baltimore Boston Chicago London Philadelphia Sydney Toronto

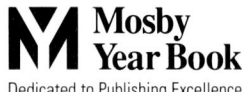

Editor: Anne S. Patterson
Assistant Editor: Maura K. Leib
Project Manager: Peggy Fagen
Designer: Elizabeth Fett
Production: Suzanne C. Fannin

The authors and publisher of this book have made every effort to provide accurate information consistent with standards of practice at the time of publication. Readers should consult other information sources, particularly concerning new or unfamiliar drugs or procedures, and give due consideration to the context of clinical situations and to new developments. The authors, editors, and publisher cannot be held responsible for typographical or other errors that may be found in this work.

Copyright © 1992 by Mosby–Year Book, Inc.
A Mosby imprint of Mosby–Year Book, Inc.

Mosby–Year Book, Inc.
11830 Westline Industrial Drive
St. Louis, Missouri 63146

All rights reserved. No part of this publication may be reproduced, stored in a retrieval system, or transmitted, in any form or by any means, electronic, mechanical, photocopying, recording, or otherwise, without prior written permission from the publisher.

Printed in the United States of America.
International Standard Book Number 0-8016-

Permission to photocopy or reproduce solely for internal or personal use is permitted for libraries or other users registered with the Copyright Clearance Center, provided that the base fee of $4.00 per chapter plus $.10 per page is paid directly to the Copyright Clearance Center, 27 Congress Street, Salem, MA 01970. This consent does not extend to other kinds of copying, such as copying for general distribution, for advertising or promotional purposes, for creating new collected works, or for resale.

92 93 94 95 96 GW/WA/WA 9 8 7 6 5 4 3 2 1

Contributors

THOMAS J. BAKER, MD
Assistant Clinical Professor of Surgery (Plastic)
Department of Surgery
University of Miami School of Medicine
Miami, Florida

RICHARD G. GLOGAU, MD
Associate Clinical Professor of Dermatology
University of California
San Francisco, California

WILLARD L. MARMELZAT, MD
Emeritus Clinical Professor of Medicine (Dermatology)
University of Southern California Medical School
Los Angeles, California;
Visiting Professor of the History of Medicine and Dermatology
Tulane University School of Medicine
New Orleans, Louisiana

> To Helaine

"Share Your Experience"

Francis L. Lederer, M.D.
Professor and Chief, Department of Otolaryngology
University of Illinois College of Medicine, 1933-1968

In Memoriam

During the preparation of the manuscript for this book, I was informed of the extremely untimely deaths of both Sam Stegman, M.D., and Ted Tromovitch, M.D. These men were pioneers and giants of dermatologic surgery. Their original laboratory studies of the histology of chemical skin peeling remain a major portion of the backbone of the basic science of this procedure. Both were deep thinkers and thorough investigators, and their input has substantially increased our pool of knowledge of exactly "what happens" during a chemical skin peeling procedure.

When the format for this book was first conceived, I asked Sam if he would contribute the chapter on the histology of chemical skin peeling and, with his usual magnanimity, he agreed. His able associate, Richard Glogau, M.D., has kindly filled Sam's very big shoes by writing that chapter, drawing on much of the work that Sam intended for inclusion.

Dermatologic surgery is now without two of its staunchest voices and most productive talents. This book is dedicated to their memory.

Preface

Since my introduction to chemical skin peeling, in 1969, as a guest in the operatorium of Richard Ariagno, M.D., of Chicago, I have been fascinated with and infatuated by the procedure. Later, as I became involved in practicing the procedure and then teaching the procedure through lectures and writings, I realized that there was a relative paucity of "step by step" illustrations—particularly in color—of the actual technique. Perhaps because the procedure had been practiced generally outside the academic community, and even by nonphysician/lay practitioners, there seemed to be less information about this procedure for the young, inexperienced practitioner than for most other procedures in cosmetic surgery.

It seemed that, in fact, much peeling was somewhat of a cult practice perfomed in rented hotel rooms or practitioners' homes and for which little documentation of technique and results existed. I realized the need for a textbook particularly strong in illustrations by which the entire process of patient selection, evaluation, treatment, aftercare, and management of complications could be portrayed.

I recalled my delight as a resident in owning a copy of the *Atlas of Otorhinolaryngology and Bronchoesophagology* authored by several of my teachers. Those professors at the University of Illinois Medical Center—Paul Holinger, M.D., Francis Lederer, M.D., and Richard Buckingham, M.D.—were convinced that students and practitioners needed to see as much as read. And yet, could one see "everything" in a relatively short practice lifetime? Certainly not. But a well-illustrated book could present several lifetimes worth of visual experience.

Remembering my delight in learning from visual example as well as written text, and drawing on my interest in medical photography, I have sought to assemble an array of photographs that best illustrated the before, during, and after of chemical skin peeling. These were needed for my own quality control efforts in my practice, as well as for teaching of other physicians in the medical community. As I developed this library of illustrations for my lectures, there came the decision to compile a detailed photographic summary of this procedure. The decision to write a textbook, after encouragement by the publisher and a colleague, Richard Bennett, M.D., was relatively easy since, in fact, the library had already been composed. My hope was that the book would allow the novice practitioner to benefit from my many years of experience and speed the route to excellence.

Excellent journal articles have been written on chemical skin peeling, and specific chapters in some textbooks are extremely helpful. But perhaps this book can somewhat fill a special role in the teaching of future practitioners of this fascinating and increasingly popular art.

ROBERT KOTLER

Acknowledgments

To my office staff, literally partners in this production, goes much appreciation for their patience, personal sacrifices, and devotion to the cause.

Suzanne Sirotkin, our practice administrator, coordinated the variety of activities necessary to bring this project to fruition. The manuscript was prepared by Barbara Passard; the bibliography by Susan McComas and Betty Campana; photo processing and cataloging was managed by Nancy Whisman, O.R.T., Monica Granados, and Felipe Rangel. Technical support was provided by Lauren Ashley Kotler and Lindsey Alexandra Kotler.

Tae-Yeun Lee, R.N., my multitalented surgical assistant of many years, in her usual efficient manner, acted as "producer and director" for the intraoperative photos. Not one photograph was taken without her aid.

Joyce Crump, Head Librarian at the Los Angeles County Medical Association Medical Library, and Beverly Garner, Medical Librarian of Century City Hospital, helped locate and retrieve many of the original references needed.

My two Mosby–Year Book editors, Eugenia Klein and Anne Patterson, kept me "on target" with grace and charm. Maura Leib, Peggy Fagen, and Liz Fett of Mosby–Year Book did a masterful job of coordinating the text, photographs, and legends, using faxes and overnight mail.

To my many gracious patients who endured "just one more photo for my peel book," thank you. Without you, there would be no textbook.

ROBERT KOTLER

Contents

Introduction Bits of History, Bits of Mystery—A Historical Review of Chemical Rejuvenation of the Face, 1
Willard L. Marmelzat

1 An Overview of Chemical Skin Peeling, 41

2 Histology of Chemical Peels, 52
Richard G. Glogau
   Historical Investigations, 53
   Clinical Correlations, 54

3 Peeling Agents, 60
   Phenol, 60
   Trichloroacetic Acid (TCA), 62
   Jessner's Solution, 64
   TCA/Jessner's Combination, 65
   TCA/CO_2, 66
   Resorcin, 67
   Alpha-Hydroxy Acids, 67

4 Indications and Patient Selection, 71
   Patch Testing, 77
   Pretreatment Use of Retinoic Acid, 81
   Consultation and Informed Consent, 81

5 Anesthesia, 96

6 The Procedure, 100
   Preoperative Preparation, 100
   Chemical Application, 101
   Occlusive Dressing Application, 114

7 Dressing Removal and Aftercare, 120
   First 48 Hours, 120
   Neck Swelling, 125
   Aftercare for the Next 4 Days, 126
   "1 Week Visit," 128
   Skin Care After Rejuvenation; Long-Term Management, 130

8 Complications, 132
   Combining Peeling with Surgery, 132
   Cardiac Arrhythmias, 134
   Atrophy, 135
   Scarring, 135
   Texture Change, 151
   Pigmentation Change/Demarcation Line, 154
   Persistent Redness/Telangiectasia, 165
   Infection, 169
   Toxic Shock Syndrome, 170
   Acneiform Dermatitis, 171
   Emergencies of Dark Nevi, 172
   Itching and Burning, 172
   Milia, 174
   Hirsutism, 175

9 Repeeling, 176

10 Neck and Chest Peels, 182

11 Facial Peeling in Men, 190

12 Technique: Step-by-Step, 198
   Preparation Before Procedure, 199
   Application of Peeling Agent and Occlusive Dressings, 200
   Mask Removal, 201
   Retaping Deeply Wrinkled Areas, 202
   Postpeel Follow-Up, 203
   Results at 5 Months, 204
   Long-Term Results, 204

A Discussion with Thomas J. Baker, M.D., 206

References, 218

Chemical Rejuvenation of the Face

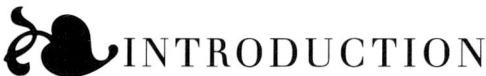INTRODUCTION

Bits of History, Bits of Mystery— A Historical Review of Chemical Rejuvenation of the Face

WILLARD L. MARMELZAT

To trace the history of any disease, medical procedure, or drug often is difficult and sometimes impossible. There are many reasons for this. No written records exist from the prehistoric period. Vast amounts of ancient medical history have been lost forever. Despite centuries of study of extant works by physicians, members of allied professions, medical historians, archeologists, iconographers, classicists, and philologists, some knowledge still lies silently undeciphered in clay tablets, dusty papyri, and unfound treasures that await the archeologists' picks.

Other problems sometimes confront the historiographer. Medical terminology is confused, making accurate interpretations and reliable drug identifications impossible. Diseases change, become milder or more severe, occasionally spontaneously disappear. Operative and medical procedures are lost, only to be rediscovered and rerediscovered many times.

We are dealing here with a manual, relatively simple, *elective* cosmetic method to improve highly visible and undesirable permanent cutaneous signs: facial wrinkles and residual facial scars that may follow ailments such as acne, smallpox, and chickenpox. Thus it would seem that our task is straightforward. But this is not so. This subject may not require dealing with poorly understood systemic diseases, but it has its own complexities; to my knowledge, a history of phenol peeling for facial rejuvenation has not previously been published.

Lest we moderns be harsh, amused, or perhaps disgusted in judging the procedures and preparations of our predecessors, we must constantly try to realize the state of medical knowledge, or lack thereof, under which physicians worked for millennia. We must always try to appreciate and to understand both the medical and social milieus and to consider the doctor in his *own time.* No easy matter. We must also constantly be beware of incorrectly attributing modern knowledge to our predecessors, knowledge that they did not have and that they could not have possessed. In John Riddle's fine phrase, we should avoid "bestowing modern medals upon ancients." Let any hubristic 1991 physician heed the words of Dr. Oliver Wendell Holmes:

> "Little of all we value here
> Wakes on the morn of its hundredth year
> Without both feeling and looking queer."

It would seem that the history of skin peeling would logically begin with the discovery of phenol in Germany as the first third of the nineteenth century ended. At this time the basic sciences, such as pathology, physiology, biochemistry, and pharmacology were in their infancy. Modern organic chemistry had begun to develop. It would be almost four more decades before bacteriology would arise from the work of Louis Pasteur and Robert Koch. Joseph Lister's surgical antisepsis with carbolic acid (phenol) soon would appear on the stage and revolutionize medicine. Modern aesthetic plastic surgery and dermatology, as we know them, developed near the end of the century.

As we shall see, during the nineteenth century the treatment of skin ravaged by time—visible wrinkles and pigmented spots—was, in general, not considered the province of the medical profession. Neither was the cosmetic treatment of acne, chickenpox, or smallpox scars. Although the general populace accepted such defects as products of aging or the prevalent diseases, the *haut monde* did not. Toward the end of the century, the upper classes flocked to cosmeticians or "beautifiers," who had an armamentarium of "wonderful" cosmetic procedures, paints, dyes, and perfumes. Vanity, ah vanity!

Vanity, however, was not new. Vanity, cosmetics, and attempts to rejuvenate aged skin had long been inseparable triplets. Where, then, should we begin our story, a story so filled with mystery and with fascinating long periods of silence? Perhaps we should go back four millennia to ancient Egypt and meet the "old man" who wanted to be transformed into a youth.[1]

When we look at the earliest historical period in sun-drenched Egypt, we learn from the medical papyri that the use of cosmetics was highly developed; unguents, pomades, creams, oils, rouges, powders, nail paints, and eye paints were valued—and not just for beautification. Oils and unguents were used, by all classes, to keep the skin supple and to maintain its elasticity and youthfulness.[2,3] This, I believe, is the first attempt to delay cutaneous aging from the desiccating rays of the Sun God.[4,5] It is both fascinating and paradoxical that the very first description in recorded history of an attempt to rejuvenate aged skin involves the male of the species and not the female.

We are grateful that some unknown scribe added an ointment recipe to the famous Edwin Smith *Surgical Papyrus,* the oldest medical document in existence. The ointment is described in *The Beginning of the Book of Transforming an Old Man into a Youth.* In a rational, professional manner, not unfamiliar to us, the scribe furnishes the recipe ingredient, a large quantity of *hemayet* fruit, about two *quar.*[6]

Then, step by step, in minute detail, the author describes the complex technique for preparing the final wrinkle-removing recipe. This consists of preparing the specified amount of the *hemayet* fruit by the following processes: progressively bruising, drying, threshing, adding water at various stages, boiling, washing in the river, test-tasting, grinding, cooking, kneading, bleaching, and removing surplus oil by dipping and sieving and placing the treated mixture in a clay-coated *hin*-jar. The final product, a paste, is placed in a costly alabaster vase.

The scribe's concluding paragraph, "Directions for Use,"[7,8] is a gem:

> "Anoint a man. It is the remover of wrinkles from the head. When the flesh is smeared therewith, it becomes a beautifier of the skin, a remover of blemishes, of all disfigurements, of all signs of age, of all weaknesses which are in the flesh. Found effective myriads of times."

Skipping approximately one and a half millennia, (to about) 300 BC, we come to sunny Greece. The ancient Greeks had inherited much medical knowledge from Egypt. This they refined and expanded. Here and there are tantalizing tidbits, such as recipes and instructions for treating wrinkles, brightening the complexion, and furnishing a youthful and robust appearance. The Greek ladies of the *haut monde* began to use overnight face masks consisting of meal that was washed off the next morning with asses' milk. Such beauty masks "guaranteed" that skin blemishes, pits, scars, and wrinkles would be removed. We know how effective this facial recipe was. Then, as now, the placebo effect frequently worked!

Over the next few centuries, we hear of facial masks made from imported mineral-rich earths that were mixed with a variety of plant substances. Subsequently, the Romans applied various types of lead. On occasion, mysterious deaths occurred.

We have now come to the first century of the Roman Empire—the height of its power. In Classical Rome, as they had in Greece, men and women increasingly were obsessed with cosmetics. The face, as well as the body, had to be free of wrinkles. Furthermore, although many Roman physicians would not hesitate to deliberately incise an abscess, we can understand why they would shy away from surgically removing acne comedones, papules, or cysts. To run the risk of iatrogenically producing scars in a common condition would not be helpful to a physician's reputation.[9]

Cleopatra VII (69-30 BC), whose very name down to this day conjures up visions of allure and beauty, wrote *Book on Beautification.* Apparently a cosmetic recipe formulary, this work was quoted by Galen and often by other Roman writers. Mention of her recipes can be found in Aretaeus (ca. 150-200 AD), in Paulus (625-690 AD), and down to the thirteenth century.

Cornelius Celsus (25 BC-25-50? AD), the great Roman encyclopedist, stated his disinterest in cosmetology[10-13]:

> "To treat pimples and spots and freckles is almost a waste of time, yet women cannot be turned away from caring for their looks.... Freckles are, in fact, ignored by most; they are nothing more than a roughened and indurated discoloration.... But pimples are best removed by the application of resin to which not less than the same amount of split alum and a little honey has been added.... Freckles are removed by resin to which a third-part of rock salt and a little honey has been added."

Pedanius Dioscorides (40?-80 AD) of Anazarbus was the foremost ancient authority on drugs. He is considered the father of modern pharmacology.[14] Dioscorides' highly original pharmacologic work, *De Materia Medica*, became the standard treatise on drugs for the next 15 or so centuries—in the East no less than in the West.[15]

Of interest is that Dioscorides mentions cosmetic remedies that removed wrinkles, gave color, cleaned the face, and made it shine. Hear Dioscorides on the virtues of almond oil[16-18]:

> "It takes away spots on the face and wrinkles [when combined] with honey, white lilly root [*Lilium candidum*] and Cyprium foot salve.

> "Bruise the leaves [of the croton plant; *Ricinis communis*, or croton oil] and put with flour for assuaging tumors and inflammations of the eye. It is good for milk-swollen breasts and it aids erysipelas. When laid on by itself or with vinegar ... an oil is made from its seed and rough berries.... It is not to be eaten but is useful ... for plasters.... it is beaten and applied to cleanse pimples *[ionthi]* and abscesses. Its leaves are bruised with flour and applied to some tumors and phlegmons ... either by itself or with vinegar."

Pliny the Elder (Caius Plinius Secundus) (23-79 AD) described here and there various tidbits of information that are cosmetically significant. For instance, he rubbed the skin with pumice, then applied ointment *(psilothrum)* or pitch *(dropax)*. He stated that among the requirements for facial beauty were a full row of white teeth, two good eyes with long dark lashes, darkened, well-shaped eyebrows that met in the midline between the eyes, and, of course, a complexion that was soft in texture and of good color.

To remove cutaneous excrescences, various combinations of frankincense, niter, myrrh, special imported salts, and resinous tree exudates were used, as well as white lead and a host of plant products. All these served to lighten the skin and remove wrinkles. Each ingredient was supposed to have its own purpose in healing blemishes, removing wrinkles, softening the skin, making it clear, and giving it good color. Oftentimes fragrances were added.

According to Pliny, Poppaea (?-65 AD), Emperor Nero's wife, originated another facial treatment, a bread dough poultice that, when soaked with asses milk, was applied to the face. The next morning it was washed off with milk. She took a herd of asses with her whenever she traveled. (We have seen that the Greek ladies had introduced a similar but simpler mask, using meal.)

The iron hand of Galen (129-210? AD), the chalcenteric polymathic Pergamene, was to grasp medicine's throat for at least 15 centuries. Galen emphatically stated that cosmetology was not a part of medicine. Then, reluctantly, because the royal ladies demanded it (he was the personal physician of Marcus Aurelius), Galen devoted many pages to reviewing the cosmetic literature, sometimes giving credit to previous writers, frequently "borrowing" large swatches of cosmetic writings from his predecessors without giving acknowledgment.[19]

The Roman satirical poets and epigrammists had a ball deriding the cosmetic craze that had swept Rome. In their jibes at Roman high-class society, Roman poets Martial, Juvenal, Horace, and many others hint at first-century cosmetic practices:

> "Is this thing which she cares for so gently really a face or an ulcer?" (Juvenal)

> "Hair you bought and teeth and rouge and wax to make you peel; you would have bought an eye as well—there wasn't one for sale." (Lucilius)

> "The face you showed the world is laid at night. Not in your bed but in your hundred rouge pots." (Martial)

> "Blackberry hued Lycoris feels delight, knowing Cerussa makes her dark face white." (Martial)

> "You try to conceal your wrinkles by the use of bean-meal. But you plaster your skin, Polla, not by my lips. Let a blemish which is small, simply show. The flaw which is hidden is deemed greater than it is." (Martial)

> "You dye your hair, but you will never dye your old age. Or smoothe out the wrinkles of your cheeks. Then don't plaster all your face with white lead so that you have not a face, but a mask; for it serves no purpose. Why are you out of your wits? Rouge and paste will never turn Hecuba into Helen!" (Dio Chrysostom)

The Greek writer Plautus has left us a dressing-room scene in which the superannuated courtesan Scapha gives instructions to her young mistress Philematium in how to use cosmetics properly:

> "Phil.: Give me the white lead.
> Sc.: What do you want it for?

Phil.: To whiten my cheeks.
Sc.: You want to whiten ivory with lamp-black!
Phil.: Then give me the rouge.
Sc.: I won't. You're pretty enough. Do you want to patch up a very pretty piece of work with more painting? Your age ought never to touch paint, white lead, or white paint, or any other such stuff.... Now those old hags who smear themselves with ointment, ancient, toothless, refurbished creatures, who try to hide their blemishes with paint, smell, when their perspiration mixes with their ointments, like a lot of different kinds of broth which a cook has poured together. You don't know what it smells of except that it smells bad."

We pass over the Byzantines. It is possible that several commentators made occasional remarks about smoothing the skin and improving the complexion. Paulus (fl. A.D. 640), the last of the great Byzantine medical compilers, does mention methods to remove wrinkles. To my knowledge, this subject in this particular period has not been studied.

We enter the Middle Ages. The harshness and diminished quality of life associated with early medieval times severely limited the use of cosmetic arts and their development. As the church more and more controlled the Christian West, the use of cosmetics in Europe declined progressively.

One instance of cosmetic revival in countries where cosmetic arts had practically ceased is illustrated by the Crusades. During their forays into the eastern Mediterranean, the crusaders rediscovered useful cosmetic materials in eastern countries and brought them home. This revived the interest in cosmetics. In these early modern centuries—from the Renaissance, indeed to the French Revolution (1789) and continuing into our times—interest in cosmetic fashions continued to rise and fall. For instance, during Elizabethan times cosmesis became very fashionable. The resurgence in popularity was not limited to women, who used both sensible and sometimes strange treatments; for instance, they applied urine (their own!) to the face. To show respect for the red-headed queen, Elizabeth I of England, or perhaps to curry favor, men dyed their beards dark red.

Elizabeth herself, to preserve the appearance of youth, took to painting lines on her face, following the outlines of the superficial veins, a practice that she convinced herself ameliorated the affects of weather and age.

During the seventeenth and eighteenth centuries, after a long decline, cosmetics again began to be used excessively. Like the Romans before them, ladies of the *haut monde* employed cloth patches to cover smallpox pits and wrinkles. They applied full-face masks and placed minute wax prostheses on their wrinkles and scars. Of course, should the Elizabethan lady become overheated for some reason, her wax prostheses would melt.[20]

It is worth noting that John Goodyer (1655) translated the famous treatise, *The Greek Herbal of Dioscorides*.[21] From 1652 to 1655 the great botanist of Petersfield had laboriously written out the entire Greek text with an interlinear English translation on 4,540 quarto pages. This was, and apparently still is, the only attempt to produce an English Dioscorides. As we have seen, Dioscorides of Anazarbus in Cilicia had been the chief source of pharmacologic knowledge for more than 15 centuries. Here are some examples of how wrinkles may have been treated in Goodyer's version of Dioscorides:

174. Chia. Chian earth.

"But of ye Chian, that which is white, & drawing to an ashy colour & that which is like to ye Samian is to be taken: but it is crusty, & white, but differing in ye forms of ye making up. But it hath ye same virtue that ye Samian hath. And it makes ye visage, and more ye whole body to be without wrinkles and clear, & in a bath it scours instead of Nitre" (p. 658).[22]

141. Phrugios Lithos. Pumice with alum

"The Phrygian stone, which ye Dyers in Phrygia use (whence also it is named) groweth in Cappadocia. That is ye best which is paler & indifferently heavy, not firm by ye compacture of ye body, having between partitions of white, like as Cadmia. But ye stone is burnt thus: having moistened it with the best wine, cover it with live coals & blow it continually; and if it change the colour being of a more deep yellow, taking it out, quench it with ye same wine, & putting it again into ye coals do ye same things, then burn it ye third time, looking to it crumble not, & vanish into soot. But both ye raw & that which is burnt, hath an effectually binding faculty, & besides a cleansing and a somewhat incrustating one, & an healing one of ambustions [burns] Cerate; & it is washed like as Cadmia is." (p. 650)[23]

An amusing, eighteenth-century method of proto–face lifting follows[24]:

"Marechal de Richelieu 'lifted' his face, since at the age of eighty this libertine still hungered madly after the pleasures of love and tried to disguise his decrepitude by a then original method. Every morning he ordered his servant to pull up the skin of his forehead and cheeks and attach the resultant folds firmly to a pad which he wore pinned on the hair of his head" (p. 102).

By mid-eighteenth century, attempts to cover cosmetic ravages caused by disease and time with such substances as lead carbonate face powders became increasingly popular. By that time it apparently was recognized that leaded face masks could lead to death. Nevertheless, their popularity continued through the nineteenth century, at times falling from favor, at other times making comebacks.

In this whirlwind flight over the premodern centuries, I have stopped at sporadic intervals to see if, by chance, any of the major figures in the immense literature used a full-face peeling procedure or formulation that would be comparable to today's effective methods. Although physicians did have some powerful caustic drugs such as croton oil, cantharides, and others, I have thus far found no evidence that they used them for cosmetic face peeling. A study of the literature of all premodern centuries would, in my opinion, take a team of scholars many years.

The heart of our story, the phenol face peel, begins with Friedlieb Ferdinand Runge, the famous German chemist. In 1834 Runge discovered carbolic acid (phenol) by mixing cresols he obtained from coal tar. He named the result carbolic acid. In 1842 the French chemist Auguste Laurent prepared phenol in a pure form from coal tar. This he named phenolic acid *(acide pheniquechemisten)*, or phenol-hydrate. Charles Frederick Gerhardt had already coined the name phenol in 1841. The first synthesis (by use of the oxidation of benzene to phenol) was done by Sterry Hunt in 1849 by using silver nitrites and aniline hydrochloride. In 1867 August Kekule prepared phenol by melting potassium benzene sulfonic acid with potassium hydrate. (Since about 1860, large-scale crystallized production has been used in industry. Phenol was not known before the coal tar industry and the coal tar chemists.) A collection of reports on phenol was presented at the 1867 Paris Exhibition.[25] (Phenol is now prepared synthetically by a recent process that utilizes chlorobenzene as the starting point.)

From the time of Robert Willan (1757-1812), the "father"[26] and generally accepted founder of modern dermatology in the beginning years of the nineteenth century, it seems there was little interest in attempting to improve facial freckles, artificial facial-staining, pockmarks, and certainly wrinkles. The dermatologists were engrossed in managing and classifying cutaneous diseases. Innovative plastic surgeons were pioneering revolutionary new techniques for far more important congenital and acquired deformities. Cosmetic removal of pits and wrinkles did not interest them. The implied consensus seemed to be that cosmetology did not belong in medicine, an opinion, incidentally, that dates back 2,000 years to Celsus and Galen.

The silence, however, was not complete. Pierre Rayer (1793-1867) was one of the century's major dermatologic figures. He addressed freckles in his masterpiece, *A Theoretical and Practical Treatise on the Diseases of the Skin.*[27] Rayer states that lentigo, more generally known under the name of *freckle,* is never made the subject of medical treatment. He differentiates lentigo lesions from those of ephelides. He recognized that freckles have a direct relation to sun exposure. He concludes by quoting Celsus: "To treat pimples and spots and freckles is almost a waste of time, yet women cannot be turned away from caring for their looks."

The French master also comments on artificial stains of the skin[28]:

> "Various substances applied to the surface of the skin stain it different colors. The females of our great cities especially, are, many of them, in the habit of using rouge, with a view to restor-

ing the brilliancy of their complexion, when wrinkles and the lapse of the years begin to abate its color and freshness.... The study of these ... practices, and the discussion of several of the species of artificial masculation of the skin, are almost foreign to the object of this work".

Rayer describes and discusses the practice of tattooing but does not treat tattoos.[29]

A generation later the scene shifts to Vienna. Enter the Viennese master dermatologist Ferdinand Hebra (1816-1880), held by some to be the "father" of modern dermatology, and a charismatic teacher who attracted students from the world over. Hebra's experimentations laid the foundation for experimental dermatology. The master's clinical teaching "was performed with a great deal of Sherlock Holmes–style showmanship that delighted the Dr. Watsons present" (Crissey and Parish).

I have found no evidence that Hebra treated wrinkles. However, he did not hesitate to treat freckles and even melasma by using exfoliative agents in various original combinations. He employed such drugs as spurge-olive, croton oil, cantharides, mustard seed, and sulfuric acid in moderate amounts. He also used stronger preparations that contained acetic, hydrochloric, and nitric acids, borax, the caustic alkalis and their carbonates, and corrosive sublimate. In addition, he noted that freckles could be removed or lightened by repeated painting with tincture of iodine and lead. He cautioned,[30] however, that

> "these methods are very troublesome and cannot be carried out in all cases.... A collyrium, whose chief constituent is corrosive sublimate, and which it is said the ladies of the seraglio employ for the removal of freckles, has long been known.... If, however, we wish to remove the pigment patches within as short a time as possible, we must make use of a concentrated solution of corrosive sublimate, five grains to the ounce of distilled water, alcohol, or collodion. In order to avoid possible inconveniences and even injury, we proceed with all due precaution...."

Hebra then describes his specific procedural methods:

"Place the patient in bed, prepare compresses closely fitting on the affected parts of the face or of the body, and, after the face, for instance, has been cleansed previously by washing with soap, the soap removed with water, and the face thoroughly dried, we apply the compresses dipped in the above-mentioned fluid, so that they are not creased, but lie firmly and smoothly. We have then to be careful that no stratum of air insinuates itself between the skin and the compresses.

"These pledgets are now carefully and continuously kept uniformly moist; for which purpose we do not now and then remove them and dip them in the fluid, but we make use of a clean dossil of charpie, by means of which we continually reapply the fluid to the pieces of lint; of course we scrupulously guard against any of the fluid going into the eye, or the nose, or the mouth, or running down the neck, because we should then destroy the epidermis in places where we had no intention of doing so. This dressing is applied uninterruptedly for four hours, during which time, therefore, the pledgets remain *in situ,* and are kept properly wet with the fluid.

"When we remove the compresses at the end of the time mentioned, in many cases the epidermis will be seen to be lifted up in large blisters; in others, the skin is merely reddened. In the first case, we prick the blister in order to let out its contents, and to keep its cover, the epidermic layer, still on the skin. Moreover, in any case in which a blister is formed, or the skin merely reddened, we strew a sufficient quantity of starch on the place affected, and then wait patiently for some days till the layer of epidermis which has been raised from its substratum has separated in the form of a brown or black crust. The newly-formed epidermis, which afterwards becomes visible, will assuredly exhibit a lighter and finer colour."

Among his multiple activities, Hebra invented topical preparations. One of them, "Hebra's ointment," stayed popular for decades. Of special interest to us is the innovative Hebra's introduction of the mull. This furnished a new topical therapeutic technique. In the popular and authoritative multiauthored *Handbuch* edited by H. von Ziemssen,[31] Hebra's eminent medical colleague, the mull[32] is described as follows:

"Unna has recommended recently a new form of medicinal substances with fats in which mull fabrics impregnated with ointment mixtures are employed as bandages for diseased parts. This method, which is constantly being improved, appears to be suited for extensive employment."

In 1866, one Arnold J. Cooley, an English pharmacist, published a book for the layman, *The Toilet in Ancient and Modern Times.*[33] Cooley tells us that the removal of old scars "is a matter of greater difficulty and time than their prevention" (p. 222). He uses tepid glycerinated, ioduretted lotion applications, gentle massage with warm iodized oils, a glycerinated solution of bichloride of mercury and warm sea-water baths. "When more immediate effects are desired, a more active line of treatment must be adopted, and with *corresponding caution*" (p. 222). He does not mention phenol.

Cooley's caveats have an amazingly modern ring:

"Methods... which grew more rapid and certain [than milder preparations], but being dangerous in non-professional hands, I have purposely omitted.... If the cautions in the text... be disregarded by the reader he will only have himself to blame.... the application of tincture of iodine, acetic acid and nitrate-solution to a very delicate skin is sometimes liable to considerable irritation.... use them only at half-strength the first time....

apply them only to a small surface of the skin at one time... never... to a large surface at one time.... try them the day before their use on the soft fleshy tissue of the fore-arm, by way of experiment" (pp. 223-224).

Cooley gives us interesting information about smallpox:

"Small-pox—'variola' of the medical profession—is a malignant, contagious disease, which, happily for society, owing to the general practice of vaccination, is now comparatively seldom met with, although, at no very remote date, it was very common and fatal in these realms. Its medical treatment, owing to the severity and danger of the disease, does not properly fall within the province of the present work. The prevention and removal of its ill effects on the personal appearance will, therefore, be alone spoken of here....

"As small-pox is still not an infrequent disease, the interest in the subject of the prevention and removal of its permanent effects on the skin continues unabated, as may be seen by the frequent inquiries about it in the popular periodicals of the day. When we recollect how many beautiful faces are disfigured by small-pox, and how many gentle and deserving beings have had their prospects in life thus blasted, it is surely important to be able to rob this fell disease of more than half its sting....

"Small-pox is not, however, a rare disease; since in this metropolis alone, about one thousand persons die annually of it. The 'lives of six to eight hundred' of these persons 'might be saved by an (efficient) Act of the legislature.'" *(Medical Times)*

Cooley presented various plans to prevent permanent skin disfiguration by smallpox pustules that result in pits and scars. He indicated that the most certain method was to exclude light and air. On the third day a facial mask in which holes were cut for the nostrils, eyes, and mouth was applied after it had been thickly coated with mercurial ointment. The procedure was repeated daily, or every other day—always by candlelight—and continued until the pustules disappeared. Another "highly spoken of" therapy was to coat the entire face with gold leaf or to apply gold-beater's skin dusted over with a dark powder such as lamp-black, or black-lead. Such procedures were intended not only to treat the pustules but also to keep the face in darkness. Mature pustules were punctured to prevent "peeling." Meanwhile, general measures were taken to keep the patient cool, such as placing the individual on a cool, hard bed in a cool, well-ventilated apartment that admitted little light, and by serving "antiseptic" cooling drinks.

Cooley's applications included tincture of iodine, acetic acid, sufficiently strong to cause erythema and some desquamation of the cuticle, silver nitrate solution, and others.

Cooley was pessimistic about treating wrinkled and loose skin. He indicated that it was an "attenuation of the cutis or true skin—they cannot be regarded as a disease of the skin; but are the result of long-continued bad health, anxiety and study and of general emaciation and old age" (pp. 224-225). He offered only measures to promote the general health and urged frequent washings with soap and warm water, followed by applications of mild cosmetic preparations, and ingesting cod liver oil. In conclusion, he said that this therapy "is all that the art can do for the purpose."

It is interesting to compare two landmark dermatologic works that were published during the decade 1871-1881: Tilbury Fox's *Skin Diseases* (1871)[34] and Henry G. Piffard's *A Treatise on the Materia Medica and Therapeutics of the Skin* (1881),[35] the latter the first dermatologic book published in America that was limited to therapy.

Fox's formulary consists of 190 compounded prescriptions. In these we find various drugs, or their precursors, that were used in twentieth century cosmetic peeling formulas: carbolic acid (phenol), borax, glycerine, cantharides, almond oil, and others. Fox never used phenol in excess of a 20% strength and for various dermatoses and dermatitides. He does not mention cosmetic facial peeling.

Piffard's book, written 10 years later, is organized as a modern textbook, which indeed it was. Of interest to us are two drugs. First is the drug oleum tiglii *(Croton tiglium)*. We know this as croton oil, an ingredient in today's phenol peeling formulas (p. 79). Piffard describes different types of inflammatory actions that occur both within the "epidermic pustule" and also the "dermic pustule," which involves the entire thickness of the skin and the tissues beneath. (Rarely, the inflammation is so severe as to result in destruction of a portion of dermic tissue with a resulting cicatrix) (pp. 79-80).

Piffard's discussion of acidum carbolicum (carbolic acid, phenol) contains the following interesting sentences:

> "If strong carbolic acid be applied to the surface of the skin, an immediate tingling and burning sensation is experienced; the spot affected becomes white, the neighboring skin displays a red areola, and the symptoms are similar to those attending the application of a powerful caustic. In the course of a few days there is exudation from the surface attacked by the acid. The irritation persists for a fortnight or three weeks." (p. 6)

Piffard goes no further. He does not discuss cosmetic use of phenol peeling in treating acne or scars from chickenpox or smallpox. Nor does he mention wrinkles.

One searches through the published medical texts during the next five decades for the mention of phenol exfoliation in cosmetically removing facial pits, scars, and wrinkles. The reward: *Silence*—a surprising, disappointing, total silence. Why?[36] There lies one of the major mysteries in this story. Possibly in some long-discontinued journal lie elusive revealing clues. If so, I have missed them.

My hunch is that at some time during the 1880s or 1890s, possibly earlier, lay operators or "beautifiers" had commenced cosmetic peeling with phenol. This is difficult to prove. For the very nature of lay medicine and the folklore of the "wise old women" has always been to transmit drug recipes and medical procedures by the *oral* tradition—father to son and mother to daughter—and to commit practically nothing to writing. Until recent decades sometimes valuable medical information entered formal medicine purely by serendipity. It is not my intention in this introductory essay to deal with the part played by nonmedical individuals in phenol peeling. This subject would take a large volume, brimming with bizarre, violent, and controversial events—indeed worthy of a lurid Hollywood scenario.[37]

In 1892, Edmund Saalfeld, a Berlin dermatologist, commenced to publish a series of articles on cosmetics in the *Therapeutisches Monatsheft*. These later appeared separately in pamphlet form. He then published a small book, *Kosmetik*, which was well received.[38] Saalfeld begins thus:

> "Only a short time has elapsed since the Art of Cosmetics has obtained recognition in medical circles. This special branch of Dermatology has indeed been left too long in the hands of quacks, and even today in many newspapers one is able to see how much mischief is done in this department. How many advertisements of remedies for a bad complexion are daily to be seen in the papers, and yet of what value are these?" (p. 1)

Saalfeld's book covered a wide range of dermatologic conditions (bad complexion—seborrhea and acne vulgaris; cornification anomalies; new vessel formations; hypertrichosis; premature alopecia; pigment anomalies; sweat secretion anomalies; and cosmetic massage) and their treatments by various means. It was translated into Dutch. A second edition was translated into English and was published by the well-known American publisher, Paul B. Hoeber.

Saalfeld's comments on wrinkles are worth quoting:

> "Creases, furrows, and wrinkles manifest themselves not only in older people, but sometimes also very early in young persons. In order to render them less conspicuous, ladies usually employ powder or paint. Not only can these inconvenient signs of age be so concealed, but they can even be banished for a short time by subcutaneous infiltration with sterilized, physiological saline solution. Perfect filling-up of the hollows, moreover, can be attained by paraffin injections [see note 39].... Should one not care to employ either this [the paraffin injections] or the saline solution . . . massage [which is described at great length] . . . trial may be made of Bier's suction glasses . . . a longish cup . . . the margin of which is covered with an indiarubber [sic] border; suction is performed for half an hour several times a day . . . by consecutive applications of this treatment . . . wrinkles become less apparent." (pp. 164-168)

Saalfeld warned against the use of elastic rubber masks, which, when closely applied during the night to the face, were supposed to smoothe the facial skin and to remove crow's-feet and wrinkles. He warned that patients place unrealistic expectations on a procedure in which furrows are smoothed out and court plaster or nonirritant plaster applied, creating a mask to be removed the next morning. He also disapproved of "enamelling" the wrinkled face, neck, and shoulders, as well as using electric gadgets on the face.

Because of the recent interest in manual massage and vibration apparatuses for beautifying purposes, Saalfeld explained in great detail how these methods were to be employed on facial furrows, folds, and wrinkles (pp. 163-167).

He quotes Hebra's method of treating freckles: "saturating a previous placed mask of linen, the mask being moistened with sublimate lotion, the blister being pricked at the lower margin with resultant collapse, the epidermic crust falling off within a week, the newly formed skin being white and pigment-free" (p. 117-118). Saalfeld states that he had never tried Hebra's method. His including it proves the lasting influence of the great Hebra.

Saalfeld recommended phenol for various reasons: for instrument sterilization, in several acne prescriptions, and as a cauterizing agent for treating warts. He also used phenol to treat hypertrichosis by dipping the needle used in electrolysis in a 3% carbolic lotion before each insertion.

Of special interest to us is his statement that when "the ephelides are not too numerous you can best remove each sort separately by limited cauterisation with pure carbolic acid" (p. 110).

The scene now shifts from Europe to the early years of twentieth-century America and to the persona of a 25-year-old neophyte, New York physician George Miller MacKee. Thus begins an almost completely American story. In 1903 MacKee had commenced experimenting and treating acne pits and scars with phenol exfoliation for cosmetic reasons. We shall meet him later when he finally published on the subject in *1952*—one half century later!

We move cross-country to San Francisco, 1917. In that year there appeared the first American article on phenol. Douglass W. Montgomery's (1859-1941) article, "Phenol," was published in the *Journal of Cutaneous Diseases*, the foremost journal of dermatology in the country.[40] Montgomery, a pioneer San Francisco dermatologist, wrote extensively, including articles on the history of dermatology.[41] His phenol article begins thus:

> "Carbolic Acid applied locally acts as a caustic, an antiseptic, an analgesic and anti-pruritic, and a decolorizer of pigmentary discoloration, such as freckles. Its caustic action may sometimes extend to being escarotic [sic], but usually attendant circumstances, *such as enclosure under a bandage* [my emphasis], must be present in order for it to do so. Carbolic acid when applied over a large surface may, by absorption, cause the constitutional symptoms of phenol poisoning." (p. 157)

In a discussion of the use of phenol as a caustic, Montgomery wrote that

"pure carbolic acid has been recommended in a great number of cutaneous diseases.... I have employed it frequently in alopecia areata, lupus erythematosus and psoriasis.... Carbolic acid is employed, painted on pure for the removal of pigmented spots on the skin such as freckles.... Some time ago, surgeons used pure carbolic acid followed by washing with alcohol, for disinfecting their hands. For the skin of many people this was too strenuous a procedure, and other antiseptics have been found equally effective and not so detrimental." (p. 158)

In an amazing passage expressed as a reflective side note, Montgomery recalled that, on one occasion,

"a Scotch woman called, expressing great delight at seeing me, and saying that in my early days of practice I had befriended her by securing her employment as a nurse. She then told me she had failed to achieve a living in San Francisco and had gone to Los Angeles, where she had been equally unfortunate. She then tried chicken ranching, which also proved a failure. After this she went to New York, where by some means she secured rooms on Fifth Avenue, and put out her shingle as a 'Beautifier'. From then on the road had been smooth 'wi' lots o' munny'.

"In a burst of confidence she divulged to me her sole remedy, carbolic acid. She painted it on, and then covered the spot with the vitelline membrane of an egg." (p. 158)

Here is another instance of occlusive procedure after phenol application—about which we have heard before and will hear many more times again in our story.

Montgomery relates another amusing aside:

"One of my first cases on beginning practice was a woman, who got an extensive and very painful ulceration of the anal opening and rectum, through being treated for hemorrhoids with phenol injections by a quack. I have never forgotten the incident, because it was very remunerative at a time when I needed sustenance." (p. 159)

Thus, in the first account of the Scottish patient, we learn that lay peelers ("beautifiers") were peeling faces with phenol way back in the 1880s. Montgomery relates that his Scottish patient had learned the technique from someone and was practicing phenol beautification on Fifth Avenue, New York, more than a decade before young Dr. MacKee began his cutaneous experiments with this particular chemical exfoliative drug. As we shall see, MacKee apparently became the first physician in America to employ phenol cosmetically on the face.

Montgomery used phenol as an antipruritic in 0.5% to 2% strength for its antiseptic and analgesic properties. His references include articles concerning fallacies regarding phenol and gangrene of the finger caused by 5% phenol ointment. Of great importance to us is that in this article Montgomery did not state whether he or other physicians had used phenol for facial peeling.

The scene shifts to Southern California. In *The Medical Journal and Record* of 1927 there appeared the following article, "Truth and Fallacies of Face Peeling and Face Lifting."[42] Its author was an almost unknown physician, H. O. Bames, a middle-aged Los Angeles plastic surgeon (1885-1963). This article, Dr. Bames' first publication, was probably the *first* article on cosmetic phenol peeling published in America and, to my knowledge, possibly the first paper on this subject published anywhere.

Hear H. O. Bames as he begins his article:

"Youth and beauty in one hour by plastic surgery. The school girl complexion restored by a face peel.

"Thus read the advertisements of the daily papers. And among the news items one finds that England's most acclaimed actress has had her face lifted and America's brightest star has had her face peeled, while among women of all classes and ages, the desire to perpetuate youthful appearance is a topic of never-ending interest." (p. 86)

Bames explains that the medical profession is interested in life conservation and health. It has never desired to be associated with anything "done merely for beauty's sake." However, the public of all classes demands this type of work (plastic surgery). Thus "arose the greatest drawback to all cosmetic work." He complains that irregular lay practitioners who "promise anything and everything" do not appreciate the risks involved. We must remember that irregular practitioners do not possess superior knowledge; they merely apply principles that have been worked out by bonafide members of the medical profession. Bames' article continues:

"Just to what extent he [the lay practitioner] will walk where the regular fears to tread will be shown in this article. The information will be a revelation to most practitioners. But for the purpose of safeguarding their patients, family physicians should be fully conversant with the *modus operandi* of the rejuvenators."

Bames writes that everyone believes that underneath the skin's surface, which ages, roughens, and shrivels, there exists a beautiful, youthful complexion. Thus, if that layer [the epidermis] could be shed, we would again appear youthful. "Thus arose the peel."

Bames describes two kinds of peels: a light peel and a deep peel. (The simplest one is sunburn: when skin shreds come off, "a good healthy skin is revealed." Frequently, however, undesirable freckles quickly follow.) Bames' light peels consist of resorcin in alcohol. He describes a technique of application with a camel's hair brush and soothing ointments. Bluish, dusky discoloration follows. The new skin is fresh and

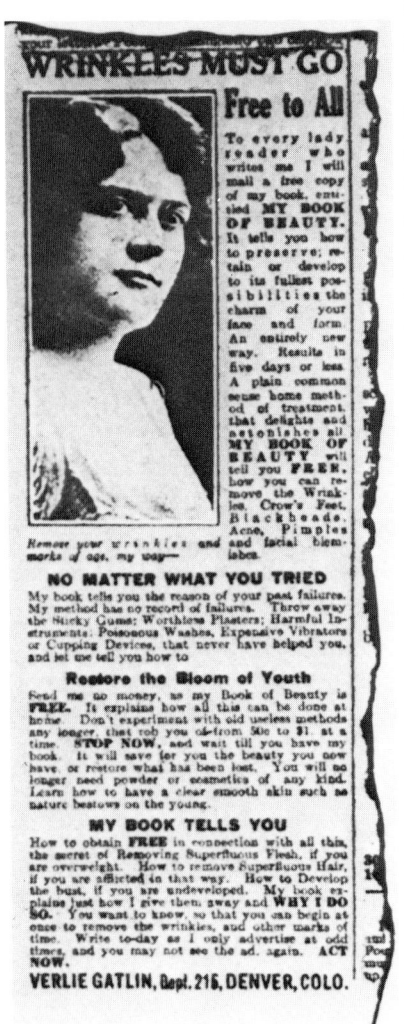

Figure 1.
(From *Nostrums and Quackery,* ed 2, Chicago, American Medical Association, 1912.)

clear, often much improved by this process. According to Bames, after the light peel (for bleaching), new freckles will not reappear, which might make the individual look younger. This light peel would not be satisfactory for wrinkles because "while it might improve the complexion it does not affect the wrinkles and lines appreciably." This will require a *deep* peel designed to take care of the marks of age.

Bames then described his procedure for the deep peel: 50% to 80% phenol (carbolic acid) is applied to half the face on the first visit, the other side treated 1 week later. Pain and numbness follow for a few minutes; alcohol stops the corrosive action of phenol. [The treated area] *"is covered airtight with adhesive plaster* [emphasis mine]." Inflammation sets in. Moderate discomfort to agonizing pain follows. Within 3 days, sloughing occurs and the plaster falls off, showing a very raw skin. "Were the treatment to stop here, we would have the same results as from the light peel, namely, a cleared complexion. But when it is desired to eliminate all wrinkles we must continue." The operator sprinkles the surface with aristol (thymol iodide) daily. When this combines with skin secretions, a hard dry crust forms. The skin shrinks and causes scar formation in the subcutaneous tissue; 5 days later, this crust comes off and soothing salve is applied. "All lines, bags and wrinkles" have been eliminated.

According to Bames, it may take 4 weeks to 3 months to treat the face and neck. For several months, the skin is tender to slight changes in temperature. Red patches appear in warm weather, purplish in cold. Bames concludes, "But finally it becomes normal again; in time it may develop so far toward normal that it will sag and wrinkle again as before; but a clear, almost parchment-like complexion may be yours for some time."

Bames mentions the dangers of face peeling:

"This is the process when everything goes well; what are the risks? 1. You may die from phenol poisoning within 24 hours; others have done it. 2. You may get chronic nephritis from delayed phenol poisoning. 3. Due to uneven contraction of the scar tissue formed you may have your mouth drawn to one side and an eyelid to the other, or sufficient scar tissue may form to destroy all expression and give you a masklike appearance. 4. The escharotic action may destroy the skin unevenly and you will have visible scars; this is particularly apt to take place in the neck, hence many 'peelers' will not 'do' the neck. 5. But you *may* come out all right. [Notice *may.*] Is it worth it? Who can answer for everybody?"

Bames definitely considered phenol peeling a part of plastic surgery:

"The woman who feels herself slipping or passé will grab after the one chance in ten of coming back. Disregarding all pain, all risk and sparing no money, and as long as she is informed that regular plastic surgery can do for her everything she had hoped to accomplish by the deep peel, and can do it with a minimum risk, and the assured outcome as to appearance, how can we blame her for grasping after the long chance of a deep peel."

Although Bames' article contains no bibliography, he makes no claim for originality. In fact, Bames gives the impression that facial rejuvenation by phenol peeling was a well-known and sought-after procedure.[43] Where did Bames obtain his knowledge and formula? Possibly during one of his European study trips after World War I (during the period 1919-1927), during which time he studied plastic and possibly aesthetic surgery with the well-known French plastic and aesthetic surgeon, A.M.L.F.E. Noel.[44,45]

The well-known Dutch dermatologist, M. K. Polano, furnishes valuable historical information about chemical peeling in a recent journal[46]:

> In the first decades of this century chemical peeling was practiced by dermatologists in Europe. In general use were a resorcinol paste of Unna (zinc paste, 40 gm, resorcinol, 40 gm, ichthammol, 10 gm, petrolatum, 10 gm) and Lassar's prescription (β-naphthol, 10 gm, sulfur, 40 gm, sapo viridis [tincture of soap], 25 gm, petrolatum, 25 gm). Resorcinol is a less irritating hydrocarbon than phenol. The indications were "rejuvenation" of a wrinkled skin with irregular pigmentation and actinic keratoses. Unna's paste was applied for three to four days. When the skin became brown and shriveled, a mask of zinc gelatin (Unna's boot) was applied. After an overnight stay, the mask, with the adherent dead skin, was removed and a smoothing application was given.

Polano adds that R. O. Stein's contribution to Jadassohn's monumental *Handbuch* revealed that chemical peeling was gradually being abandoned at that time.[47,48]

In 1941 Joseph J. Eller and Shirley Wolff published in the *Journal of the American Medical Association* what has been considered the first article on skin peeling and scarification in the United States.[49] (However, H. O. Bames' article preceded that of Eller and Wolff by 13 years.) They first discuss how the peeling procedure is performed on chloasma, marked freckling, excessive oiliness, recalcitrant cases of acne vulgaris, and rosacea, as well as its use to improve skin tone. For pitted scars from acne vulgaris, smallpox, and chickenpox, the authors used the following chemicals: salicylic acid, acetone, resorcinol, formaldehyde solution, betanaphthol, glacial acetic acid, mercurial salts, sulfur, solid carbon dioxide, and phenol. They describe one office-performed procedure in which the major exfoliating ingredient was resorcinol. (No phenol is included.) Their peeling formula contained a mixture of the following ingredients:

	Gm or cc
Resorcinol	60.00
Salicylic acid	30.00
Lactic acid	30.00
Oil of rose	0.195
Ethyl hydrate	240.00

The two phenol-containing lotions that Eller and Wolff used only for home use consisted of a mixture of the following ingredients:

Salicylic acid	6.00
Phenol	30.00
Alcohol (95%)	64.00

or

Salicylic acid	3.00
Mercury bichloride	1.50
Phenol	22.50
Alcohol (95%)	22.50

Eller and Wolff's remarks on phenol are limited to a few lines:

> "Phenol lotions are used when an intense reaction and deep peeling are desired. The number of applications will be determined by the sensitivity of the skin, and it is advisable at first to apply one coat only, to note the reaction. The number of applications should be limited to four and may be given over a period of an hour." (p. 937)

During the 1940s, phenol peeling by means of full-face application to remove acne pits and scars was being practiced by some dermatologists. However, few results were published, to my knowledge, other than Eller and Wolff's 1941 *JAMA* paper and that of Joseph C. Urkov, the next significant contributor to this story.

In the February 1946 issue of the *Illinois Medical Journal* there appeared an article that has received little attention. Its author was Joseph C. Urkov (1894-1957), a Chicago plastic surgeon.[50,51] Urkov states that the techniques and exfoliative agents presented in his study "have been used in the treatment of over two thousand treatments during a period of fifteen years" and that "in no instance has it not been possible to list the case as 'improved.'" Other than occasional transitory symptoms there had been no evidence of toxic absorption. "Considerable experimentation" was involved in the development of Urkov's techniques. His hope was that his work might provide a valued addition to the armamentarium of plastic surgeons and dermatologists.

In his techniques of "superexfoliation" for shallow pits and scars, Urkov used milder formulations that contained no phenol and performed full face peelings. Urkov employed "a rubberized adhesive tape" to occlude the entire area. This was removed by the physician 24 hours later. (Note the use of occlusive dressings once more.)

This plastic surgeon then proposed a highly unique but time-consuming and cumbersome procedure for the treatment of individual pits or depressed scars. One drop of tincture of cantharides is placed *into* the pit of the defect. When this dries in 2 to 3 minutes, a second drop is applied. The pit is sealed off with plain flexible collodion. Twenty-four hours later, the resulting blister is punctured. Then at home the patient applies zinc stearate powder for 1 week and a light liquid petrolatum the night before returning for another office visit. At this time the physician removes the crust, which reveals a reddened pit. According to Urkov, the central scarring has been removed. The old scar tissue at the pit bottom also has been removed.

One week later, pure phenol on a cotton-swab applicator, which has been moistened with a few drops of phenol, is applied to each previously treated pit. Urkov treats each pit individually. The phenol is blotted with a fan. Escharotic whitening develops. Then electrocautery is used to "plane off the edge of each pit by drawing it smoothly around the rim." The cautery is to be "not red hot but slightly less than warm." Thus the extruding rim is planed off to the level of the adjacent skin. The operator applies elastic adhesive as a dressing to each individual pit. This is removed in 24 hours. The author states that not only have the pit rims been leveled off but a growth of new healthy tissue has been provoked.

Urkov treated deep lines and wrinkles differently, omitting the use of cantharides in the aforementioned first step. In wrinkles, there is no scar tissue to be removed. Here he was not dealing with pits and scars caused by cutaneous diseases. Urkov's procedure for treating each wrinkle individually follows:

First day. Liquefied phenol is applied to each wrinkle. The wrinkle edges are cauterized. Then adhesive plaster is used as an occlusive dressing.

Second day. Plaster is removed. A mixture of phenol and alcohol, 30 drops each, is brushed over each forehead wrinkle edge. The cautery smoothes out the forehead. Plaster adhesive occlusive dressing is applied.

Third day. The face is treated with a moderate formula. However, instead of occluding the entire treated area with adhesive, the patient is instructed to occlude each treated wrinkle with individually shaped strips of adhesive plaster, designed for each wrinkle of the right and left cheek, the forehead, and the chin. These are removed the next morning. Zinc steroid powder is then applied until the next patient visit. At this time, liquid petrolatum is applied.

Seventh day. The patient returns for the final peeling of all wrinkled areas. Presumably a moderate exfoliative solution is used.

Precautions in phenol use are specific. Rarely are more than 20 to 30 drops used over each wrinkle. The phenol is never applied over a large area and never to the neck.

Urkov argues that his method offers a safe and effective alternative to the practice of face lifting. His unique report is probably the third *published* paper in America that advocated phenol as the exfoliating agent in face peeling. It may have contained the first published report of postoperative occlusion by the use of strips of adhesive tape. It is possibly also the first publication to describe phenol as part of a complicated technique designed to ablate *wrinkles.* By 1946 phenol application was "old hat" for treating pathologic scarring due to acne, chickenpox, and smallpox. George Miller MacKee had been using phenol for this purpose since 1903.

The lack of a bibliography in Urkov's article suggests the originality of his method. Yet an air of mystery remains concerning his combinations of various modalities, some hearkening back to the nineteenth century (his use of electricity and cantharides), and his treating each lesion or wrinkle individually.

There is no doubt that Urkov's methods were cumbersome and time-consuming for both physician and patient, a fact that he does not point out. (Sometimes patients were required to make seven office visits within a 2-week period.) Although his unique and unorthodox methods were briefly tried by a few dermatologists, apparently no physician adopted his techniques of treating pits, scars, and wrinkles.

In 1950 an article appeared in the *British Journal of Dermatology* by L. Winter, a Budapest surgeon.[52] Winter treated 100 patients with a "new" method of permanently removing freckles. He used 20% to 30% pure carbolic acid in ether. His procedure consisted of the application of phenol, which caused immediate but not unbearable burning. Freckles became dark brown, and slight edema was seen. He applied no dressings. Next day, more freckles became visible and surrounding skin was copper-colored. No blisters occurred. Forty-eight hours later, erythema and edema had disappeared; the skin gradually dried and shriveled until the fifth or sixth day. Then it cracked and peeled off, the freckles being removed with the scales: "Underneath a rosy, slightly bluish tint, tender skin is found like that of a new-born infant."

For 2 weeks postoperatively, "a simple, greasy application should be used on the skin and, subsequently, gradually increasing doses of ultraviolet light are suggested. As far as is known, no successful method of permanently removing the freckles has hitherto been recorded." Winter concludes that the "removal of freckles is permanent. Even in cases treated eight years previously there's been no occurrence."

Winter did not advise the use of sunscreens. In contrast, as we have just seen, he used ultraviolet-produced artificial actinic rays as part of his peeling process. This flies in the face of procedures that were being used before 1950 and of current postoperative advice to the patient.

The publication of Winter's article as a new treatment for freckle removal is difficult to understand. Freckle removal, as we have seen, was an old procedure. Yet, the article has no references. Thus its publication in a prestigious British journal is surprising. Winter employed phenol in a 20% to 30% dilution, which would increase the chance of internal absorption and the likelihood of systemic complications. One might speculate that this article might have played a part in MacKee's decision years later to finally publish in the *British Journal of Dermatology*.[53]

Enter George Miller MacKee (1878-1955). MacKee, a poor young man, was the first outstanding dermatologist to receive his entire dermatologic education in the United States. Young MacKee began to experiment with phenol application for the cosmetic improvement of acne scarring in 1903. He rose with amazing rapidity to a position of eminence. Within 6 years, at the age of 31, MacKee became the editor of the premiere

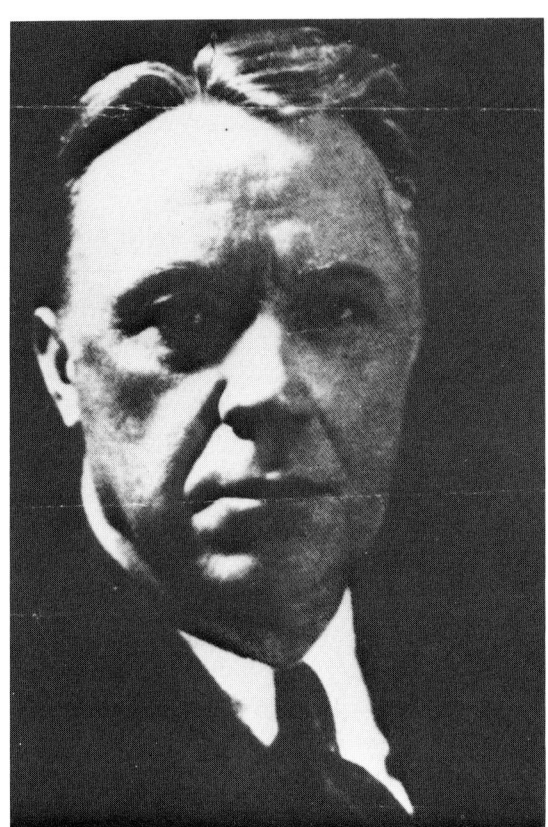

Figure 2.
George Miller MacKee, M.D.
1878-1955.

dermatologic journal in the land, the *Journal of Cutaneous Diseases*. He held this key editorial position from 1909 to 1919 (MacKee is cited more than 100 times in the 1916 volume alone!).

From 1903 until the mid 1930s, MacKee experimented with phenol, first on himself, and then performed a full-face peel on an early, nationally known office partner whose face had been badly pitted and scarred by acne. Over the years as his knowledge grew, MacKee treated carefully selected patients in his enormous private practice. From the beginning years throughout his career MacKee only peeled with pure (88%) phenol.

How back in 1903 did MacKee obtain the idea to peel the face for cosmetically improving acne scarring and pitting? Could it have spontaneously arisen in his fertile and innovative mind? Could he have known Piffard's very brief description a quarter of a century earlier of what happens when phenol is applied to the skin? (MacKee never failed to cite sources; giving full credit was his hallmark.) Could he have heard from European colleagues of this particular cosmetic technique? Or perhaps from American lay peelers and "beautifiers?" We have not yet found the answers. Perhaps we never shall.

Now come possibly the most enigmatic questions of all. Why did MacKee wait almost half a century (until 1952, 5 years into his retirement) to publish his initial and only paper on the topical application of phenol? Why did this distinguished author, who had for decades served with distinction on the editorial boards of the *three* foremost American dermatologic journals, choose to publish in the *British Journal of Derma-*

tology? Less puzzling is that he should choose to publish with a co-author whom he had known for years, a cherished associate whom we are soon to meet.

An attempt to offer speculative answers provokes many possibilities. MacKee was an internationally respected dermatologist and teacher with an unsullied reputation. For decades, quackish lay operators had been operating in the New York vicinity. Horrible results from phenol peeling had led to lawsuits against the ill-trained, commercially driven lay operators. Their scandalous activities had even been reported in the national media. Reputable physicians would have wanted to distance themselves from any association with the activities of lay peelers.

Another reason why MacKee may not have published on phenol peeling earlier was that compared with the important research and multiple publications with which he was constantly involved, phenol peeling was not of comparable significance. One might also speculate that during World War I, the Great Depression, and World War II, economic factors may have adversely affected the public's interest in cosmetic procedures. Numerous East Coast dermatologists whom I have interviewed concerning MacKee's reluctance to publish on phenol peeling agree with my speculations.

MacKee's seminal 1952 paper, the initial publication of his results, will be discussed shortly.

In 1936 a frail, charming, 51-year-old Parisian émigré arrived in New York City. Thus the totally forgotten lady dermatologist, Florentine L. Karp (1885-1987), enters our phenol story.

This physician's modest manner and retiring personality belied her earlier adventurous life. Born in St. Petersburg, Czarist Russia, the young Karp had obtained her medical education at the Faculté de Médicine de l'Université de Genève, Geneva, Switzerland, graduating in 1911. Returning to Czarist Russia, she commenced working as a general practitioner on the Tashkent railway and remained in Russia during much of the Bolshevik Civil War. Her railroad position enabled her to escape, eventually arriving by a long circuitous route in Paris in 1921 or 1922.

France during that period was very chauvinistic vis-à-vis female physicians, no matter their credentials. We do not know at what institutions Karp obtained her specialized knowledge of cutaneous diseases. But this she did. She maintained a practice in her home, and this was possibly where she developed unique formulas that in 1936 she brought with her to the United States.

While serving a mandatory internship at the New York House of Detention for Women, Dr. Karp met Dr. MacKee. Greatly impressed by Karp, MacKee immediately invited her to work in his office and arranged her appointment to the venerable and famed New York Skin and Cancer Hospital where he had been chairman for more than a decade. Almost certainly their mutual interest in chemical face peeling for acne pits and scars played a significant part in their friendship. MacKee and Karp became close professional colleagues and warm friends until the day MacKee died 19 years later (1955). Under MacKee's chairmanship a special phenol peeling clinic was established at the New York Skin and Cancer Hospital sometime in the early or mid-1940s. Karp was in charge. For some years, probably into the early 1950s, she gave detailed lectures and precise demonstrations of the phenol peeling technique to successive classes of "matriculates," as postgraduate students were called at this postgraduate dermatologic institution.

Over the years a number of future dermatologists became familiar with this peeling process. Anyone who was seriously interested was readily welcomed to observe and then to assist in Karp's weekly phenol clinic. Here this gentle woman in her quaint Russo-French accent expertly taught the art of facial peeling.

Although Karp published original papers on other subjects, why did she not publish anything on phenol peeling until 1952 and then as a junior co-author of MacKee? Probably for the same reasons that her chief chose not to do so.

MacKee was a man who well deserved the loyalty he enjoyed. His loyalty to most of his associates for over half a century is legendary. No one was more loyal than Karp, the unknown dermatologist to whom MacKee had given a dermatologic home—just as he opened the doors of the New York Skin and Cancer Hospital to many displaced dermatologist colleagues from the Third Reich.

Now we come to the classic 1952 publication in the *British Journal of Dermatology and Syphilology* by George Miller MacKee and Florentine Karp.[54] Consisting of but 3½ pages, the authors' report is a model of conciseness. The first three sentences confirm my earlier statements that MacKee had started to use phenol applications cosmetically almost one-half century previously:

> "Although no method has yet been devised that will eradicate post-acne scars, there are a number of procedures that may effect improvement. Of these phenol has given us the best results. (One of us—G. M. M.—has been using it for this purpose since 1903.)"

In this article MacKee and Karp emphasize that they carefully selected their patients and give determining caveats. They avoided treating black or dark-skinned patients because of the possibility of depigmentation, but they said ordinary "brunettes" were candidates for the procedure. They used this procedure for treating only patients with acne, and rejected those with allergy to phenol or coal tar, and those with constitutional diseases (nephritis, severe anemia, tuberculosis, or diabetes). They were cautious with patients who had had x-ray treatment.

Key excerpts (the order of presentation is slightly revised) from MacKee and Karp's article follow:

> "We employ phenol liquefactum U. S. P. [as the sole peeling agent].... immediate severe buring sensation [occurs] which lasts about 45 seconds.... the skin assumes a milk white color.... [Numbness occurs]... about 10 minutes [later].... burning sensation returns... for about 45 minutes.... it may be 60 to 90 minutes before... complete comfort. Thereafter there is

no pain ... only a tight dry feeling for the next 5 or 6 days....
Procaine hydrochloride injections mitigate pain, but most patients prefer the pain to multiple injections. Occasionally, demerol hydrochloride or morphine derivative is necessary.

"When phenol is applied there is almost immediate coagulation of albumen, which apparently prevents penetration and absorption. Preoperatively and postoperatively in a number of patients, urine testing, blood chemistry, and phenol evaluations were done. Essentially, results were negative. Slightly increased conjugated phenols of low toxicity were occasionally found. Such occasional elevated phenol determinations might be caused in various ways, one of which may be a breakdown of coagulated proteins of the skin."

In specific detail, the authors describe their technique: soap and water cleansing of the face, castor oil instillation to protect the eyes. Each cheek, the chin, and the forehead should be painted with the phenol solution as rapidly as possible. After 30 to 60 seconds, 95% alcohol is applied. Successive skin changes occur, white to gray-brown and finally to red. Moderate edema may occur, lasting for 5 or 6 days, but never vesiculation, bleeding, or exudation.

The postoperative directions to the patients were to stay indoors until exfoliation is complete. Five or 6 days postoperatively, they were to apply warm mineral oil for 2 hours, then steam the face for 2 hours with hot towels. The crusted skin exfoliated in large flakes, thus leaving the skin smooth and pink. Intraderm tyrothricin or a similar remedy was applied twice daily for 2 weeks. For 1 month, avoidance of direct or reflected sunlight exposure and application of a sun-protective cream or lotion were prescribed.

MacKee and Karp's results were successful. They had treated 112 patients with a total of 540 treatments over a 10-year period: "Many private patients, who received the phenol treatment years ago, have been seen by the senior author [MacKee] 10 to 30 years later." Their phenol procedure had not caused phenol allergy, sensitization, or any permanent poor results, keloids, ulceration, sloughing or infection, atrophy, hypertrophy, wrinkling, hyperkeratosis, or epithelioma. "Every patient shows definite improvement. Most patients were improved 80 percent."

The first two sentences of the authors' section on histopathology are important and revealing:

"Microscopical examinations were made one half-hour to two months after mild and strong applications. The two photographs show the results of one such study."

This passage indicates how thoroughly the authors followed the healing process histopathologically at different intervals after phenol application. It also reveals their courage, spirit of inquiry, and experimental uniqueness, in that they had performed similar histopathologic studies in more than one patient. Two photomicrographs show a male patient from whom a biopsy specimen had been obtained from the upper right portion of the back 1 month after his having had six monthly phenol applications. Who after all, physician or patient, would want a biopsy specimen taken from the face after it had been cosmetically treated? These two photomicrographs are highly significant for several reasons. To my knowledge, they represent the *first* such attempt to correlate histopathologic changes with the clinical findings of patients who have undergone phenolic peeling; second, I believe that these comparative microscopic studies are historically important. They illustrate the necessity of *control* in scientific experimentation—the very hallmark of modern scientific inquiry.

The authors describe their slide representing posttreatment microscopic changes:

> "The epidermis is flattened with obliteration of many rete pegs and papillary bodies. It is slightly thickened. The horny layer is thin and composed of loose lamellae. The granular layer has from two to four rows of cells. The basal cell layer is well defined. *The collagen bundles in the dermis are much denser and more compact than normal and are arranged more nearly parallel to the epidermis, especially in the upper corium* [my emphasis]. There are many scattered fibroblasts, particularly in the upper, and to a less extent, in the mid-corium ... numerous small, thin-walled, dilated vessels in the upper and mid-cutis.... The capillaries of the sub-epidermal zone are very small and sparse.... there were no follicles or sebaceous glands.... The fine elastic fibres of the upper corium are absent. The coarser fibres of the mid and deep corium are present and, apart from some fragmentation, reveal no abnormalities."

MacKee and Karp's "Explanation of Results" displays their depth of insight:

> "A combination of several factors may be responsible for the improvement. One factor may be an inherent quality that favours maximum response. Another may be improved circulation and physiological activity effected by the inflammation. A third factor may be the exfoliation, which is presumably most pronounced at the margins of the pits. It is probable that the principal factor is the change in the true skin, consisting mainly of collagen hyperplasia and a more *horizontal arrangement of the collagen bundles* [my emphasis]. This may cause elevation of the floor of the pits. However, more experimentation is necessary before the question can be answered with complete satisfaction."

It might be of interest to mention my brief acquaintance with Dr. MacKee during 1948-1949 and closer professional relationship with Dr. Karp when I was concluding my dermatologic training at the New York Skin and Cancer Hospital. At that time, it was my privilege to serve as Karp's assistant in the phenol peeling clinic. It was my impression that Karp may have been experimenting with different peeling formulas in her private practice. MacKee had always employed pure phenol as his peeling agent. He continued to use this solution, which he never varied during his entire career. In the clinic Karp also used plain phenol primarily but on occasion used other preparations.

The following excerpts are taken from my notes at that time:

Phenol treatment of acne scarring

Formula 1	Phenol 88% liquefied	
Formula 2	Phenol crystals	80 parts
	Glycerine	10 parts
	Water	10 parts
Formula 3	Acetic acid	
	Boracic acid	
	Salicylic acid	
	Glycerine	āa 15.00
	Citric acid	1.625
	Phenol 88% liquefied	qs 480.00

CAVE (Latin, "beware"): Use Formula 3 with great caution. This is a much stronger keratolytic preparation. Use *only* in very deep scarring. It should be applied around the scars and never uniformly applied over the entire face. Only Formula 1 and 2 are to be applied over the entire face. Obtain careful history, especially as to whether patient has had atopy, kidney, liver, heart disease, or any other serious disease. Determine phenol level in urine before the procedure and 24 hours after the treatment.

Procedure 1: Face to be washed with soap and water or benzene.
Procedure 2: Place a few drops of castor oil in patient's eyes to protect them from phenol vapors.
Procedure 3: Apply Formula 2 on a cotton swab. Numbness appears and the entire treated area turns white. Approach as near as possible to the eye. Take cotton ball moistened with 95 percent alcohol to remove excess phenol. If the forehead has no scars, apply the phenol solution very lightly. White color lasts for about 10 minutes, then turns brownish. At this time, severe pain often occurs, coming and going from 45 seconds to two hours.
Procedure 4: Using cotton balls, cover the face with a thick coat of talcum powder.
Post-operative patient instructions for home use: Apply talcum powder q.i.d. for six days. On seventh day, apply warm mineral oil for two hours. Remove with hot Turkish towels. Entire crusted skin falls off in pieces. Patient must stay indoors for one week. No sunshine or wind. Do not wash face at all. Patient may shave. Apply talcum powder.
Return to clinic for second visit.

This procedure can be repeated every eight weeks for about four treatments, perhaps more."

In Karp's phenol clinic during the years 1948-1949, we had noticed, in passing, that fine rhytides improved and also that freckles and various benign keratotic lesions were ablated by phenol peeling. However, no patient was selected and treated with phenol for these problems. In almost every case the sole criterion for selection for cosmetic phenol peeling was that the patient suffered from disfiguring acne pitting and scarring. A few cases of chickenpox scarring and one case of smallpox scarring were treated. (When MacKee and Karp later published in 1952, they made no mention of wrinkle improvement or that freckles or other superficial benign cutaneous lesions could be ablated in patients with pitted skin who underwent phenol exfoliation.)

Although essentially similar, the technique taught in Karp's clinic varied in certain details from that presented in the 1952 article co-authored with MacKee, which, in my opinion, did not present some of Karp's ideas. For instance, the article does not note Karp's 1948-1949 final procedure (the aforementioned procedural step 4) of using cotton balls to cover the face with a thick coat of talcum powder, although the patient is advised to dust with talc frequently during the first 6 days after peeling.

Could the practice followed in the clinic of applying a generous coating of talc as a postoperative "dressing" and the patient's "frequent" dusting during recovery at home be considered to have served an *occlusive* function? If so, was it a forerunner of the modern technique of occlusion by adhesive taping? The controversy—occlusive versus open postoperative dressings—after phenol chemexfoliation continues to be debated in the contemporary literature.

Karp specifically used procaine hydrochloride with adrenaline in her clinic. The co-authored article mentions plain procaine. Karp's Formula 3, employing five drugs in addition to 88% phenol, and its manner of use also does not appear in the 1952 article. In the clinic she also used Burow's solution and cold cream as part of the postoperative care. Although these differences may be minor, lesser points have been debated in the subsequent literature. The answers remain part of a minor mystery in our story.

Karp developed another formula, evidently after 1948. To my knowledge, it was never used in the phenol peeling clinic. She named this peeling preparation the *Phoenix Formula*.[55] Apparently this preparation became her formula of choice. Various dermatologists referred their scarred patients to her for the peeling procedure. The *Phoenix Formula* consisted of the following:

	Gm or cc
Acid citric	0.3
Sodium salicylate	1.0
Glycerine	2.0
Water	1.0
Phenol crystals	30.0

Proper preparation required a specific technique devised by Marcus Ross, a talented pharmacist with a special interest in preparing difficult and unique dermatologic prescriptions for many East Coast dermatologists.

Karp successfully practiced dermatology until her one hundredth birthday because her loving patients refused to let her retire. She died at the age of 102 (December 17, 1987), about 1 year before I commenced this historical study.[56]

In 1953 Abner Kurtin's article, "Corrective Surgical Planing of the Skin," was published.[57] Dermabrasion, as the procedure is now known, took dermatology and plastic surgery by storm. This was a better way to improve acne pits and scars. Actually, Kurtin reintroduced Ernst Kromayer's dermabrasion procedure, which Kromayer had introduced into medicine in Germany in 1905.[58]

Kromayer used motor-driven rotary steel burrs to remove tattoos or acne scars by skin abrasion. He later described his techniques in *Cosmetic Treatment of Skin Complaints* (1930).[59] Of interest is that Kromayer did not consider skin abrasion as a method for removing wrinkles. Subsequent investigations since that time have confirmed the superiority of phenol applications for ablating fine wrinkling. Why had no one since 1903 (or 1930) employed Kromayer's mechanical abrasive technique until Kurtin reintroduced it decades later? Another mystery.

Between 1954 and 1960 the literature on phenol application is sparse at best while dermabrasion became more and more the preferred procedure for acne scar removal. The history of dermabrasion and its predecessors—sanding techniques—does not concern us here. After the 1952 MacKee-Karp publication, I found no American publications on phenol peeling for the rest of the decade. Dermabrasion had largely displaced it.

(It had been agreed in the late 1950s that phenol was a better procedure for rejuvenating the skin by removing wrinkles, whereas dermabrasion was a better method for removing pits and scars. This is generally agreed upon today.)

Then, as the sixth decade of the twentieth century dawned, at least one group of American dermatologists continued to prefer phenol peeling over dermabrasion. In a 1960 article, "Dermal Defects: Treatment by a Chemical Agent,"[60] physicians Frank C. Combes, Perry A. Sperber, and Milton Reisch argued that chemical peeling, especially the use of liquid phenol to improve skin texture and to remove minor blemishes, is more effective than mechanical dermabrasion in the treatment of acne scarring:

> "Mechanical dermabrasion done over a wide area of the face frequently causes a dead-pan appearance. Although it has been practiced for the past 50 years, recent improvements in technique have not completely achieved the desired results and the method still does not contribute anything to skin texture.... Therefore, for a number of years, we sought some chemical exfoliation of the skin which would *actually improve its texture* [my emphasis] as well as remove minor blemishes."

The authors had tried Urkov's method of controlled exfoliation and found the procedure "to be troublesome and tedious, though apparently effective." They had been impressed by the method of MacKee and Karp, who used liquefied phenol with satisfactory results. Combes and colleagues proposed a phenol that was neutralized with water or with a hydroalcoholic solution. The resulting material, which they termed *BDC*, was a solution containing 85% phenol, specially buffered to reduce its irritating qualities so that its use as an exfoliant was accompanied by only little discomfort. This was an exfoliant that when applied was only slightly uncomfortable.

According to the authors, a different reaction occurred when it was placed on the skin. The resulting swelling and crust formation separated in about 8 days. In contrast, the crust produced by liquified phenol (which had been used by MacKee and Karp) took 2 weeks to separate. According to Combes and co-workers:

> "The method is used for all types of atrophic and hypertrophic scars and pits (except keloids), acne vulgaris and conglobata, benign keratoses, comedones, milia, patulous pilosebaceous follicles, chloasma, simple freckles, adventitious pigmentation, facial dermoptosis, oculolateral folds, some superficial telangiectases and pigmented nevi. *It improves the general texture of the skin and above all tightens facial contours*" [my emphasis].

The authors apparently had treated at least 105 patients. They performed blood and liver function tests, as well as urinalyses, 24 hours before and after treatments. They conclude that

> "the improvement may persist for years and if it should ever be necessary to repeat the procedure it may be done when indicated.... In many patients there was a distinct personality change for the better following improvement of the skin."

Meanwhile, how had plastic surgeons been treating wrinkles during the first half of the twentieth century? Preliminary work had begun just before the turn of the century. As stated previously, the use of paraffin was introduced by Robert Gersuny of Vienna for this purpose in 1899[61] and had produced spectacular results. Within a few years harmful effects caused the medical profession to abandon paraffin use.[62]

Attention then turned to the surgical removal of wrinkles. Erich Lexer operated for this condition as early as 1906, but the first reported case was that of Hollander in 1912. Raymond Passot (1919) and Jacques Joseph (1921) also devised improved operations for the elimination of wrinkles. Further modified techniques were reported by A.M.L.F.E. Noel, R. O. Stein, Ernest Eitner, H. Deselaro, Ernst Kromayer, and others.[63]

During the first quarter of the twentieth century, plastic surgeons differed as to whether wrinkles should be treated by surgical operations. Some surgeons refused to operate on wrinkles under any circumstances. They believed that skin wrinkling, like hair graying, comes normally with aging and that operative intervention merely panders to the patient's vanity and is not justifiable.

Other plastic surgeons, however, thought differently: that for the patient's economic future and for psychiatric reasons, especially when wrinkling occurs prematurely, such as that following radiotherapy, surgical removal of wrinkling was often an indicated procedure.

In this connection, Harold D. Gillies, the noted British plastic surgeon—later knighted for his pioneer contributions to plastic surgery—stated in 1935[64]:

> "The desire to look young and attractive is no prerogative of any one class. The world is made up of a penn'worth of all sorts, and

it is not everybody's good fortune to grow more graceful and beautiful in advancing age. The operations for removal of eyelid wrinkles, cheek folds, and fat in the neck, are justifiable if the patients are chosen with honest discrimination."

In a delightfully reminiscent book that Gillies co-authored in 1957 with a favorite protegé and friend, the noted American plastic surgeon D. R. Millard, Jr., there is a brief mention of the treatment of acne scars by face lifting[65]:

"The deforming pits of acne and smallpox scarring can be somewhat improved by the face lifting procedure. This type of skin usually has a premature laxity. If the face is undermined close to the skin so that the individual pits can be stretched and the skin is put on tension, there is a great reduction in the dark spotty effect of the pitting."

Following this, Gillies and Millard devote four lines to sanding:

"If the pitted areas are first sanded down to a "furry" dermal base to flatten the mounds and scarify the bottom of the pits, as suggested by Iverson and McEvitt, then a later face lift will further increase the tone and smoothness." (p. 401)

For pouches below the eyes, they use *acid treatment*:

"A slight laxity of a lid is often benefited by a first-degree burn. Pure carbolic acid is painted on the lid and covered by adhesive strapping for cover and support. Its removal carries away the superficial epidermal slough. It is the aim to burn the skin just enough to achieve some tightening but not enough to produce a redness." (p. 403)

On the basis of Gillies' postoperative adhesive strapping of phenol-treated sagging eyelids for cover and support, it is believed by many contemporary plastic surgeons and dermatologists that Gillies was the first to occlude a phenolized area with adhesive strapping. However, this assignment of priority is a debatable conclusion.[66]

In 1960, Adolph M. Brown, a plastic surgeon, Leo M. Kaplan, a pathologist, and Marthae E. Brown, a dermatologist, also published an important study, "Phenol-Induced Histological Skin Changes: Hazards, Technique, and Uses,"[67] which is excerpted here:

"Although exfoliation or peeling is an accepted practice in dermatology, the method has not been too widely employed because the usual exfoliative agents have not lent themselves to a standardized technique and the results have often been unsatisfactory, unpredictable, and erratic.... Among the strong chemicals, phenol solutions are most commonly used to produce intense reaction and deep peeling, especially in treating pitted scars, pigmentations, and certain facial blemishes such as chloasma, rosacea, and xanthelasma. They have also been used in attempts to eradicate rhitides. Recently public and professional curiosity... has been aroused because their use by laymen ignorant of their toxicology and careless of the consequences has attracted attention. Lay operators... have set themselves up as being able to rejuvenate the face by one of the more dangerous of the phenols, carbolic acid.... Physicians used to be more familiar with the effects of skin absorption of phenol than they are now.... Our own work with phenols and phenol derivatives indicates that if their action is properly understood, they can be controlled to produce useful cosmetic effects safely....

"We feel [that the peeling] process can be effective over the entire face and it partially ablates intrinsic, fine rhitides. This cannot be said of dermabrasion or face peeling, the other two cosmetic procedures for smoothing facial skin.... When a properly controlled phenol solution is applied with [their] technique, the skin not only exfoliates but seems to retract slightly and to condense in cubic and surface area."

Brown and colleagues present one photomicrograph that shows the pathologic differences before and after peeling. They planned to pursue the action of phenols on experimental animals and human subjects and describe in detail histologic changes that may be regarded as permanent. In their procedure a sensitivity test is performed in order to design an effective and safe phenol solution. A typical solution is composed of phenol, saponated solution of cresol, sesame oil, and distilled water. Areas approximately 1 cm in diameter just in front of the upper portion of the ears are tested. Then they are covered with a small strip of plastic, vapor-resistant, adhesive tape, which is removed in 48 hours. During the two-step procedure on human beings, ordinary adhesive tape will not suffice, and the authors find rubber facial masks more effective:

"[These masks]... fit every contour on the patient's face.... We have used positive facial impressions in plaster of Paris, the positive impression is coated with several layers of a latex solution with gauze strips for extra strength. Slits for the orifices are cut, the mask bandaged to the patient's head with an elastic bandage to hold it snugly against the facial skin."

Enter Thomas J. Baker and Howard L. Gordon, who established the modern procedure of cosmetic phenol peeling early in the 1960s. After they experimented extensively, Baker's initial report appeared in the *Journal of the Florida Medical Association* in 1961.[68] Their formulation consisted of the following:

Phenol	5 cc
Distilled water	4 cc
Croton oil	3 drops
Septisol	5 drops

As the final step in their procedure, Baker opted to occlude all treated areas with strips of adhesive tape.[69]

Subsequently, Baker and Gordon published a number of papers, book chapters, and a text on the subject, including slight modifications of this formula.[70] Their modified formula, remarkable in its simplicity, was adopted by large numbers of plastic surgeons and dermatologists. Over the years, Baker and Gordon's formula and technique have maintained their popularity.

Shortly after this 1961 article, numerous authors debated changes in the procedure. Important contributors such as Samuel Ayres, III, C. Litton, P. A. Sperber, B. G. Gross, M. Spira, and many others made significant contributions to the literature.[71] Some physicians preferred formulas other than Baker's. A few, concerned with the possibility of phenol absorption, preferred face peeling with strong trichloracetic acid or omitting occlusion after phenol peeling. Conflicting views on whether phenol-treated areas should be occluded or not were debated in the ensuing literature. They still are.

In retrospect I think it fair to state that in large measure Thomas Baker and Howard Gordon's work during the 1960s provided the stimulus for the phenol technique to emerge from semiobscurity and take its rightful place as a respectable and valued procedure in aesthetic surgery.

In this essay I have tried to trace the story of cosmetic rejuvenation from the Egyptian papyri of 2000 BC until the present, a span of four millenia. With few signposts to guide me, I have tried to provide some answers to some mysteries and silences in this enigmatic tale. At times I fear that I have raised almost as many questions as I have furnished tentative answers. Is that not usually the way with history?

This presentation does not pretend to completeness. The contributions of some important civilizations, both Old World and New World, are not mentioned. I feel sure that I have missed or slighted some worthy individual contributors. I can only plead that I find myself in good company. So, I say with Plato, "As it is the commendation of a good huntsman to find game in a wide wood, so it is no imputation if he hath not caught it all."

SUGGESTED READINGS

These sources are intended for the English-speaking reader who is interested in Egyptian and ancient drug lore.

Estes JW: *The medical skills of Ancient Egypt*, Canton, Mass, 1989, Science History Publications USA.

Forbes RJ: Studies in ancient technology, vol 3, Leiden, The Netherlands, 1955, E. J. Brill.

Leake CD: *The old Egyptian medical papyri*, Lawrence, Kan, 1952. A pioneer contribution of the late Chauncey D. Leake, eminent pharmacology teacher, researcher, and medical historian.

For a brief survey on the history of cosmetology, see Parish LC and Crissey JT: Cosmetics: a historical review. In Abramovitz W, editor: *Clinics in dermatology—cosmetic dermatology*, Philadelphia, 1988, JB Lippincott.

Riddle JM: *Dioscorides on pharmacy and medicine*, Austin, 1985, University of Texas Press.

John Scarborough's numerous detailed and heavily referenced papers on ancient drugs cover a huge and varied span of ancient drug history: Greece (Theophrastus [third century BC], Nicander [second century BC]), ancient drug trade routes, specialized studies of various individual drugs, such as aloe, and Roman pharmacology and that of Early Byzantium. See especially Scarborough J: Criton, physician of Trajan: historian and pharmacist. In Eadie J and Ober J, editors: *Festschrift Chester Starr*, Washington, DC, 1985, University Press of America.

Von Staden H: *Herophilus, the art of medicine in early Alexandria*, Cambridge, UK, 1989, Cambridge University Press.

NOTES

1. The idea has prevailed down through the centuries that it is the female half of the human race that has been greatly concerned, if not obsessed, by its loss of youthful appearance. Conventional opinion holds that cosmetology probably began when the first prehistoric women walked the earth 3½ million or so years ago; that as civilization developed it was the female species who almost exclusively used cosmetics to attract lovers and mates, to hide or disguise the effects of advancing age, and to compensate for external visible defects.

    I would like to argue a different view. To my knowledge there is no archeologic, iconographic, or, of course, textual evidence that prehistoric humankind recognized and treated aging skin or skin scarred by natural diseases. (I exclude such religious and magico-superstitious cosmetic practices as tattooing, face painting to intimidate spirits, and ritual skin deforming.) For millions of years hominids followed a hunting and gathering existence. About 10,000 to 8,000 BC, human beings abandoned that societal pattern and settled down into villages. They took up farming and domesticating animals. An entirely new set of social values evolved—values that are vital to our story. Society changed drastically. For the first time social classes arose, with marked distinctions between them. Both sexes must have been involved. Laws regarding land, ownership, and particularly such matters as the rights of legal succession arose. With laws came conflicts. At this time, in various ways cosmetics and beautification procedures must have become closely associated with class structure. In my view, attempting to disguise or correct the signs of aging could have become important in political succession. Usually the masculine or feminine reigning leaders did not like to relinquish power. Those in power must have used almost any available cosmetologic drug recipe, subterfuge, or procedure to obfuscate the keenly observant eyes of impatient, eager, would-be successors. Déjà vu?

2. A study of the earliest medical books of the ancient Egyptians, especially the Smith surgical papyrus, the Ebers papyrus, and the Hearst papyrus, reveals a striking number of available topical drugs used both as simple or as compound preparations. Many were used or could have been used as beautifying creams, ointments, plasters, astringents, rubefacients, mechanical abrasives, therapeutic earths, and clays for clearing disfiguring skin lesions. Even a partial list is formidable. The various plant, mineral, and animal substances include alabaster powder (calcite), alum, aloe, arsenic salts, barley, bean meal, bran, beeswax, mustard, and beetles (*Cantharis vesicatoria*). There are also kaolin and earths containing various potent chemicals: copper salts, arsenic salts, antimony, lead oxides, salt (red salt in particular [*sodium carbonate*], an external rubefacient), and calamine. Plant and animal topical drugs include castor oil and seeds, onion and leek, honey, myrrh, and milk and fat from a variety of animals, some favored more than others.

    I wish to acknowledge the debt owed to the pharmacologist-medical historian, J. Worth Estes, for his chemical identification of the ancient Egyptian drugs and for determining their pharmacodynamic action.

3. *The Papyrus Ebers, the greatest Egyptian medical document*, Copenhagen, 1937, Levin & Munksgaard (Translated by B. Ebbell).

4. A full treatment of ancient cosmetology would necessarily include the contributions of the great Eastern civilizations, such as ancient India, China, and Persia, peoples of the Bible, and ancient inhabitants of the New World. I plan to address these in another study on ancient cosmetology, which is in progress. I am indebted to John M. Riddle, Wesley D. Smith, and Dale C. Smith, who furnished material for my ongoing studies in this field.

5. The Egyptians of the Ebers papyrus recognized that there are two skin layers, a superficial one and a deeper "leather" layer. Further, they also knew that beneath the "leather" layer (the dermis), there lies a loose subcutaneous layer.

6. *Hemayet* fruit has not been identified.

7. Breasted JH: *The Edwin Smith Surgical Papyrus*, vol 1, Chicago, 1930, University of Chicago Press, pp. 492-498.

8. The Smith surgical papyrus, the oldest known medical book, was written about 1700 BC with evidence showing that elements dated back to 3000 BC. This papyrus is written with a true spirit of scientific inquiry. The Ebers papyrus is slightly younger, perhaps by a century. It deals almost completely with internal diseases and drug recipes. Multiple recipes compounded from various animal, mineral, and vegetable substances, designed to cure wrinkles and cutaneous blemishes, appear in both the Smith surgical papyrus and the Ebers papyrus, and probably in

other medical papyri as well. These two papyri contain simple and compound remedies that probably represent the first recorded attempts to rejuvenate the skin by rationally applying drugs.
9. We must remember that in Classical Greece and even more so in Classical Rome, private baths for the upper classes, as well as communal baths for the poorer classes, were an essential part of everyday life. The number of baths varied from two to seven daily. What Greek or Roman, man or woman, would want to appear unclothed if his or her cosmetic defects would be exposed?
10. Spencer WG, translator: *Celsus de medicina*, vol 2, London, 1938, Heinemann, pp. 183, 185.
11. We should be mindful that Celsus *was* interested in some types of plastic surgery. He has earned the patristic title, the "father" of plastic surgery, for the first description in the West of cosmetically repairing defects of the ears, the nose, the lips, and the eyelids. (See Marmelzat WL: Celsus [AD 25], plastic surgeon: on the repair of defects of the ears, lips and nose, *J Dermatol Surg Oncol* 8:1012-1014, 1982.)
12. Celsus seems not to have been afraid to incise infected cysts, when necessary. (See Marmelzat WL: The account of Celsus' surgical management of pilar and epithelial cysts, *J Dermatol Surg* 3:287-288, 1977.)
13. Ancient Indian medicine, which possibly dates back to 800 BC, is well known for its plastic surgery achievements. In the Samhita, the Indian doctor Sushruta records in Sanskrit his remarkable techniques in successfully employing rotating pedicle flaps to reconstruct amputated ears and noses. (Nose and ear amputations were common punishments for criminal acts, for enemies taken prisoner in battle, and for adultery.)

The stories of such surgery as rhinoplasty and procedures for cleft repair and flap development have been extensively studied and are well known, which is not the case with cosmetic chemexfoliation, the subject of concern here.
14. An army physician to the Roman legions, Dioscorides from early youth was interested in and read the literature of botany. He had traveled widely before setting down in five volumes his *De materia medica*, a great scientific work with a new methodology.
15. Dioscorides' *De materia medica* lists numerous topical drugs. Among his 800 or so drugs from the plant, mineral, and animal kingdoms, he recommends many that are of dermatologic value. These vary from powerful drugs at one extreme—arsenic, copper, alum, mercury, croton oil, podophyllin, tannins, and resins—to such mild drugs as lanolin and benign plant substances at the other extreme. (See note 23, Riddle, *Dioscorides on Pharmacy and Medicine.*)

Of further interest to us is that Dioscorides may have known penicillin and tetracycline, as well as how to cure superficial premalignant tumors or superficial cancers.
16. Cyprium foot salve has not been identified (Riddle JM: Letter to author, March 28, 1990).
17. Riddle JM: Conversation with author, April 25, 1991, about Dioskurides P: *De materia medica*, book 4, chapter 161, Wellman edition, 1904.
18. Dioscorides proposed a drug directly related to modern dermatology as a peeling agent. The juice of the ammoniac plant (*Ferula tingitana*) is given for "cleaning . . . rough spots from the eyelids." In 1864 the drug galbanum (from *Ferula galbaniflua*, Baiss. & Bushe) was melted with potash lye, and an acid called resorcin or resorcinol was identified, which is known for its keratolytic antiseptic and antifungal properties. (From Riddle JM: *Dioscorides on pharmacy and medicine*, Austin, 1985, University of Texas Press, pp. 48-49.)
19. For an excellent summary of Galen's contribution to pharmacy, see Scarborough J, editor: Early Byzantine pharmacy. In *Dumbarton Oaks papers*, No 38, Dumbarton Oaks Symposium, Washington, DC, 1984, Dumbarton Oaks Research Library and Collection, pp. 215-221.
20. Parish LC and Crissey JT: Cosmetics: a historical review, *Clin Dermatol* 6:3-7, 1988.
21. Dioscorides P: The Greek herbal of Dioscorides, book 5, No 174, Oxford, 1934, University Press (Translated by J Goodyer, 1655; edited by RT Gunther).
22. See note 21.
23. The various types of earth from different islands and geographic areas both near and far in ancient times were highly popular as drugs. *Dirt* is a word that describes a variety of minerals, some of which have medicinal use. In general, each particular earth was credited with its own healing usages. Thus there are special earths called *Eretrian earth* from the city of Eretria (heavily laden with magnesite), Samian earth from the island of Samos, Lemnian earth from the island of Lemnos, and many others. For a complete discussion of the dermatologic effects of ancient earths, plants, and minerals see: Riddle JM: *Dioscorides on pharmacy and medicine*, Austin,

1985, University of Texas Press, pp. 148, 153, 156, 162-163.

Even today, 2,000 years later, facial mud and clay applications and beauty packs remain popular procedures among both the laity and cosmetologists.

24. Brain R: *The decorated body*, New York, 1979, Harper & Row.
25. Prager B and others, editors: *Beilsteins Handbuch der Organischen Chemie*, Berlin, 1928, Julius Springer, pp. 110-111. I am indebted to Professor Marcel Bickell of Bern, Switzerland, for explaining the history of phenol during the middle and latter parts of the nineteenth century.
26. In the history of medicine, the bestowal of paternity on any one figure is a risky business and, at best, a debatable proposition. For a comment on this patristic tradition, see Marmelzat WL: Philip Syng Physick, the reluctant medical student who became "the father of American surgery"—a saga for the bicentennial, *J Dermatol Surg* 2(5):380, 1976.
27. Rayer P: *A theoretical and practical treatise on the diseases of the skin*, ed 2, Philadelphia, 1845, Carey & Hart, p. 342.
28. See note 27 (Rayer, p. 347).
29. See note 27 (Rayer, p. 348).
30. Hebra F and Kaposi M: On diseases of the skin, including the exanthemata (Tay W, translator and editor), London, 1874. New Sydenham Society, vol. 3, pp. 22-23.
31. von Ziemssen H, editor: *Handbook of diseases of the skin*, New York, 1885, William Wood & Co, p. 144.
32. I have found no previous author who used a mull. (The dictionary definition of a mull is "an ointment of high melting point intended to be spread ... and used like a plaster." It also is called *steatin*. Can the application of a mull not be considered another early prototype of occlusion?)
33. Textual quotes are from Cooley AJ: *The toilet in ancient and modern times, with a review of the different theories of beauty*, New York, 1970, Burt Franklin, pp. 222-225 (originally published in 1866).
34. Fox T: *Skin diseases: their description, pathology, diagnosis and treatment*, New York, 1871, William Wood & Co.
35. Piffard HG: *A treatise on the materia medica and therapeutics of the skin*, New York, 1881, William Wood & Co.
36. The many distinguished dermatologists scattered over Europe, most directly or indirectly successors to Hebra, were thinking of far more important diagnostic, physiopathologic, and therapeutic matters than cosmetic or aesthetic surgical procedures. Special stains were being developed for histopathologic studies of basic cutaneous disease processes. For instance, Paul Gerson Unna, the founder of modern cutaneous dermatopathology, and other investigators were utilizing phenol extensively in investigating the irritative and inflammatory cutaneous phenomena.

On the clinical side, improved dermatologic classifications were being devised for the understanding of both major and minor dermatoses and dermatitides: infectious exanthemata, syphilis, leprosy, cutaneous tuberculosis (lupus vulgaris), lupus erythematosis, systemic and cutaneous forms of tuberculosis, and many others. In the decades immediately before and after the turn of the twentieth century, the discoveries of specific etiologic organisms were occurring with the frequency of exploding popcorn. Last but not least, Ehrlich produced his "magic bullet" for treating syphilis. Compared with such major diseases, a cosmetic procedure like phenol peeling was trivial.

I wish to acknowledge the noted dermatologist-historians, Karl Holubar of Vienna and Arthur Rook of Cambridge, England, for helping my search through the continental textbooks of the 1890s and early 1900s for descriptions of cosmetic phenol peeling.

37. In view of this negative statement regarding skin rejuvenation, the medical historian must in all fairness turn the coin over and acknowledge the many positive medical contributions that have been made by laymen down through the centuries. For examples of some lay contributions to medicine and their importance, see Oliver Wendell Holmes' tribute: Medicine and history: a dermatologist briefly scratches his itch to probe bits of medical history, philosophy and dermatology, *J Dermatol Surg* 2:203-204, 1976.
38. Saalfeld E: *Lectures on cosmetic treatment, a manual for practitioners*, New York, 1910, Paul B Hoeber (Translated by JF Halls Dally).
39. For an excellent historical account of the paraffin saga, see Goldwyn RM: The paraffin story, *Plast Reconstr Surg* 65:517-524, 1980.
40. The textual quotes are from Montgomery DW: Phenol, J Cutan Dis Syph 35:157-162, 1917.
41. Douglass William Montgomery (1859-1941) was born in Canada and educated at Toronto School of Medicine and at the College of Physicians and Surgeons in New York. After his graduation in 1882, he went on a 4-year postgraduate medical tour of Europe—to Italy, Heidelberg,

Würtzburg, Vienna, London, and Edinburgh. In 1886 he arrived in San Francisco where he started to practice dermatology. Montgomery served as professor of pathology (1888-92) and professor of dermatology (1892-1912) at the University of California, San Francisco, Medical School. He wrote extensively and was one of the earliest supporters of Ehrlich's salvarsan.

42. Bames HO: Truth and fallacies of face peeling and face lifting, *Med J Record* 126:86-87, 1927.

43. Bames believed that warts, moles, birthmarks, smallpox pits, and acne scars received scant attention: "Whether electrolysis, fulguration or excision should be employed, only the experience of the operator may decide. For small-pox pits, acne scars and nevi, no remedy can approach the results which can be obtained by carbon dioxide snow repeatedly applied in slush form." (Carbon dioxide slush therapy was to be rediscovered several times.) From Bames HO: Aesthetic plastic surgery, *Calif West Med* 33:2, Aug 1930.

44. Noel AMLFE: *La chirurgie esthétique, son Rôle social*, Paris, 1926, Masson et Cie. Therein may lie some mention of European cosmetic phenol facial rejuvenation.

45. I am indebted to three sources for the professional and personal information concerning Herbert Otto Bames. First, I am grateful to Dr. and Mrs. Salvador Castanares of Los Angeles. Castanares, a retired plastic surgeon, and his wife have an amazing recollection of Bames, whom they knew well. Castanares was a younger associate of Bames during the 1920s. In addition, Erica Hanson, the long-time librarian of the Hollywood Presbyterian Hospital of Los Angeles, where Bames founded the plastic surgery department, furnished valuable information concerning the many years she worked with this pioneer Los Angeles plastic surgeon.

Herbert Otto Bames was born in Balingam, Germany, in 1885. The details of his first 25 or 26 years pose a mystery. There is no record of where he obtained his schooling before he emigrated to this country or why he came to Los Angeles. It is possible that he changed his original surname. His published articles always bore his initials, H. O. That is evidently how Bames wanted to be known.

After his arrival in the United States, the first establishable fact is that Bames received his M. D. degree in 1913 from the University of Southern California School of Medicine. He was a genial and talkative man with a thick German accent, but he never talked with his pioneer colleagues about his life before getting his medical degree. From 1913 until the end of World War I, Bames practiced general medicine. During this time he apparently became interested in plastic surgery procedures and was probably self-taught. Finding the state of plastic surgery knowledge primitive (there was no American university department of plastic surgery at that time), shortly after World War I ended he sought training abroad. He frequently attended lengthy courses at the internationally known clinics of F. Burian (Czechoslovakia) and Jacques Joseph (Berlin). In Paris he studied with A.M.L.F.E. Noel, the famous Parisian plastic surgeon especially interested in aesthetic surgery. Bames referred to her as "the countess."

Bames was a charter member of the American Board of Plastic Surgery.

46. Polano MK: *J Am Acad Dermatology* 18:1149, 1988. Polano cites Stein RO: *Jadassohn's Handbuch der Haut und Geschlechtskrankheiten*, Berlin, 1930, Julius Springer, pp. 69-92.

47. For a full explanation of topical acne therapy, see Richter P: Geschichte der Dermatologie. In Johannes von Fick J, Richter P, and Spitzer R: *Geschichte der Dermatologie Geographische Verteilung der Hautkrankheiten Nomenklatur*, Berlin, 1928, Julius Springer, p. 2.

48. M. K. Polano confirmed that in 1935 his distinguished dermatologist father, M. E. Polano, and he had occasionally used chemical peeling but had abandoned it (Polano MK: Letter to author, April 4, 1990).

49. Eller JJ and Wolff S: Skin peeling and scarification in the treatment of pitted scars, pigmentations and certain facial blemishes, *JAMA* 116:934-938, 1941.

50. Urkov JC: Surface defects of skin: treatment by controlled exfoliation, *Ill Med J* 89:75-81, 1946.

51. Joseph C. Urkov was an uncertified plastic surgeon. Mysteriously little seems to be known about his life or career other than his birth in 1894, graduation from the Chicago College of Medicine and Surgery, and licensing in Illinois in 1914. His office was located at 162 North State Street in Chicago. (Christiansen RA, Director, Administrative Records, Illinois State Medical Society: Letter to author, March 27,1991.)

52. Winter L: A method of permanent removal of freckles, *Br J Dermatol* 62:83-84, 1950.

53. George Miller MacKee began his dermatologic career with the well-known dermatologist John A. Fordyce at the Bellevue Hospital Medical College and as an in-

structor at New York University. He followed Fordyce to the Vanderbilt Clinic of the College of Physicians and Surgeons, Columbia University, in 1912 where he remained as Fordyce's principal collaborator until Fordyce's death in 1925. After a short period of time, MacKee along with a dedicated group of followers, including Fred Wise, Isadore Rosen, E. W. Abramowitz, and Max Scheer—all famous names in American dermatologic history—left Columbia and transferred to the New York Post Graduate Medical School and Hospital. Dr. MacKee was appointed Professor of Dermatology and Syphilology in 1928. Subsequently he became chairman of the "old" New York Skin and Cancer Hospital, which under his guidance became an internationally celebrated dermatologic training center.

When the *Journal of Dermatology and Syphilology* became the *Archives of Dermatology and Syphilology* (which continues to this day as the *Archives of Dermatology*), MacKee served as a valued member on the editorial board of the successor *Archives of Dermatology* (1919-1987). He was on the editorial board of the *Journal of Investigative Dermatology* from 1939 to 1947. (See Frances Pascher's touching memoir for Dr. MacKee's contributions as an author, investigator, teacher, superb organizer, and especially humanitarian: Pascher F: George Miller MacKee 1878-1955: a memoir, *J Am Acad Dermatol* 9:166-172, 1983.)

54. MacKee GM and Karp FL: The treatment of post-acne scars with phenol, *Br J Dermatol* 64:456-459, 1952.
55. In Egyptian mythology the phoenix was a beautiful, lone bird that lived in the Arabian desert for 500 to 600 years. It then consumed itself in fire, rising renewed from its ashes to start another long life. It is used as a symbol of immortality. What an apt title for a rejuvenating formula!

    Unfortunately, the "phoenix formula" fell into the hands of a "countess" patient, who teamed up with some commercial business promoters. Their plan was to set up a string of lay phenol peeling parlors. The resulting scandal received national criticism.
56. I wish to acknowledge my great debt to six people for helping me construct the MacKee and Karp contributions to phenol peeling.

    First to Diane Silberling, the long-time secretary of the New York Skin and Cancer Hospital and to Dr. Alexander A. Fisher, who taught me allergy at that institution long ago (he is still teaching me about drug allergies). Their intimate knowledge and gracious willingness furnished me with information that has not been recorded. Dr. Fisher and Ms. Silberling were invaluable in suggesting vital contacts, especially Dr. John Heinlein, a former partner of Dr. MacKee; Mr. Marcus Ross, who from 1931 on prepared the phenol formulas for both Drs. MacKee and Karp; and Mr. Harold Greenwald.

    Marcus Ross met MacKee in 1931. A young pharmacist, Ross quickly became aware of the special need for cooperation between professionals in dermatology and pharmacy. More than 90% of the physicians practicing in the building where Ross worked were dermatologists (approximately 25 to 30). Many of them were destined for greatness. Ross, who still actively practices pharmacy, is a veritable fountain of dermatologic lore.

    I am particularly indebted to Mrs. John Jacob Niles Noyes, Karp's only living relative, for furnishing me the exciting details of her aunt's early life.
57. Kurtin A: Corrective surgical planing of skin, *Arch Dermatol Syph* 68:389, 1953.
58. Kromayer E: Rotationsinstrumente: ein neues technisches Verfahren in der dermatologischen Kleinchirurgie, *Derm Z* 12:26, 1905.
59. Kromayer E: *Cosmetic treatment of skin complaints*, New York, 1930, Oxford University Press.
60. Combes FC, Sperber PA, and Reisch M: Dermal defects: treatment by a chemical agent, *NY Physician Am Med* 36-42, 1960.
61. Gersuny R: Ueber eine subcutane prothese, *Ztschr Heilk* 1:199, 1900.
62. See note 39 (Goldwyn).
63. For an extended list of references on the surgical treatment of wrinkling during the first six decades of the twentieth century, see Gonzalez-Ulloa M: Facial wrinkles—integral elimination, *Plast Reconstr Surg* 29:658-673, 1962: Gonzalez-Ulloa M: Wrinkle correction—ear-island method, *J Int Coll Surg* 25:620-624, 1956.
64. Gillies HD: The development and scope of plastic surgery, *Northwestern University Bulletin, The Medical School* 35(20):31, 1935.
65. Gillies HD and Millard DR Jr: *The principles and art of plastic surgery*, Boston, 1957, Little, Brown & Co, pp. 401, 403.
66. Gillies never reported the use of adhesive occlusion before 1957. Note, however, the following 1968 statement by Batstone JHF and Millard DR (an endorsement of facial chemosurgery, *Br J Plast Surg* 21:193, 1968): "Gillies had been using the acid painting and taping technique for eyelids

many years before publishing a paragraph in the section of reduction and resection surgery" (Gillies and Millard, 1957).

My historical essay, however, has shown how very old occlusive procedures are.

67. Brown AM, Kaplan LM, and Brown ME: Phenol-induced histological skin changes: hazards, technique, and uses, *Br J Plast Surg* 13:158-169, 1960.
68. Baker TJ: The ablation of rhytides by chemical means, *J Fla Med Assoc* 48:451-454, 1961.
69. See note 66.
70. Baker TJ and Gordon HL: *Surgical rejuvenation of the face*, St Louis, 1986, Mosby–Year Book.
71. In 1963 Perry Sperber introduced a new term for the process of chemically peeling the skin in cosmetic treatment: *chemexfoliation*. This term found favor and is widely used. (Sperber P: Chemexfoliation, a new term in cosmetic therapy, *J Am Geriatr Soc* 11:58-62, 1963.)

Sperber also wrote an interesting book on chemexfoliation (Sperber P: *Treatment of the aging skin and dermal defects*, Springfield, Ill, 1965, Charles C Thomas). The historically minded practitioner will enjoy this work for its historical introduction on cosmetology.

ACKNOWLEDGMENTS

This introductory history could not have been written without the sympathy and cooperation of many persons who have been generous in sharing with me, often at considerable personal inconvenience, their knowledge, ideas, and personal remembrances, many of which date back six and seven decades.

In the Notes credit is given to those individuals who went to especially great lengths to make available to me original information that was otherwise unavailable.

I am greatly indebted to Professor John M. Riddle. Specifically for this study, he graciously translated into English the two passages of Dioscorides that I quote. I am also grateful to Professor Wesley D. Smith, who kindly furnished me with valuable data on cosmetology in antiquity.

I gathered my data from a large number of personal interviews. The following individuals opened doors for me or gave me one or frequently many interviews: the late Dr. David N. Alcon; Dr. Harry L. Arnold, Jr.; the late Dr. Samuel Ayres, Jr.; Dr. Samuel Ayres III; Dr. Richard G. Bennett; Dr. Marcel Bickell; Dr. Samuel M. Bluefarb; Dr. Harold L. Boyer; Dr. Earle W. Brauer; Dr. Marthe E. Brown; Dr. and Mrs. Salvador Castanares; Dr. John T. Crissey; Dr. J. Worth Estes; Dr. Alexander A. Fisher; Dr. Charles Flood; Dr. Andrew George Franks, Sr. (the oldest living graduate of the "old" New York Skin and Cancer Hospital); Harold Greenwald, Esq.; Dr. B. G. Gross; Ferenc A. Gyorgyey; Dr. Michael Gurdin; Dr. Bert Hansen; Dr. John Heinlein; Dr. Leo Kaplan; Dr. Robert Kotler; Mrs. John Jacobs Niles Noyes; Dr. Norman Orentreich; Dr. Lawrence J. Parish; Dr. George L. Popkin; Dr. Milton Reisch; Dr. Hilliard M. Shair; Diane Silberling; Dr. Perry A. Sperber; Dr. Dale C. Smith; Dr. Wesley D. Smith; Dr. Douglas P. Torre; Dr. David White; Richard Wolfe; and Dr. Maxwell J. Wolff.

For their patient, cheerful, and expert assistance in unearthing some of the obscure, long-buried material on skin rejuvenation, I must thank many librarians and their institutions. My greatest debts are to Katharine E. S. Donahue, Head of the History and Special Collections Division; Cynthia Becht, assistant head; and Johana Alvarez, assistant, of the Louise A. Darling Biomedical Library of the University of California at Los Angeles, Center for Health Sciences. I am equally indebted to Joyce Crump, Head Librarian, and Lori Potter, Assistant Librarian, of the Los Angeles County Medical Association Library.

Also I wish to acknowledge the help of Michael Rissinger and Erich Meyerhoff, archivists of the Ehrman Medical Library, New York University Medical Center; Nancy Whitten Zinn, head of Special Collections, The Library, University of California at San Francisco School of Medicine; Elizabeth H. Wood, head, Reference Section, and the reference librarian staff of the Norris Medical Library, Richard J. Wolfe, Rare Books librarian, Francis A. Countway Library of Medicine, Boston Medical Library–Harvard Medical Library; Ferenc A. Gyorgyey, historical librarian, Yale University Medical Library; Ann Pasquale, head of Special Collections, and Adrienne Millon-Levin, reference librarian, The New York Academy of Medicine Library.

A special thank you to Marison Mull, my tireless research and editorial assistant.

Finally, I wish to thank my wife, Ruth, who has been most supportive during this project.

CHAPTER ONE

An Overview of Chemical Skin Peeling

Chemical skin peeling is an established technique for improving or erasing wrinkles, keratoses, and areas of increased pigmentation, including freckles, "age spots," "liver spots," etc. This technique is also known as chemexfoliation, chemical facial rejuvenation, chemabrasion, exodermology, and, somewhat inaptly, chemosurgery or chemical face lifting. When skin peeling is well performed on properly selected patients, the results can be very impressive and a source of immense satisfaction to the patient and the physician.

The process of skin peeling, an aggressive and deeply penetrating exfoliative process, relies on penetration of an irritating exfoliant or escharotic agent into the skin to the dermal level, producing wounding and then sloughing of superficial skin layers. The injury, in addition to producing necrosis of the epidermis and a superficial portion of the dermis, evokes a nonspecific tissue regeneration. The result is a smooth, more youthful-appearing skin.

The history of this intriguing process has roots in antiquity and is elegantly explored by Willard Marmelzat, M.D., in the Introduction. In 1952, MacKee and Karp[74] reported on their treatment of postacne scars with phenol. MacKee noted that he had been using phenol "for this purpose since 1903." Primarily as a result of clinical and laboratory investigations by Brown, Kaplan, and Brown (1960)[32]; Combes, Sperber, and Reisch (1960)[37]; Litton (1962)[65]; and Baker and Gordon (1962),[13] the procedure became accepted by the mid-1960s.[17]

The exponential growth of cosmetic surgery in the 1970s and 1980s has made chemical peeling a frequently performed procedure.

A study performed by the University of North Carolina in 1989 surveyed members of the American Academy of Facial Plastic and Reconstructive Surgery. Those responding reported 11,040 skin peels done in 1988. The comparable number for 1986 was 8,800. In 1987, the American Society of Plastic and Reconstructive Surgeons reported 15,600 chemical peels performed by its members in 1986. In 1988, a survey of members of the American Society of Dermatologic Surgery showed that 50% of the responding members were performing chemical skin peels, compared with 13% in a 1984 survey.

Brody,[28] in 1989, cited a survey of members of the American Academy of Dermatology that showed "24% were performing trichloroacetic acid face peels, 7% were performing phenol peels, and 8% were performing more superficial peels." Brody further stated, "Without question, these numbers have increased and possibly doubled in the last 5 years...."

To appreciate the initiative and heroism of the earlier practitioners, the reader is commended to many of these earlier papers, particularly Litton's.[65] In 1962 he reported on his first 50 cases with a 2-year follow-up. Litton's study included studying the effects of phenol on local tissue by biopsy and determining the blood phenol levels. Litton confesses that he "must admit from the start that it took a lot of courage to apply this solution to the patient's face for the first time. I did not have the benefit of any other physician's advice when I first started doing the procedure."

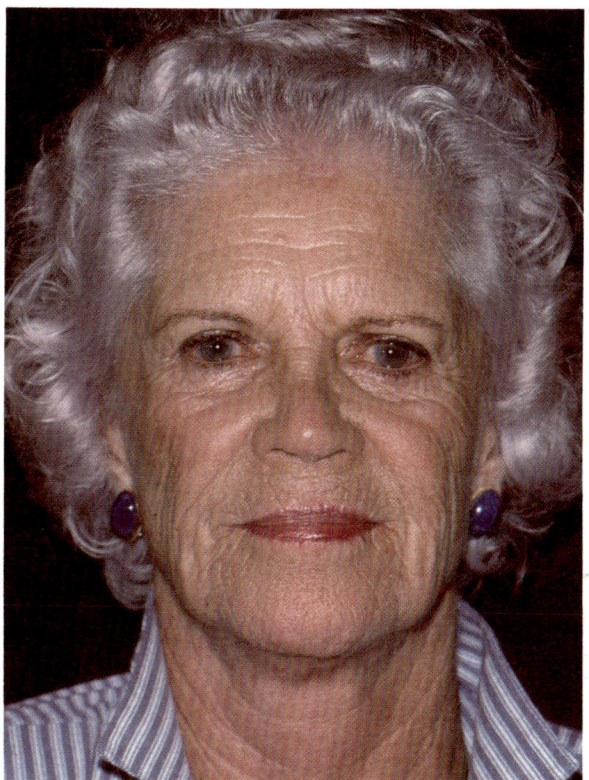 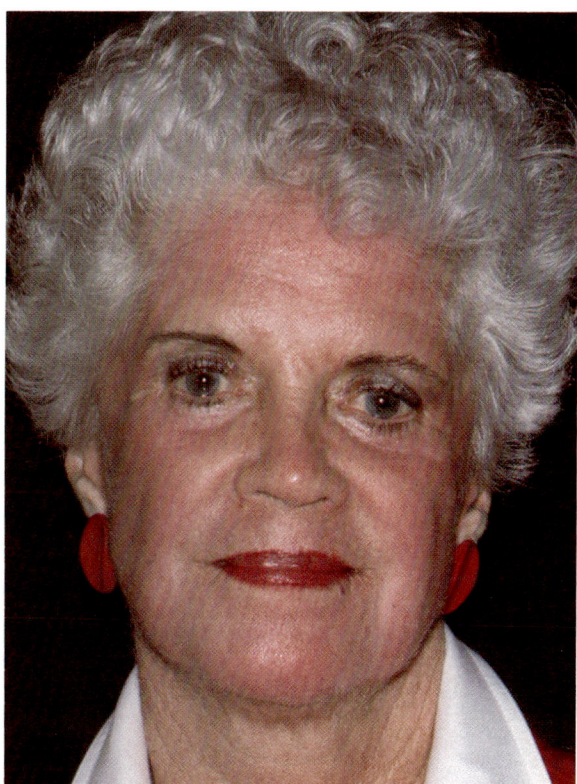

Case 1: Ideal candidate for chemical skin peeling. This 75-year-old patient's fair coloring and deep wrinkling made her an ideal candidate for a maximum technique occluded Baker formula phenol peel. The technique includes pretreatment application of 50% trichloroacetic acid (TCA) to the forehead, perioral area, nasolabial creases, and crow's-feet. Following full-face application of Baker formula, Salonpas tape was applied as the first layer to the pretreated areas and the face was fully occluded with a tape mask. The patient is shown here before treatment and 3 months after treatment in a frontal view of the face and neck at a distance of 5 feet.

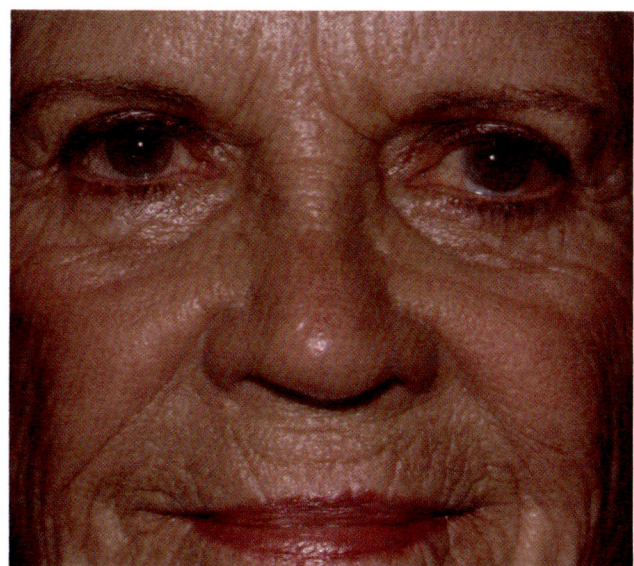 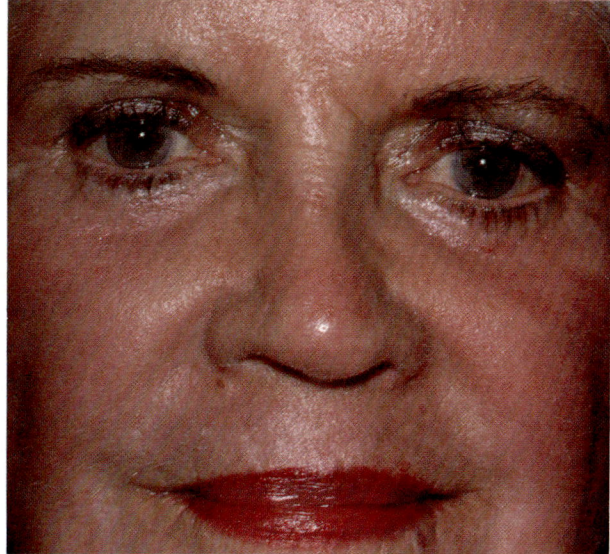

Case 1, cont'd. Close-up view of the midface before treatment and 3 months after treatment.

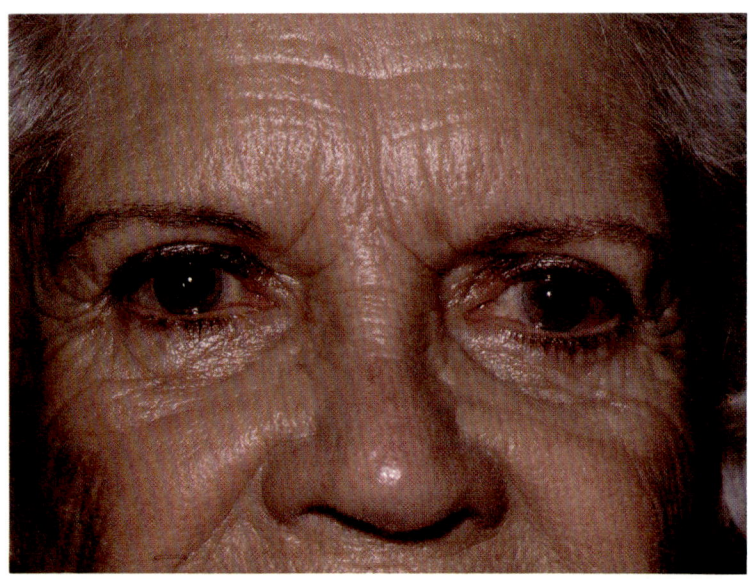

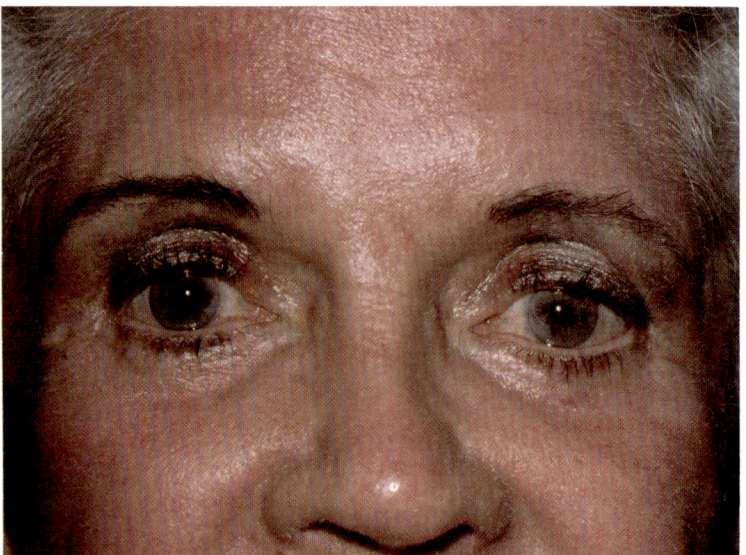

Case 1, cont'd. Close-up frontal view of the orbital area before treatment and 3 months after treatment. The telangiectasia that was still present at this posttreatment visit resolved within 6 weeks.

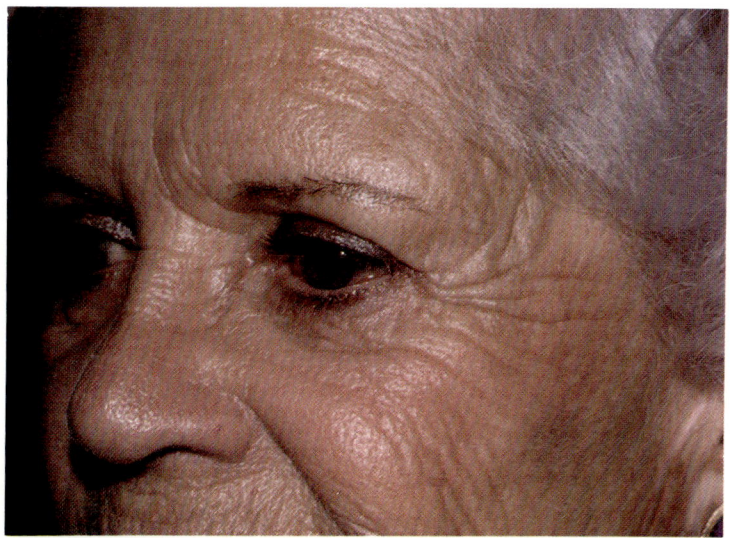

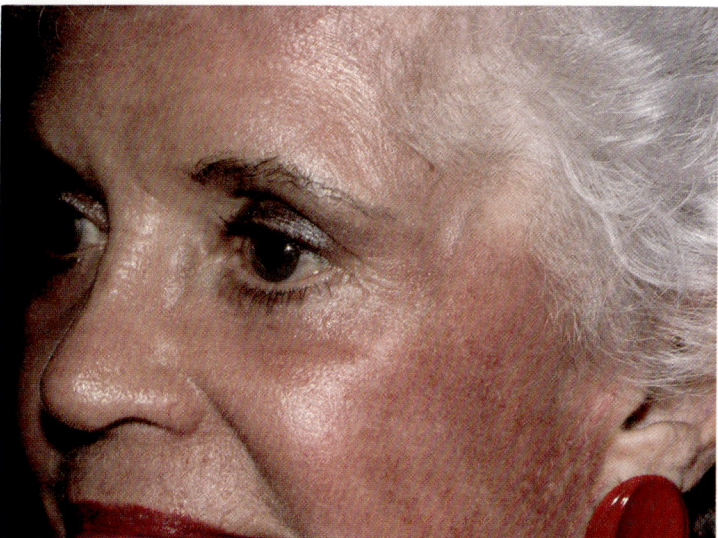

Case 1, cont'd. Close-up oblique view of the orbitomalar area before treatment and 3 months after treatment. The patient exhibited more redness than is commonly seen and reported "flushing" for a period of 1 year after the procedure.

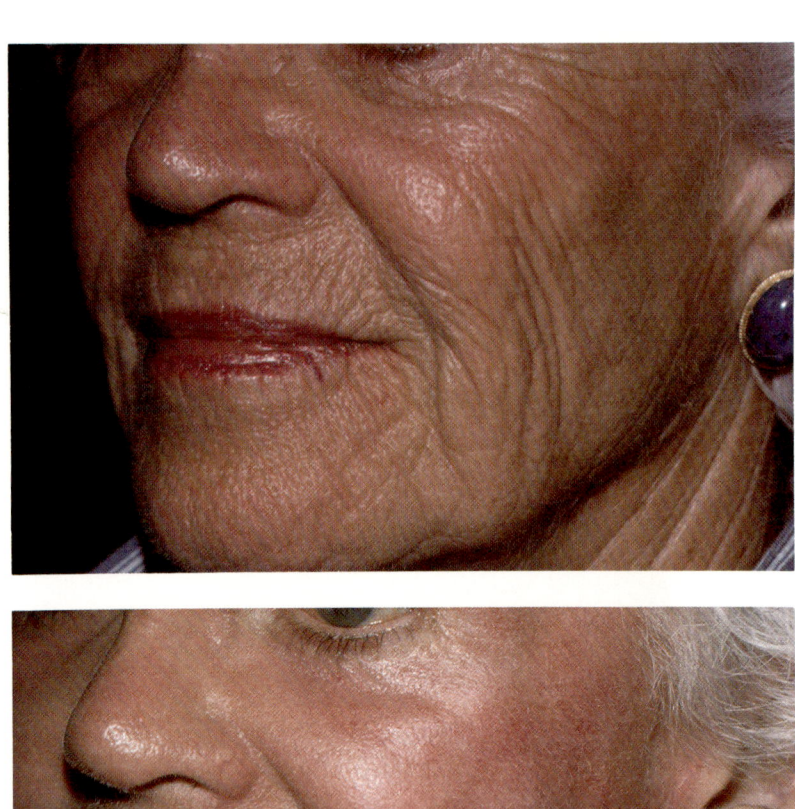
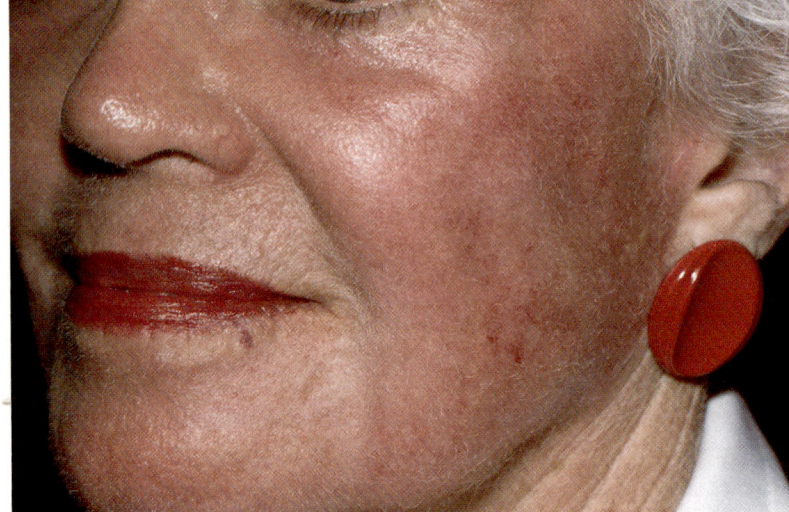

Case 1, cont'd. Close-up oblique view of the cheek before treatment and 3 months after treatment.

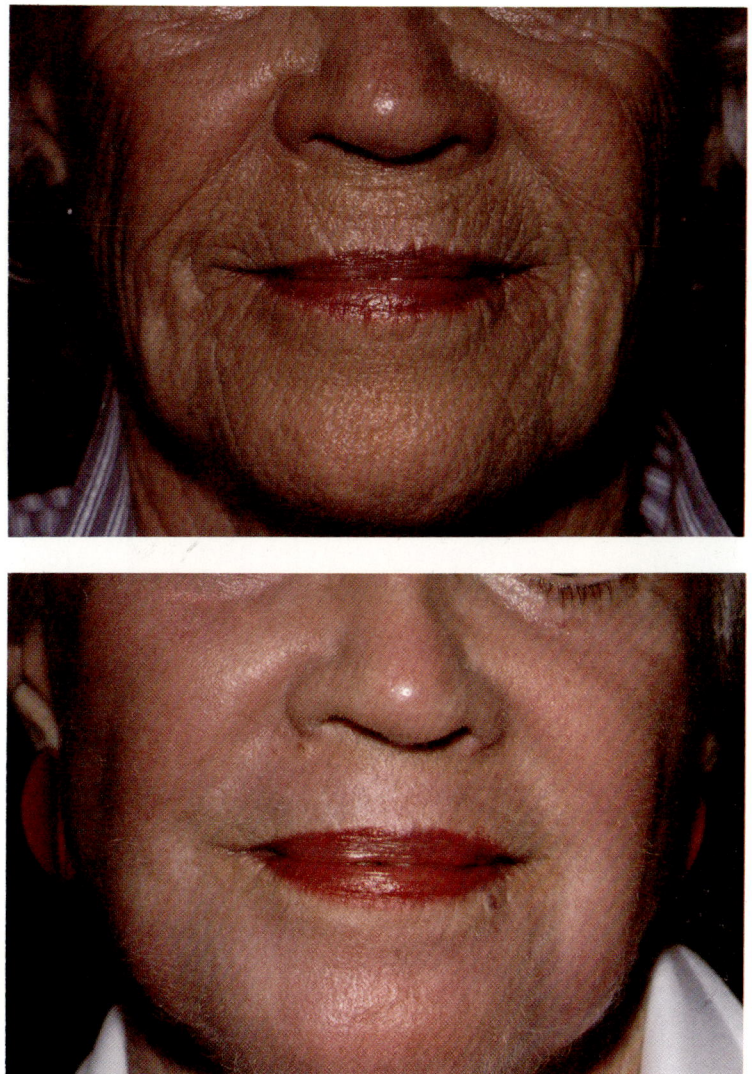

Case 1, cont'd. Close-up frontal view of the lip and chin before treatment and 3 months after treatment.

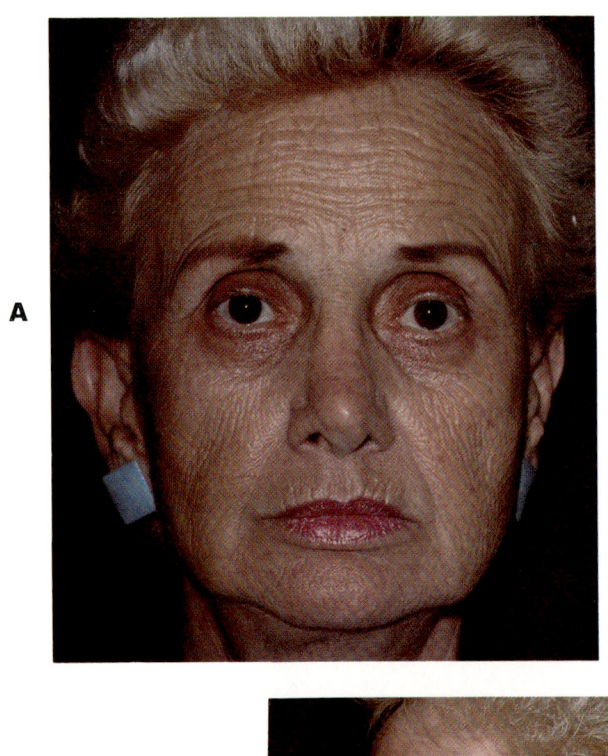
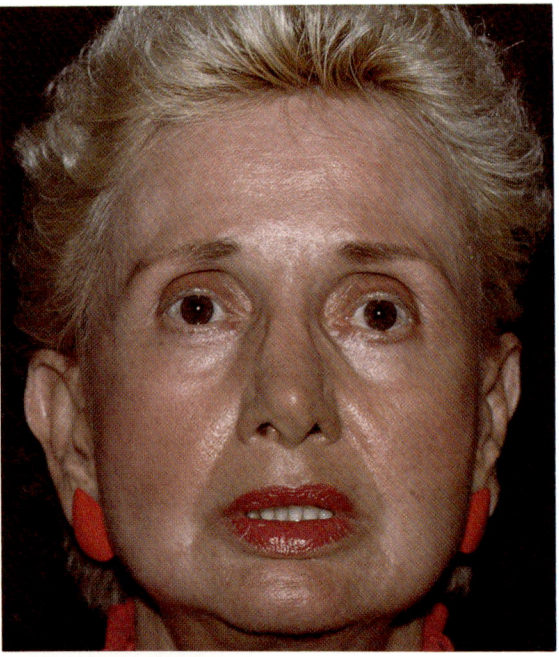
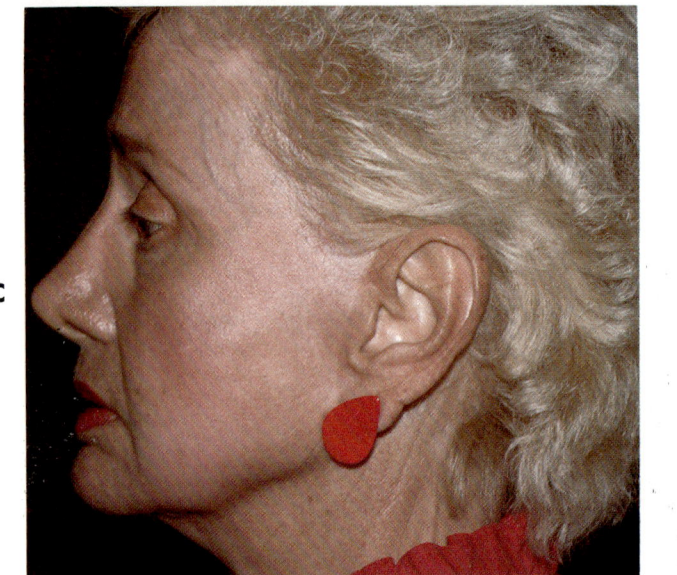

Case 2: Excellent candidate for chemical skin peeling. This 58-year-old patient has brown eyes but is otherwise an excellent candidate for an aggressive occluded Baker formula phenol peel. Deep wrinkling of the patient's upper lip, nasolabial creases, and forehead were pretreated with 50% TCA, and Baker formula was then applied over the entire face. The face was fully occluded with a tape mask, including Salonpas, as the first layer to the upper and lower lip and crow's-feet. The patient is shown **A**, before treatment and **B** and **C**, 9 months after treatment. **B**, Frontal view of the face at a distance of 4 feet and **C**, lateral view of the face.

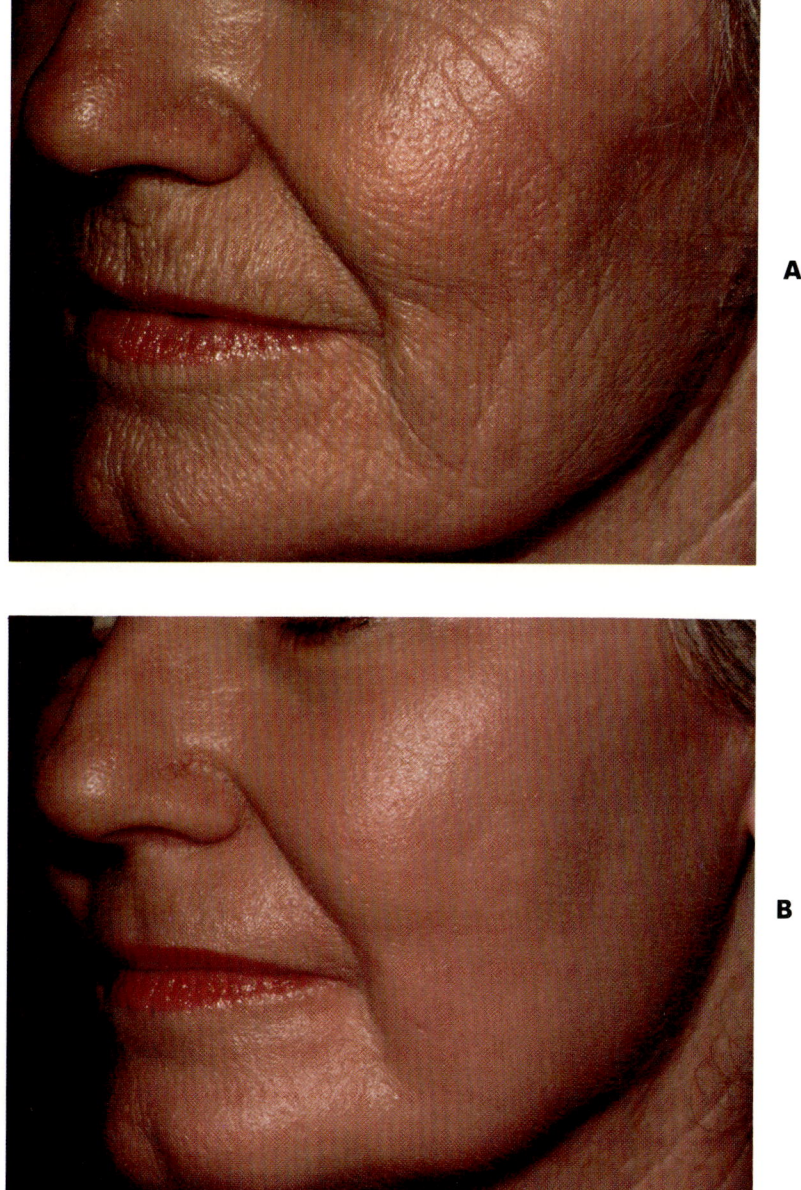

Case 3: The "perfect" candidate for chemical skin peeling. This 54-year-old patient's nearly pigment-free skin and blue eyes make her the "perfect" candidate for a maximum technique occluded Baker formula phenol peel. Deep wrinkles of the orbital area, glabella, and crow's-feet were pretreated with 50% TCA, followed by full-face application of Baker formula. The face was fully occluded with a tape mask, with Salonpas applied as the first layer to the upper and lower lip, infrabrow, and crow's-feet. The patient is shown **A**, before and **B**, after treatment in a close-up oblique view of the cheek.

50 CHEMICAL REJUVENATION OF THE FACE

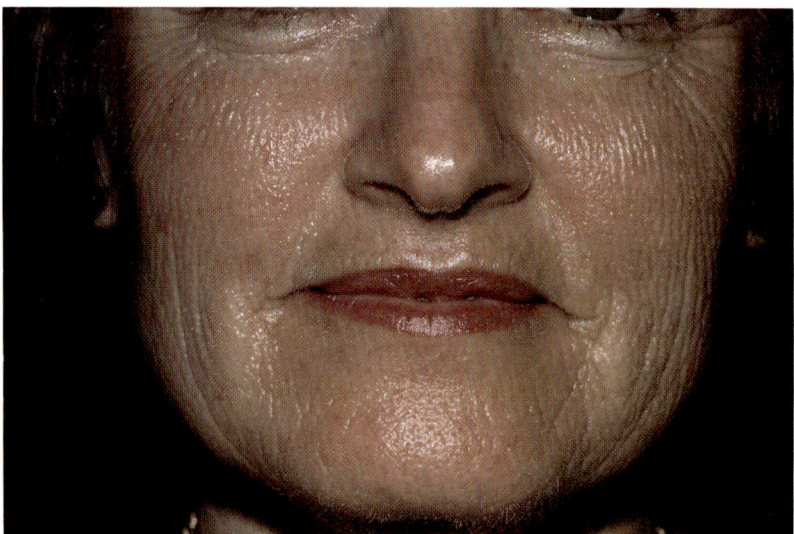

Before

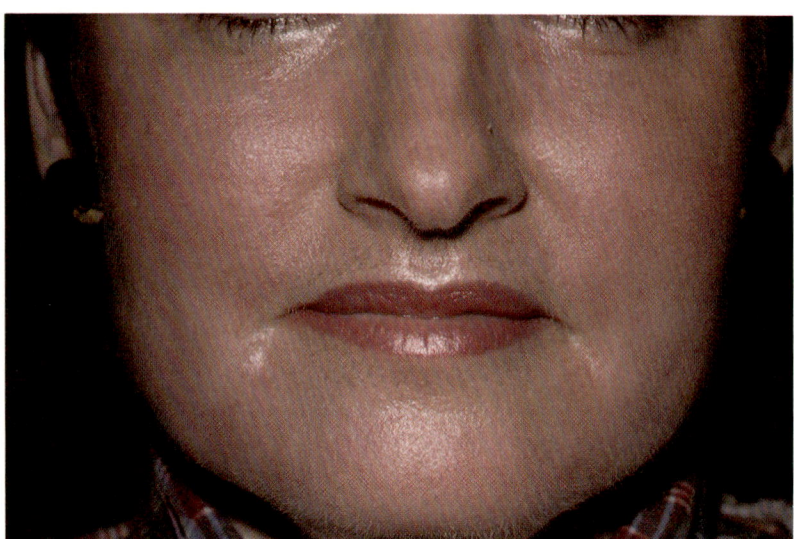

After

Case 4: Ideal candidate for chemical skin peeling to remove premature fine wrinkles. This 44-year-old patient had somewhat premature fine wrinkling of the face. Her very fair complexion and blue eyes make her an ideal candidate for chemical skin peeling, and she was treated with a fully occluded Baker formula phenol peel that included pretreatment of the upper and lower lip, forehead, and crow's-feet with 50% TCA. Salonpas was used as the first tape layer on the upper lip, vermilion border of the lower lip, nasolabial creases, forehead, and crow's-feet. The patient is shown before and after treatment in a close-up frontal view of the lip and chin.

Before **After**

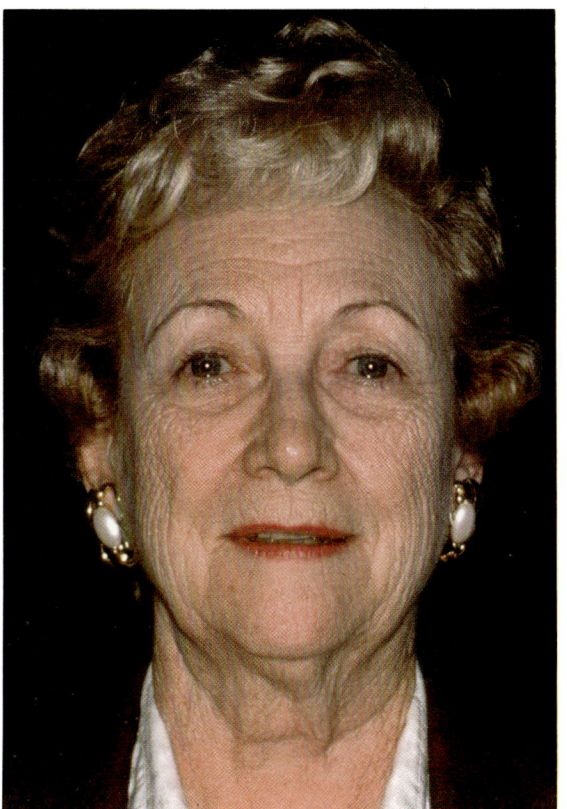 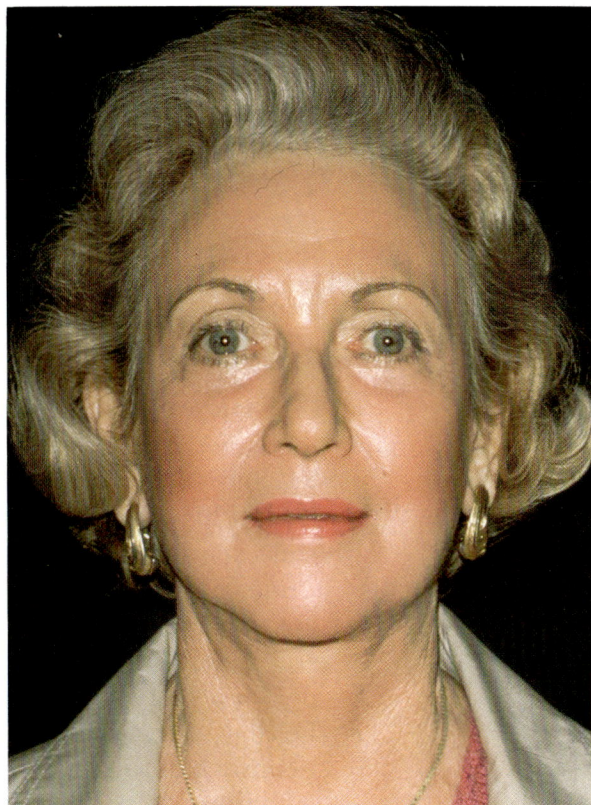

Case 5: Facial cosmetic surgery combined with chemical rejuvenation. This patient, a 69-year-old woman of Northern European ancestry, was an excellent candidate for upper and lower eyelid surgery and a face and neck lift in addition to chemical rejuvenation. Three months after her surgery she had a full-face tape occluded Baker formula phenol peel. She is shown here before and after the peel in a frontal view of the face and neck at a distance of 5 feet.

CHAPTER TWO

Histology of Chemical Peels

RICHARD G. GLOGAU

The major indication for application of chemical cauterants to the skin is premature photoaging secondary to excess ultraviolet exposure. Clinical signs of photoaging of the skin include rhytids, lentigines, keratoses, telangiectasia, loss of translucency, loss of elasticity, and sallow color.[19] To understand the effects of chemical peeling from a histologic viewpoint, it is desirable to first understand how the sun-exposed skin deviates from normal undamaged skin and how the chemical peel affects and, to some extent, normalizes the microscopic appearance of sun-damaged skin.

Elegant histologic studies utilizing 2.0 μm thick specimens embedded in glycolmethacrylate[81] have shown the sun-damaged epidermis to be characterized by a compact and laminated or gelatinous stratum corneum without clear transition to the underlying stratum lucidum. The epidermis will usually show some evidence of dysplasia and atypical keratinocytes, vacuolation of epidermal cells, occasional cell necrosis, and a diminished number of Langerhans cells. Loss of vertical polarity in epidermal cells and irregularity of the epidermal cell alignment is common.

The dermis shows elastosis with a homogenization of the upper papillary dermal ground substance, formation of amorphous masses, and breakage of fibers. There is an increase in reticulin fibers, and often mast cells and macrophages with coarse granules can be discerned. It appears that the collagen substance in the upper dermis is being slowly destroyed and gradually replaced by the amorphous material that stains poorly and is frequently associated with an increase in reticulin fibers in and around the amorphous material. The amount of elastotic material and associated fibrorhexis or fiber breakdown can be quite striking and is probably responsible for the fine rhytid formation associated with sun-damaged skin.

HISTORICAL INVESTIGATIONS

Early attempts to describe the microscopic changes in correlating with clinical improvement were spotty at best. Mackee's description in 1952 of skin from the back that had been treated monthly with phenol observed that collagen bundles in the upper dermis appeared compact and parallel to the surface.[74] Ayres found a subepidermal band of new collagen 0.3 to 0.4 mm wide with fibers aligned parallel to skin surface.[8] He made the same observations of skin that had been treated with dermabrasion.[9]

Brown, Kaplan, and Brown demonstrated thickening of the dermis with compaction of the upper dermal fibers in rabbit ears treated with phenol,[31] and termed the changes "fibrosis."

Litton made passing reference to the same phenomenon in a biopsy taken 3 months following phenol peel in 1962 and called the marked widening of the upper papillary dermis the "stratum papillare."[65]

Spira and colleagues in 1970 used the thighs of paraplegics to evaluate the impact of varying concentrations of phenol, croton oil, and occlusion in the Baker-Gordon formula. Biopsied treatment sites 3 months afterward showed dermal thickening and new collagen deposition.[99]

Baker and colleagues in 1974 examined facial skin removed in rhytidectomy from patients peeled years earlier.[17] They concluded, incorrectly, that the increased elastosis observed showed the histologic effects of the peel to be the same as those seen from chronic sun damage.

Behin and colleagues studied phenol-induced changes in the minipig in 1977.[22] They described the collagen formed in the widening dermis after 2 weeks as "scar" and noted fewer elastic fibers.

Stegman produced a single patient comparison of phenol, trichloroacetic acid (TCA), and dermabrasion in 1982,[105] which reprised an earlier animal study.[104] He described the consistent appearance posttreatment of an enlarged papillary dermis which he called "dermal scar." More importantly, he demonstrated that the depth of injury correlated with the concentration of peeling agent and could be affected by occlusion. In general he confirmed that the Baker-Gordon formula incorporating croton oil, Septisol, and phenol produced a deeper injury than either phenol alone or TCA and that Baker-Gordon's peel produced changes comparable to those seen with dermabrasion.

Kligman in 1985 utilized Baker's technique of examining rhytidectomy specimens from previously peeled patients to study long-term histologic changes, for the most part at least 10 years after treatment.[58] He noted the newly apparent wide band of thin, compact, parallel collagen bundles arranged horizontally parallel to the skin surface, usually 2 to 3 mm in width. He documented the appearance of numerous elastic fibers throughout the collagen bundles, often parallel to the collagen bundles. There was a definite diminution of the amorphous ground substance previously seen in the so-called Grenz zone of the upper papillary dermis of sun-damaged skin. Telangiectasia were noted to be confined to the deeper dermis where the peel had not reached. Normalization of the epidermal polarity and loss of atypia were also noted. Melanin was found to be present, through reduced. He noted that one could tell with relative ease where the "new" dermis and "old" dermis interfaced, marking the depth of the effect of the phenol. He believed the histologic changes "adequately account for the effacement of wrinkles and obliteration of actinic keratoses, mottling, and freckling."[58]

Brody and Hailey carefully examined the histologic effects of combining carbon dioxide slush and 35% TCA in facial peels.[30] They measured the depth of injury produced by CO_2 + 35% TCA as 0.62 mm, which correlated with Stegman's measurement of 0.5 mm for 40% to 60% TCA, 0.41 mm for open phenol, and 0.6 mm for the Baker-Gordon mixture.

Brodland and colleagues have recently published a porcine model of varying concentrations of TCA with and without occlusion.[24] They confirmed the correlation of depth of injury with increasing concentrations of TCA, but they noted that occlusion actually seemed to *lessen* the depth of injury of TCA, which they attribute to dilution effect. They noted a median depth of necrosis with 50% TCA of 0.5 mm for unoccluded sites and only 0.18 mm for occluded sites. They also noted that depth of injury was inversely related to thickness of the pretreatment epidermis.

Hayes and co-workers examined the effects of peeling after flap elevation in guinea pigs, pursuing information on the relative safety of combining the procedures.[54] Interestingly, they conclude from histologic examination of the treatment sites that the "reticular dermis responds to injury as two physiologically distinct layers, although it appears histologically homogeneous. The upper reticular dermis heals by reorganization, while the deeper reticular dermis heals by scar formation. The differing response to injury of these cell layers may in part explain the low safety margin in aggressive chemical peels."

CLINICAL CORRELATIONS

A very instructive case for physicians interested in chemical peeling was published by Rae and Falanga in 1989.[88] A 42-year-old healthy white woman developed widespread wrinkling of her skin over a 2-year period. "Histologic evaluation showed a complete absence of elastic tissue in a band throughout the middle dermis."[88] Three earlier reports in the literature were also reviewed.

A careful examination of the clinical photograph of the woman's abdomen shows very fine rhytids, particularly in the periumbilical area where gravitational draping of the skin can be seen. These wrinkles are indistinguishable from those seen in photodamaged skin. The absence of elastic fibers in this patient and the striking appearance of the wrinkling seem to suggest that the clinical improvement seen in chemical peeling, which earlier investigators have correlated with the development of the widened dermal band, can be more succinctly defined.

Clinical improvement in sun-damaged skin can be attributed to the postinjury healing response of the skin on several levels. Specifically, the appearance of numerous new elastic fibers within the upper dermal band of parallel, compact collagen bundles characteristic of postpeeled skin correlates with clinical smoothing of the skin. Obliteration and regeneration of the epidermis from adnexal appendageal structures correlate with elimination of dyschromia (mottling, freckling), atypia (keratoses), and restoration of normal vertical polarity of the epidermis. Elimination of the telangiectasia from the upper reticular and papillary dermis, essentially destruction of the abnormal papillary vascular arcades seen in sun-damaged skin, completes the triad of changes characteristic of postpeeled skin.

Clearly the degree of changes produced tends to correlate with the depth of injury produced by the chemical agent or agents. Deeper injury produces more complete clinical improvement up to the anatomic limit of the reticular dermis, where healing response shifts from reorganization to frank production of scar with excessive fibroblast and collagen proliferation. The task of the physician is to select the agents and utilize techniques that can approach this fine line without crossing it.

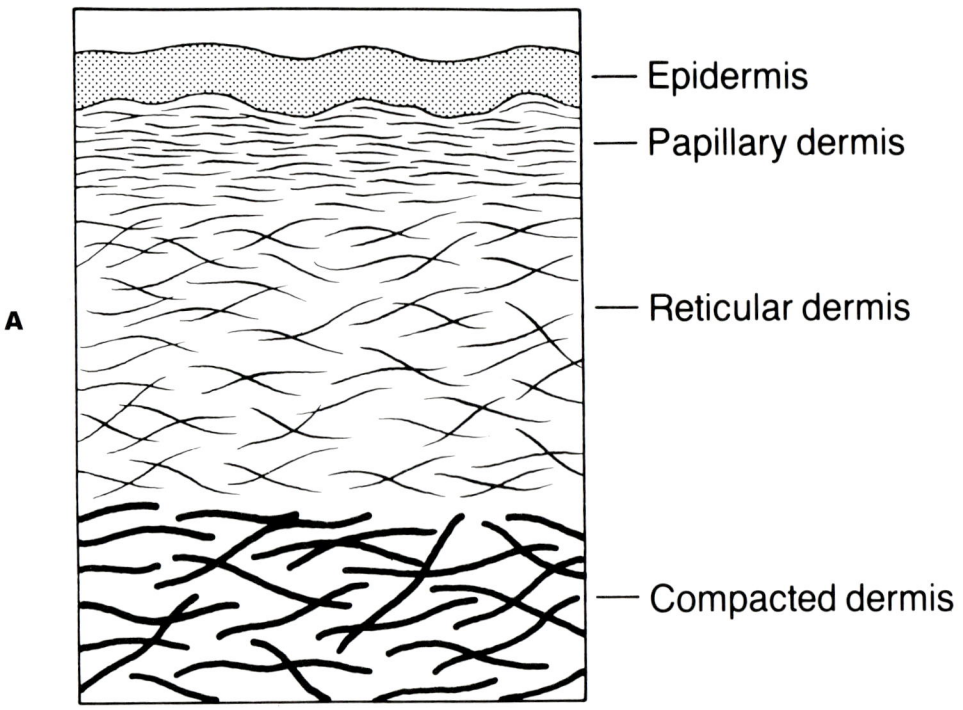

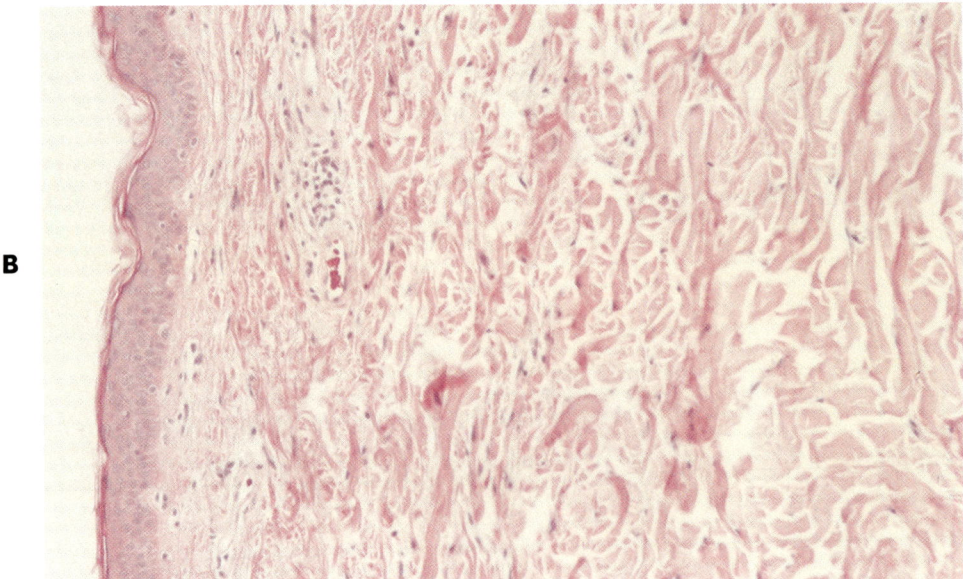

Comparison of normal and sun-damaged skin. A, Diagram illustrating the normal relationship of epidermis, papillary dermis, and reticular dermis. **C,** Section of normal, non-sun-exposed skin. (Hematoxylin-eosin stain; magnification 10×.) **B,** Diagram of sun-exposed skin demonstrating disordered epidermis, Grenz zone of Mowry-staining ground substance in the papillary dermis, amorphous elastotic material (labeled *sun damaged*) in papillary dermis. **D,** Section of sun-exposed skin showing the pale staining broad band of amorphous elastotic material in the papillary dermis. Hematoxylin-eosin stain; magnification 10×.)

SUN DAMAGE

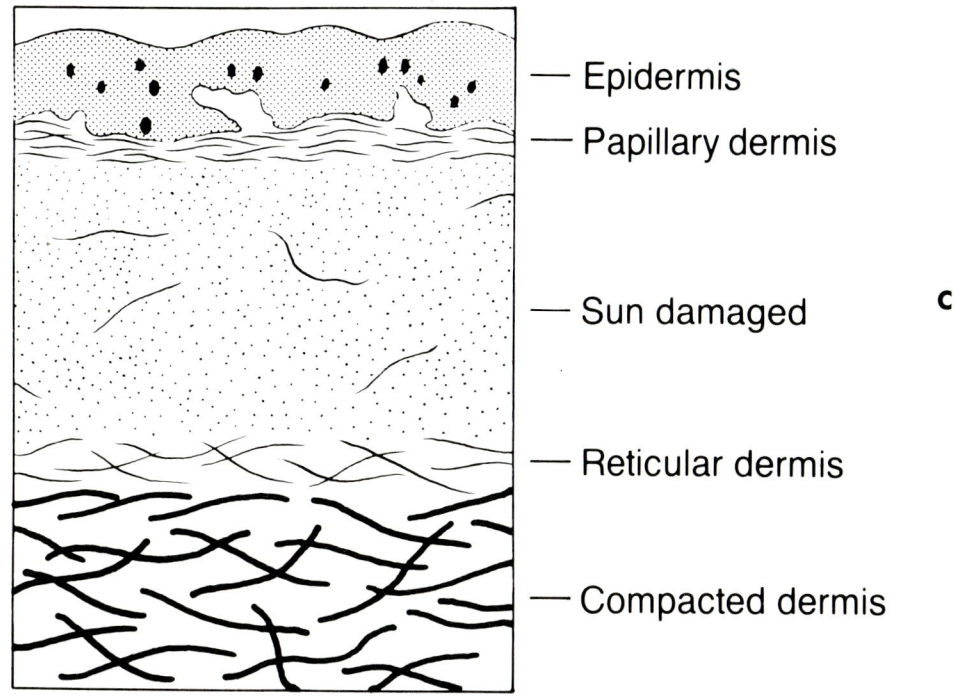

C

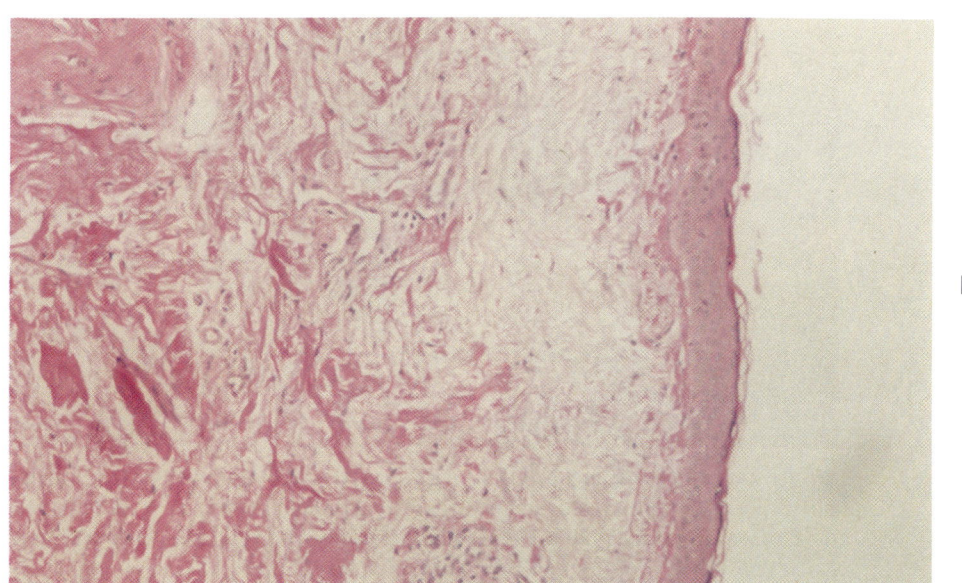

D

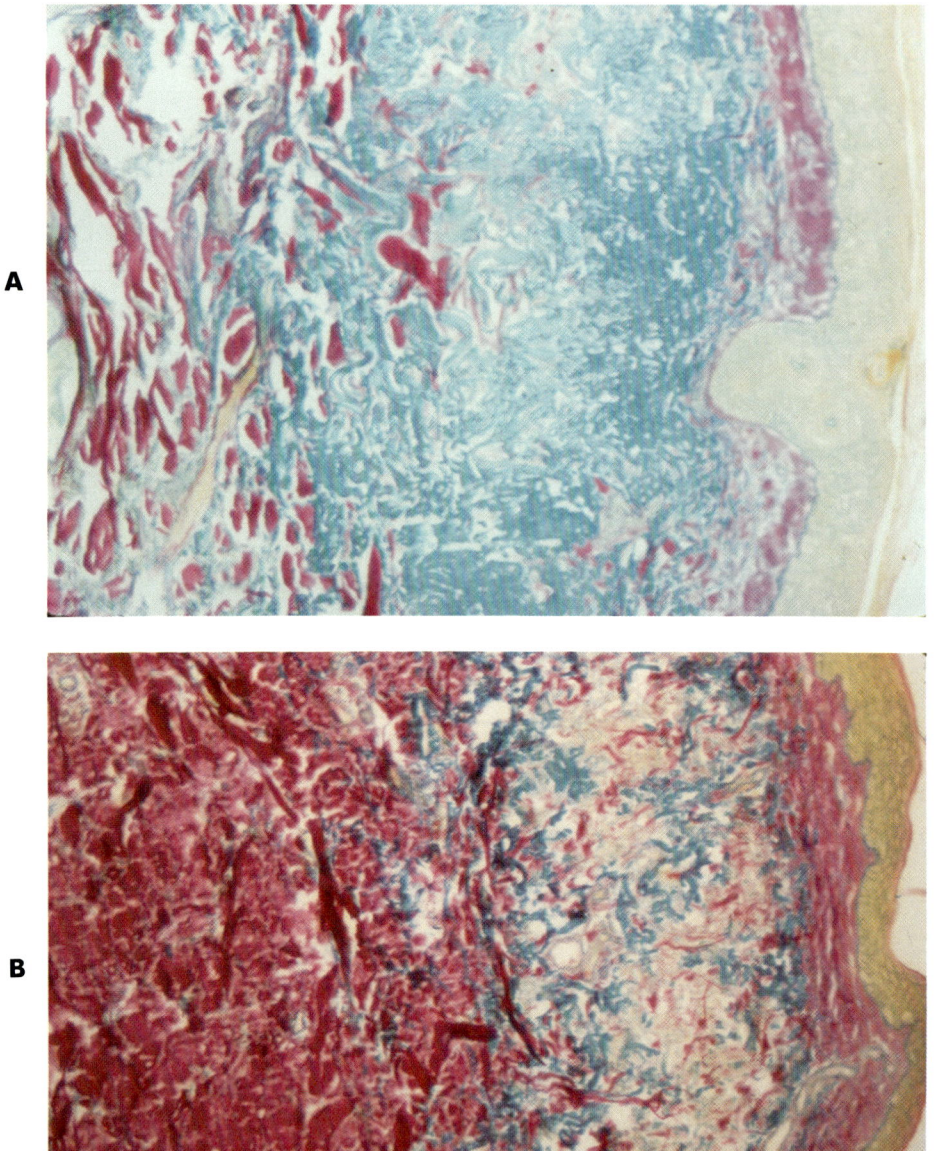

Single-patient comparison of sun-damaged skin versus skin treated with phenol Baker's formula and dermabrasion. Control sun-exposed skin. **A,** Note elastotic mass in papillary dermis. **B,** 120 days after plain phenol peel with occlusion; sun-exposed skin of neck. Note how the elastotic mass has been replaced with new compact collagen, presumably with elastic fibers scattered throughout, which are demonstrable with an elastin stain such as modified Gomori. (Colloidal iron stain; magnification 10×.) **C,** 120 days after Baker's formula peel; occluded sun-exposed skin of neck. Here changes are seen similar to those produced by plain phenol, but the band is wider and the depth of injury greater. (Colloidal iron stain; magnification 10×.) **D,** 120 days after dermabrasion; sun-exposed skin of neck. The changes are comparable in quality and depth to those produced by the Baker's occluded peel. (Colloidal iron stain; magnification 10×.)
(From Stegman SJ: *Aesthetic Plast Surg* 6[3]:123-135, 1982.)

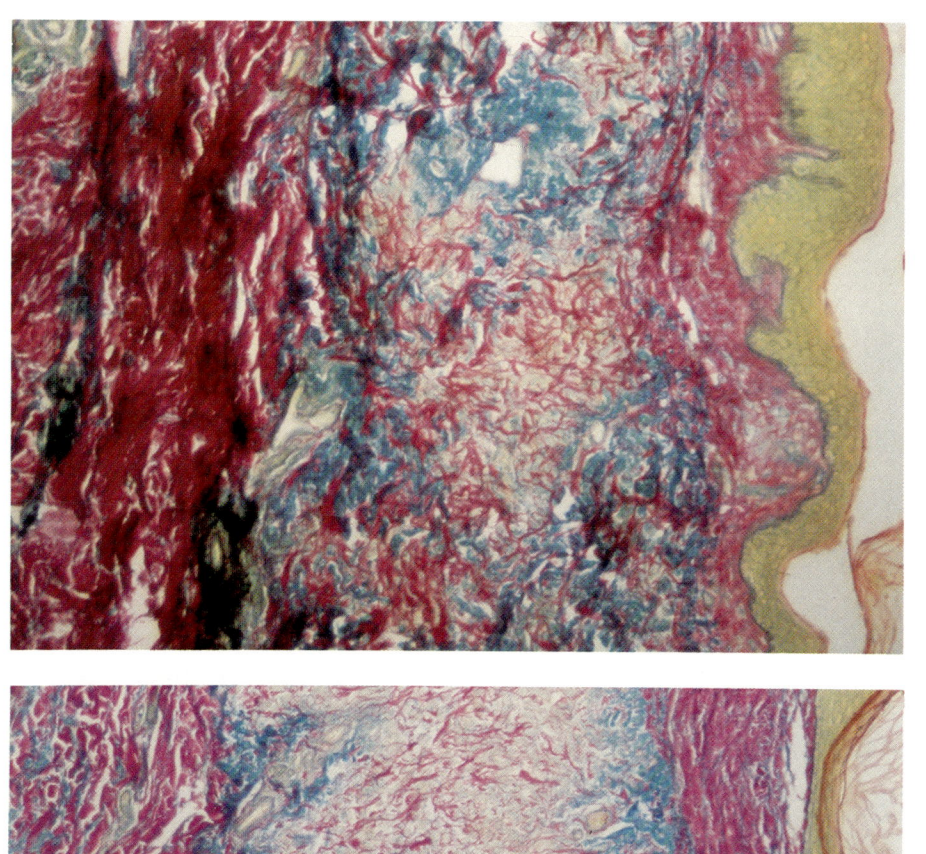

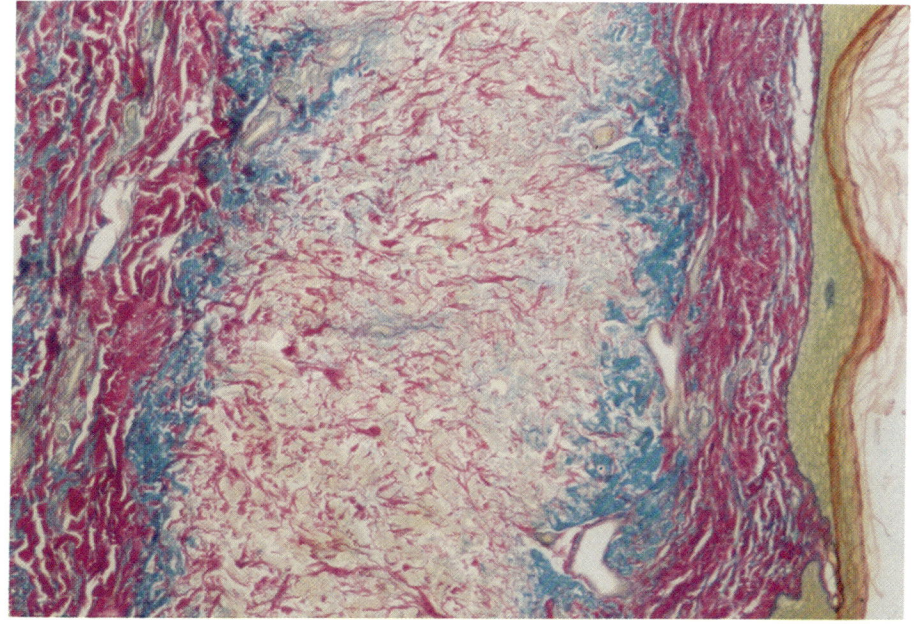

CHAPTER THREE

Peeling Agents

I recommend a single issue of the *Journal of Dermatologic Surgery and Oncology* (Vol. 15, No. 9, September, 1989),* which was devoted exclusively to chemical peels. Editor Harold J. Brody, M.D., conducted a review of the various peeling techniques. The spectrum included phenol peels, trichloroacetic acid (TCA) peels, TCA/Jessner solution peels (Gary D. Monheit, M.D.), TCA and carbon dioxide peels (Harold J. Brody, M.D.), and alpha-hydroxy acid peels.

Collins,[35] in his excellent review of chemical skin peeling in 1987, cited Eller and Wolff's (1941)[45] "menu" of peeling agents that included salicylic acid, acetone, resorcinol, formaldehyde, phenol, betanaphthol, glacial acetic acid, mercurial salts, sulfur, and carbon dioxide.

To date, the most commonly used agents are TCA and several formulas of which phenol is the main ingredient. In 1980, Gross and Maschek[52] listed several different phenol-based peeling solutions. Today, perhaps because of the simplicity of preparation and reliability of results, the formula of Baker[14] remains the most commonly employed phenol-based prescription:

> Phenol USP 88%, 3 cc
> Tap water, 2 cc
> Croton oil, 3 drops
> Septisol (liquid soap), 8 drops

PHENOL

Phenol (C_5H_5OH) or carbolic acid is an aromatic hydrocarbon derived from coal tar. Since the formula does not contain the carboxyl (COOH) group, it is at variance with the structure characteristic of organic acids. This hydroxyl group indicates it is closer to being an organic base or alcohol, rather than an acid.[65]

In high concentrations, phenol is a protein precipitant, causing

---

*Journal Publishing Group, 245 Fifth Avenue, Suite 2401, New York, NY 10016.

extremely rapid denaturation and coagulation of the surface keratin.[65] Phenol denatures the surface keratin proteins, loosely combining with them to form larger molecules with different physical and chemical properties. The coagulum created is, in essence, a protective barrier to further phenol penetration. Increasing the concentration of phenol enhances the keratocoagulation and hinders dermal penetration. When phenol is diluted, deeper penetration and greater systemic absorption occur, increasing the danger of adverse reactions.[32]

Addition of water as the diluent serves to adjust the concentration of phenol. While the Baker formula represents a phenol end concentration of approximately 50%, this 50% phenol solution is chemically stronger than the "stock" USP 88% solution. At concentrations of over 80%, phenol is keratocoagulant, "precipitating the surface protein and thus preventing an extension of the peel solution into the deeper layers of the skin."[76] At a concentration of 50%, however, phenol becomes keratolytic and disrupts sulfur bridges in the keratin layer. It may thus produce greater dermal destruction.[64]

Hence, contrary to the usual chemical pattern, dilution of phenol with water makes the resultant mixture *stronger*, not weaker. The "dilution to effect" relationship is observed clinically. An aqueous mixture that has a final phenol concentration of 50% produces a deeper wound than full strength (88%) phenol.[108]

Phenol is an extremely stable compound. Test solutions kept for over a year demonstrate full potency with no apparent decomposition. However, when not in use, the solution should be stored in a dark place in a tight, light-resistant container.[5]

Toxicity

Litton[65] studied absorption of phenol from the skin. He noted that the maximum blood level was achieved within the first hour and thereafter it declined. The highest blood level was 0.68 mg/ml. In attempting to establish what the toxic level is, he noted that there had been a case reported of a blood phenol level of 23 mg/ml in a man after ingestion. The victim survived.

Litton[65] and Wexler and others[118] noticed that after phenol is absorbed into the bloodstream, it is rapidly conjugated with glycuronic acid, or sulfuric acid, and excreted by the kidneys; or it is detoxified by oxidation to hydroquinone or pyrocatechin; or it can remain as free phenol in the bloodstream and excreted as such by the kidneys. The signs and symptoms of phenol poisoning are usually those of a central depression, fallen blood pressure, headache, and/or nausea. No hepatorenal complications from medical uses are reported in the literature, but theoretically they can occur.[118] There can be a direct toxic effect on the blood vessels of the myocardium, which usually causes the fallen blood pressure.

Pure phenol is a protoplasmic poison particularly affecting the central nervous system. It is readily absorbed from all mucous membranes, wounds, and intact skin.[82]

Deichmann[39] studied detoxification excretion of phenol and stated that "phenol is removed from the animal body by three processes: excretion, oxidation and conjugation." Mullins[83] and Lettieri cited Deichmann and Witherup's[40] work in toxic blood levels of phenol in animal studies. Their experiments demonstrated that the amount of phenol absorbed by rabbit skin depends on the amount of skin surface treated, not the concentration of the aqueous solution used.

Additive Agents: Croton Oil and Septisol

Croton oil is a commercially prepared extract of the seed of the plant *Croton tiglium.* This viscous liquid is capable of significant skin injury by itself, including inflammation, desiccation, and collagen destruction.[65] As an active agent in the peeling solution, croton oil acts to irritate the skin and cause additional maceration.

Septisol, a liquid soap, reduces surface tension and aids penetration of the phenol and croton oil into the skin.

When the suspension of phenol and accessory ingredients is absorbed into the skin, the keratocoagulation creates a chemically altered cutaneous layer that is a barrier to further phenol penetration.

TRICHLOROACETIC ACID (TCA)

Trichloroacetic acid is the other commonly used peeling agent. It also coagulates skin protein. Concentrations between 20% and 50% are commonly employed. The consensus is that concentrations above 50% to 60% may risk such intensive tissue injury that scarring may result.[107] As with phenol, penetration is enhanced by occlusion of the skin surface.

In my experience, TCA in concentrations to 50% has not been as effective as phenol in eliminating moderate to deep wrinkles. I have found it useful as a light peeling agent on the face and have used it on both face and neck (untaped) to remove the tanlike chronic discoloration associated with long-term sun exposure. In the severely sun-damaged patient, the contrast between a peeled face and unpeeled neck may not be acceptable and, hence, the desire to create a zone of transition by literally lightening the color of the neck skin. This concept will be discussed in the "Neck and Chest Peels" section of Chapter 11.

Brodland and Roenigk,[25] in an excellent review article on trichloroacetic acid peeling, primarily for severe actinic damage, listed a variety of "variations in TCA chemexfoliations." These included:

> TCA plus tretinoin preoperatively and postoperatively
> TCA plus 5-fluorouracil
> TCA plus dermabrasion
> TCA plus phenol
> TCA plus CO_2 slush

They indicated that their standard concentrations of TCA were 20%, 35%, and 50%. Although the paper dealt mainly with the management of premalignant actinic damages of the face and scalp, the principles of peeling are well established and recommended to the reader. In comparing phenol peeling with TCA peeling, they stated:

> "The margin of safety associated with TCA chemexfoliation... is one of its primary advantages. Unlike phenol, TCA is neutralized by serum in the superficial dermal plexis when absorbed percutaneously and, therefore, is nontoxic to the heart, liver, and kidneys. This characteristic obviates interoperative cardiac monitoring and makes TCA better for use in elderly patients and those with medical problems."

They further noted that:

> "Unlike phenol peels, the depth of exfoliation with TCA can be adjusted by varying the concentration of TCA on the basis of anatomic location, thickness of the skin, and thickness of the lesions treated. Phenol may cause serious complications such as hypertrophic scarring, full thickness skin loss, and ectropion, but these adverse effects may also occur with inappropriate use of TCA."

The following were listed as advantages of TCA chemexfoliation:
- Procedure possible in patients with medical problems
- Easy adjustment of exfoliation depth by varying concentrations of trichloroacetic acid
- No allergic reactions
- No systemic toxicity
- Rare scarring
- Wound healing time shorter than with 5-fluorouracil or phenol
- Treatment not dependent on patient compliance

Paul Collins, M.D.,[34] described well the chemistry and clinical aspects of TCA peeling:

> "A 50% TCA concentration is obtained by mixing 50 gm TCA (USP) crystals with 100 mL distilled water. A 35% solution is achieved by decreasing TCA to 35 gm and mixing with 100 mL distilled water. The solution should be stored in a dark glass bottle correctly labeled as to ingredients and concentration. Shake contents of the bottle prior to use and seal immediately afterwards. Evaporation will increase the concentration of TCA.

> "The light or superficial repetitive peel is performed with concentrations ranging from 10% to 25% for 'refreshing' the skin. This aids in removal of fine, subtle lines, softening the appearance of enlarged pores, smoothing the skin surface, improving skin texture, and lightening hyperpigmentary disorders. It can be used in individuals with dark complexions. This TCA solution will produce a superficial shedding of the stratum corneum after a single application. However, repetitive peels, weekly or biweekly, will also induce a mild dermal inflammatory response in addition to a deeper peel. In combination with retinoic acid and/or lactic acid, rapid improvement of the skin texture can be appreciated.

"Deep TCA peels produce a refreshing of the skin and do not eliminate but soften deep rhytides. The sallow complexion of actinic damage is replaced by a ruddy, smooth appearance. It is important that the patient understands this concept prior to peeling. A woman will find that cosmetics can be applied easily and uniformly. A pleasant, healthy, facial 'glow' that brightens the skin is the object. TCA peeling can be performed with TCA concentrations of 35%-50% in the same way TCA-S (superficial) was applied. The patient is instructed not to apply cosmetics on the day of the peel. Again, meticulous skin preparation and cleansing are necessary. All rhytides are stretched out to ensure that acid penetrates into the folds. Acid is vigorously rubbed into the unfolded rhytid prior to application to the general area. The acid is applied to the vermillion, earlobes, and brow, and feathered into the hairline. Frosting occurs quickly and dilution often does not take place, thus allowing a deep burn to develop. Neutralization of the acid with the onset of frosting is necessary to limit the depth of the burn on the neck. Here alcohol neutralization must occur within 15-30 seconds after acid application to be effective, as the protein coagulant effect of higher concentration TCA is more rapid."

JESSNER'S SOLUTION

Resorcinol	14 gm
Salicylic acid	14 gm
Lactic acid	14 cc
QS AD ethanol	100 cc

JESSNER'S SOLUTION

Stagnone[103] describes his technique of peeling with Jessner's solution exclusively:

"This formula and modifications of it have been used widely by lay peelers and in prestigious beauty salons on Fifth Avenue and in Beverly Hills. The author's modification of the method described by Horvath follows. As with TCA, the first treatment consists of an even, light coat applied with a wrung-out gauze sponge. The same burning and color changes occur, but the method varies in that washing is not essential. Many patients fan themselves for a few minutes until the burning and stinging sensation subsides. Occasionally, sponging with water is necessary. As with TCA, treatments are given weekly or less often. Assuming a slight-to-moderate reaction to the first treatment, two coats of solution are applied in the second treatment. Three coats are applied at the third treatment. At subsequent treatments, depending on the previous reaction, three coats are applied with heavier pressure and wetter sponges.

"The depth of the reaction is gauged by the degree of flushing and whitening. With the Jessner's formula, the depth of peeling is controlled by the number of coats of solution applied. In addition, the operator stretches the skin while rubbing and overcoating areas to increase the depth. Light peeling with Jessner's is limited to the face. The possibility of toxicity from resorcinol absorption has caused this limitation. When treatment is indicated on the trunk as well as the face, TCA is used on the trunk. The advantages of Jessner's over TCA are that there is no danger of using the wrong concentration of solutions, no need to neutralize the solution, and therefore no need to time the duration of applications. There are fewer chances for mistakes, and the results appear to be comparable. A disadvantage is the limitation of its use only to the face."

TCA/JESSNER'S COMBINATION

Gary D. Monheit, M.D.,[80] has popularized a variance of the TCA peel which he refers to as a "medium-depth chemical peel." Monheit favors Jessner's solution and TCA.

"Jessner's solution is thought to break the intracellular bridges between keratinocytes and thus destroy the barrier function of the epidermis. If applied alone to facial skin after degreasing, it will create a partial epidermal exfoliation that heals within 3 days. This should functionally remove the epidermis as a barrier for the penetration of TCA. Resultant histopathology shows the partial removal of the epidermis with Jessner's solution, which allows greater penetration of the 35% TCA. The TCA solution can thus penetrate through the papillary dermis, and its destructive burn induces new collagen formation that accounts for whatever degree of lessening of crinkles or improved texture is seen after the peel.... The chemicals have no specific influence on collagen bundles other than destruction.... The use of Jessner's solution enables a 35% TCA peel to be more efficacious."

Monheit further favors the combination over a higher concentration of TCA by stating that:

"The risk of scarring using TCA solutions of concentrations higher than 45% is significant and well documented. Thus, it is advantageous to use the combination of 35% TCA and Jessner's solution to reduce the risk of scarring in a medium-depth peel. The combination of both solutions creates a peel procedure that is safe, simple, and effective."

TCA/CO_2

Brody and Hailey[30] have championed the use of solid CO_2 combined with trichloroacetic acid, allowing for an intermediate depth of peeling. "We found the need for an intermediate procedure to improve patients, that would achieve greater depth but still not approach the toxicity of phenolic compounds." By combining solid CO_2 treatment with application of 35% to 50% TCA, Brody and Hailey were able to achieve peels of an intermediate depth between superficial TCA peels and those with Baker's phenol.

Brody described the technique as follows:

"After cleaning the skin with povidone-iodine, solid CO_2 is applied in block form, to further strip the stratum corneum and oil from the skin and to blunt scar edges. The ice is dipped in a 3:1 solution of acetone and alcohol to prevent it from sticking to the skin. Varying pressure is applied to create microepidermal vesiculo-bullous lesions where desired, and pressure designations of CO_2 mild, CO_2 moderate or CO_2 hard are recorded on the patient's chart. All areas of the patient's face and neck may be iced if desired, with patient tolerance and defect size being the chief limiting factors.

"Following application of the CO_2, TCA is applied liberally with cotton applicators. After five minutes, a soothing emollient is applied, usually bacitracin or a live yeast cell ointment.

"Considerable edema occurs for the first few days, but discomfort is generally relatively mild. Erythematous areas become brownish as the crust forms. I encourage my patients to wash twice daily, with antiseptic compresses to minimize crusting. Crust separation usually begins between the fourth and eighth day and is complete within fourteen days, depending on CO_2 pressure and TCA strength."

Brody noted that sometimes there is considerable serous exudation, eczematization, and pruritus, requiring treatment with topical or oral corticosteroids. He warned that some protection is imperative for minimizing hyperpigmentation and suggested that hydroquinone gel is useful as a postpeel prophylactic, especially in dark-skinned or noncompliant individuals.

Brody reported, "We have peeled in excess of three thousand patients using this modality and have enjoyed an excellent degree of success."

The only contraindications involve patients with skin types IV through VI (dark Caucasians, Orientals, Blacks), patients in constant sunlight, those with a history of herpes simplex infection, or those with "unrealistic expections."[26]

RESORCIN

As described by Unna in 1882, resorcin has been widely used for a century in France. Stagnone[103] described Letessier's technique. (See box below for formula.)

> "Unna's paste contained 10%, 20% or 30% resorcin and was applied in gradually increasing concentrations. Letessier has modified Unna's paste to contain 50% resorcin and uses it for chemical peeling. The paste is applied with gloves, first on the forehead and then on the whole face, to a level slightly below the horizontal margin of the mandible. Eyebrows, ears, and mucosal surfaces of the lips are avoided. The paste is spread by gentle massage to ensure a homogeneous peeling. After the paste dries, a mask forms that is removed with a spatula or tongue depressor. The paste is first removed from areas where skin is thinner and lastly from the forehead. The residual gray film forms a 'resorcin membrane', causing difficulty in opening the mouth and with cheek movements. Desquamation begins about the fourth day and ends about a week later leaving a pink, freshened skin. Histologically, Letessier describes superficial epidermal separation and an increase in mitoses in the stratum germinativum with increased glycosamines in the intercellular spaces, and a resulting thicker epidermis. In the dermis a prolonged vasodilitation and a proliferation of fibroblasts with an increase in fibrillar collagen cause a thickening of the papillary dermis. Except for the vasodilitation, the dermal changes were noted to persist at 4 months. Letessier reports these changes result in a more homogeneous and youthful appearance of the skin."

LETESSIER'S MODIFICATION OF UNNA'S PASTE

Resorcin	40 gm
Zinc oxide	10 gm
Ceyssatite	2 gm
Benzoin axungia	28 gm

ALPHA-HYDROXY ACIDS

Recently, there has been a flurry of clinical and basic science interest in the alpha-hydroxy acids as peeling agents. These show promise as light peeling agents for the younger age-group. Activity in this area follows the great interest in retinoic acid as an effective, albeit mild, exfoliating agent.

James J. Stagnone, M.D.,[101] wrote an excellent article entitled "Superficial Peeling" in the *Journal of Dermatologic Surgery and Oncology*. He described indications for superficial peeling as rejuvenation of the skin, acne, pigmentary changes, moderate wrinkling, actinic damage, and scarring. His definition of light peeling is that which is performed with 10% to 35% TCA, Jessner's solution (p. 64), modified Unna's paste (p. 67), alpha-hydroxy acids, azelaic acid, and retinoic acid. Stagnone noted that

> "with the exception of azelaic acid and retinoic acid, which you use on a daily basis, and resorcin, which is used after longer intervals, light peeling techniques involve weekly or less frequent applications. In general the shorter the interval between peels and the deeper the effects, the sooner maximal benefits will be obtained. The shortest interval, in our experience, is one week and we perform weekly treatments for 1-2 months initially. There is no absolute number of treatments, so patients may receive 20 or more light peels over a period of a year. The number of light peels a patient can receive is unlimited unless complications occur. Regardless of the problem—acne, pigmentary changes, or actinic damage—partial recurrences are likely. Patients have the option to return for additional light peels at the interval that they perceive is necessary to keep their problem under optimum control. The average return rate for a course of 2 or 3 weekly light peels is twice a year. Many patients sustain their improvement with regular use of retinoic acid and sunscreens and are seen annually until they are comfortable with self-treatment."

Stagnone noted that some alpha-hydroxy acids are found in foods. They include glycolic acid (sugar cane), lactic acid (sour milk), malic acid (apples), citric acid (fruits), and tartaric acid (grapes). In low concentrations, the alpha-hydroxy acids diminish corneocyte cohesion whereas in high concentrations they cause epidermolysis. Repeated and regular applications to the face diminish fine facial wrinkles significantly. In the treatment of wrinkles, the skin surface is thoroughly moistened with a solution of 50% to 75% alpha-hydroxy acid once weekly or every 2 weeks for 6 months. The solution is left on the face for 1 to 5 minutes. Initially, there will be an erythema associated with a moderate burning and tingling sensation. The solution is washed off with water or with a 5% to 10% solution of sodium bicarbonate. High concentrations of alpha-hydroxy acids are used during an office visit and can be supplemented by twice daily application of 5% to 10% concentrations of alpha-hydroxy acids by the patient at home. The mechanism for this antiwrinkle effect is unknown, but because alpha-hydroxy acids are naturally occurring nontoxic organic acids that are well tolerated, they may eventually supplant other peeling agents.

Johnson, Griffin, and Van Scott reported on alpha-hydroxy acids as peeling agents at the 1989 annual meeting of the American Academy of Dermatology. Lactic acid, glycolic acid, and pyruvic acid are nontoxic and easily neutralized. Glycolic acid and pyruvic acids at high concentrations can be used as superficial and medium-depth peeling agents. The versatility lies in altering the concentration and time of application as a means to control the depth of injury. The time of application can be controlled by altering the time until the operator neutralizes them with water. These operators employed retinoic acid 2 weeks prior to the procedure as a routine part of pretreatment preparation. As of the time this book went to press, these researchers have not published articles on the subject, although Drs. Griffin and Van Scott have been investigating the subject for over 2 years. The following is the preliminary report of Dr. Griffin*:

> "At this time, I am doing two basic types of peels with these agents. I do a light chemical peel with 70% glycolic acid. This is a very superficial peel, involving at most the lower layers of the epidermis and possibly the upper papillary dermis. This peel needs to be repeated and this can be done at one-month intervals. The number of repetitions may be as many as five, a fact which I make well known to my patients. This peel is not meant to be deep and is not meant to change the texture of the skin by inducing scarring. One sees gradual but definite improvement of fine wrinkles and pigmentary changes due to sun exposure. Between peels, I have patients use Neostrata skin smoothing cream, an approximately 30% alpha-hydroxy acid preparation. This light peel is well tolerated, heals in 4 to 7 days, and at this writing, I have not had side effects from it. As with all alpha-hydroxy acids, glycolic acid must be diluted with 100% alcohol. A good cleaning and degreasing procedure with acetone should be done prior to peeling in every 'nook and cranny' of the face.
>
> "The second type of peel is a pyruvic acid peel. This is a medium-depth peeling agent. I have used pyruvic acid as a full-face peeling agent in concentrations of 60% to 80%, once again diluted with 100% ethyl alcohol. I have also attempted to use pyruvic acid in the treatment of solar lentigines on the shoulders and back with some success. I am looking to use pyruvic acid mixed with croton oil and an emulsifying agent in the same concentrations as in the Baker formula for treatment of deep wrinkles over the lip. To this writing, I have not found a patient whom I felt to be a good first candidate for this procedure. Dr. Van Scott and I have done test spots on our arms with this formula and found it to heal more quickly and evenly with earlier reformation of the epidermal rete than with 80% pyruvic acid used alone. I am anxious to use 60% to 80% pyruvic acid to replace phenol in the Baker's formula as soon as possible.
>
> "Postoperatively, I have my patients apply ice packs for the first 24 hours to minimize swelling. In addition, they use antibiotic ointment, usually bacitracin, and then soaks and ointment after 24 hours. I tell the patients not to allow the crusts to dry. In addition, I have placed patients on prophylactic erythromycin. The

---

*Personal communication.

crusts come off in approximately 7 to 10 days with pyruvic acid peels.

"Initially I thought neutralization with water was important. However, at this time I feel that, once whitening occurs, the procedure has reached its full effectiveness. Patients tend to be relieved of stinging and burning by cool compresses, however, the true relief comes when the antibiotic ointment is applied. Generally I wait 30 minutes or so before applying the antibiotic ointment.

"In general, I think alpha-hydroxy acids are safe peeling agents. I am particularly favoring the repeated light glycolic acid peeling since the improvements are definite but the textural changes of the skin are very subtle. Dr. Howard Murad in Los Angeles is also performing repeated glycolic acid peels."

Recently, Howard Murad[84] has proposed glycolic acid treatments "for smoothing the skin and for what one might call 'preventive maintenance' against changes associated with aging or photo damage." With this approach, Dr. Murad explained in an interview, a glycolic acid concentration of 50% to 70% is applied to the face every few weeks. The face is first prepared with gauze application of chlorhexidine gluconate (Hibiclens) wash without scrubbing. The acid is then applied with cotton-tipped applicators, and these are changed often. The acid is left on for 3 to 7 minutes, then neutralized and washed off, using a water-soaked soft gauze pad.

Before initiating glycolic acid therapy, Dr. Murad emphasized, a careful history should be taken to judge the possibility of an allergic reaction and the likely sensitivity of the patient's skin.

As the clinician gains more experience, Dr. Murad went on, either Jessner's solution or acetone can be used for prepping. Either one makes the patient's skin more sensitive to glycolic acid and improves the peel. Also, he said, with repeated applications, the glycolic acid can be left on the face longer to enhance results.

The patient is given a supply of glycolic acid, either an 8% cream or a 10% gel formulation, which is applied twice daily to the areas between office visits.

The alpha-hydroxy acids (AHAs), including glycolic acid, said Dr. Murad, block hyperkeratosis. "Hence," he went on to say, "they maintain a smoother skin surface, keep follicular canals from becoming occluded, and restrain the development of various types of dermatoses. Because of this action, the AHAs are unexcelled for treating and preventing rough, dry skin and in treating and preventing age spots, most of which are keratoses rather than lentigines."

CHAPTER FOUR

Indications and Patient Selection

The most common indication for chemical skin peeling is age-induced and environmentally induced wrinkling of the skin. However, not all those who fit these criteria are acceptable candidates. Texture and color must be considered since the process is less predictable with thick, oily skin. In addition, phenol peels have a propensity to alter the melanocytic population of the skin; hypopigmentation or hyperpigmentation may occur. I shall paraphrase Stegman* by stating: "With respect to color changes following deep phenol peels, the only safe prediction that can be made is that there will be a color change, either lighter or darker. Which will occur may be uncertain." In Chapter 8 the management of hyperpigmentation is reviewed in greater detail, but generally, lightening rather than darkening can be expected to occur following a deep phenol peel.

Classically, the ideal candidate is described as a female who is thin-skinned, fair complexioned, with fine wrinkling. Patients with blue or green eyes and blond or red hair have the ideal pigmentary constitution. Likewise, the classic unacceptable candidate for phenol peeling has thick, oily skin of black, yellow, or brown color. While some practitioners claim to be successful in treating such patients, I would caution the novice against using phenol.

Acne scarring, particularly the "ice pick" variety, is notoriously resistant to improvement by chemical skin peeling. In my practice, fewer than 10% of acne-scarred patients requesting peeling are deemed acceptable. In those cases, fair complexioned patients with shallow pitting who often demonstrate spotlike postinflammatory hyperpigmentation may anticipate a reasonable result. Just the erasure of the frecklelike postinflammatory hyperpigmentation improves the appearance. Such dark spots mimic the shadows cast by the actual depressed scars and hence worsen the overall appearance.

*Personal communication.

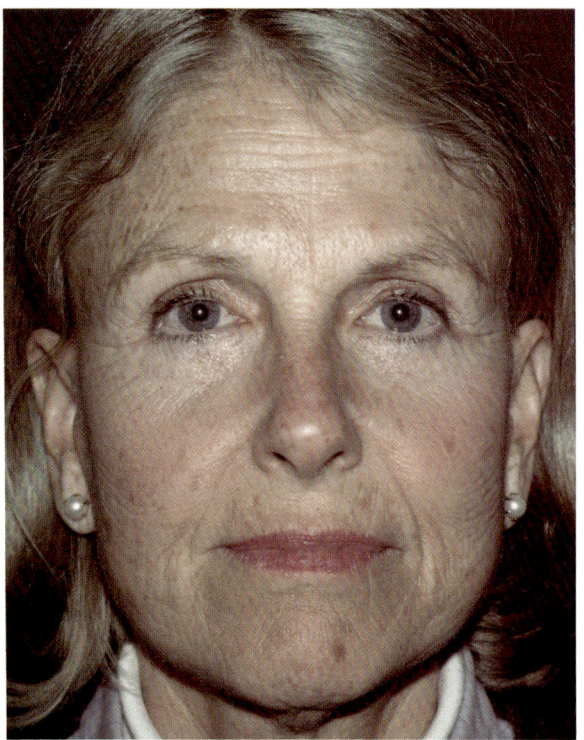

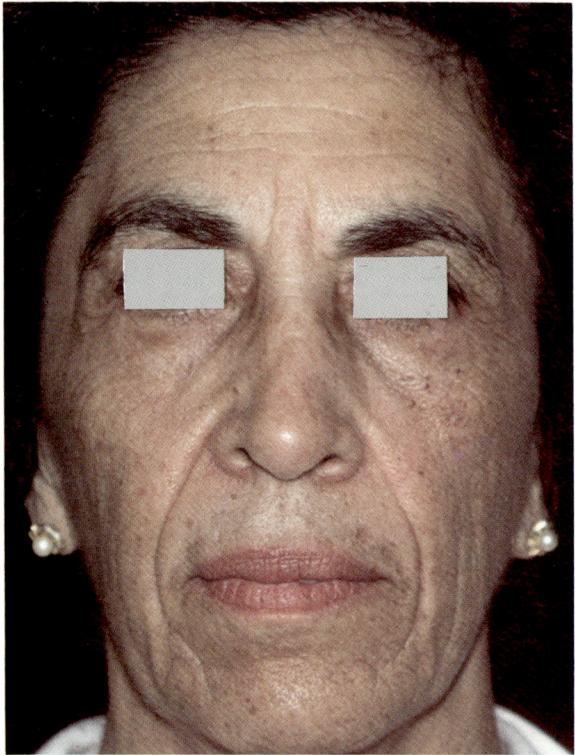

Patient selection. The first patient is an ideal candidate for chemical rejuvenation: she has thin, fair skin, fair hair, and blue eyes. She sought treatment to remove the fine wrinkling and hyperpigmentation caused by years of sun exposure and was selected for a chemical skin peel. The second patient is a poor candidate for chemical rejuvenation: she has dark skin, dark eyes and hair, and is of South American ancestry. She was rejected as a candidate for this procedure.

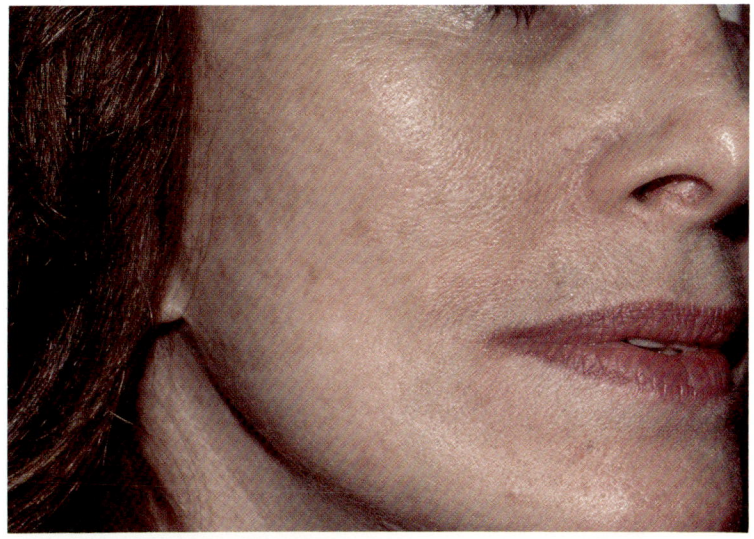
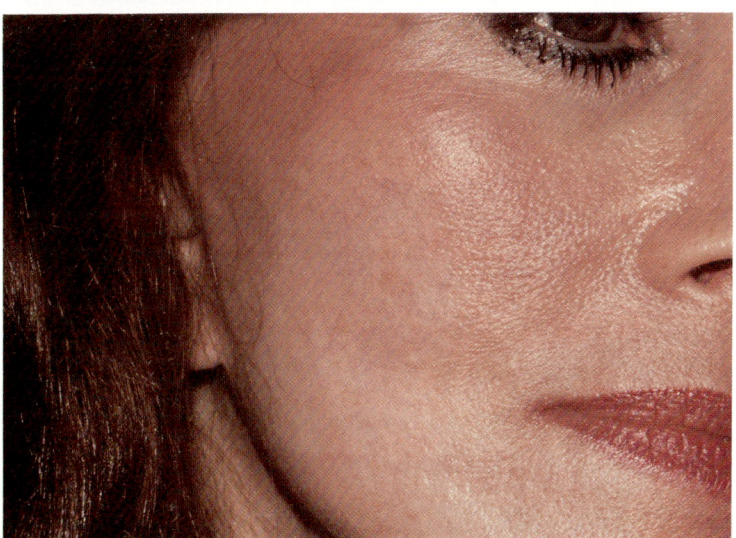

Good candidate for chemical skin peeling to remove mild postinflammatory hyperpigmentation. The patient is shown before and after treatment in a close-up oblique view of the cheek. A good result was obtained with an unoccluded Baker formula phenol peel.

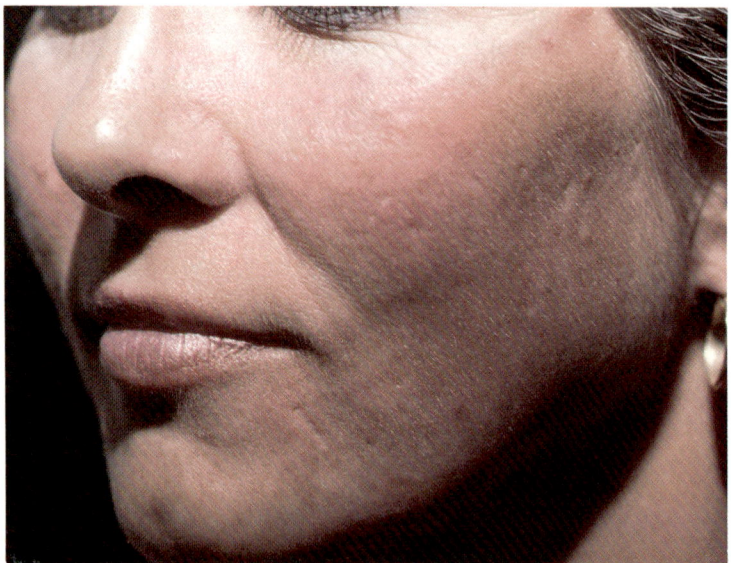

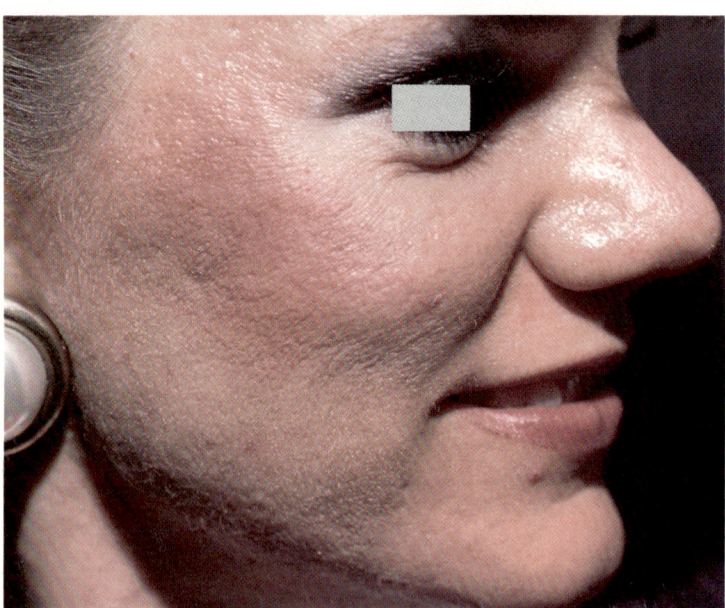

Poor candidates for chemical skin peeling. These patients were both disqualified as candidates for chemical skin peeling. The first patient sought treatment to remove acne scars, and although her fair complexion and blue eyes normally would make her an ideal candidate for chemical skin peeling, the nature of her scars and a demonstrated history of hyperpigmentation contraindicated the procedure. The second patient sought treatment to improve skin texture. However, her dark eyes, thick, oily skin, and significant acne scarring were strong contraindications for chemical skin peeling.

The issue of candidacy based on skin color must be strongly considered in the male patient since makeup camouflage of color disparity is usually not an option.

In evaluating the patient at consultation, we obtain a general medical and surgical history. We also require that a "skin peel questionnaire" be completed. I consider the racial ancestry a crucial factor since, particularly in many metropolitan areas, many patients present a mosaic of the American emigration history. It is not unknown to see a patient having each grandparent with a different ethnic or racial background. American Indian ancestry is not necessarily recognized separately, but those individuals have a strong potential for pigmentary problems.

FACIAL REJUVENATION PATIENT QUESTIONNAIRE

1. Are you now taking or have you ever taken birth control pills?   Yes   No

    If yes, when started? _____ When stopped? _____
2. Do you ever get "herpes" skin eruptions or cold sores?   Yes   No
3. Of what ancestry are you? (English, Russian, etc.)

    Maternal grandmother _____ Maternal grandfather _____

    Paternal grandmother _____ Paternal grandfather _____
4. Do you regularly sunbathe?   Yes   No
5. If so, do you tan easily?   Yes   No
6. If you do tan, is the tan even or blotchy?   Even   Blotchy
7. Do you now have or have you ever had kidney problems?   Yes   No
8. Have you ever had X-ray treatment to your face and/or neck for acne or any other reason?   Yes   No
9. Have you ever had dermabrasion or a chemical peel?   Yes   No
10. If so, when, where, and by whom? _____
11. Are you currently using or have you ever used Retin-A?   Yes   No

    If yes, when started? _____ When stopped? _____
12. Are you currently using or have you ever used Accutane?   Yes   No

    If yes, when started? _____ When stopped? _____
13. Are you currently using or have you ever used thyroid pills or female hormone pills or injections?   Yes   No

    If yes, when started? _____ When stopped? _____

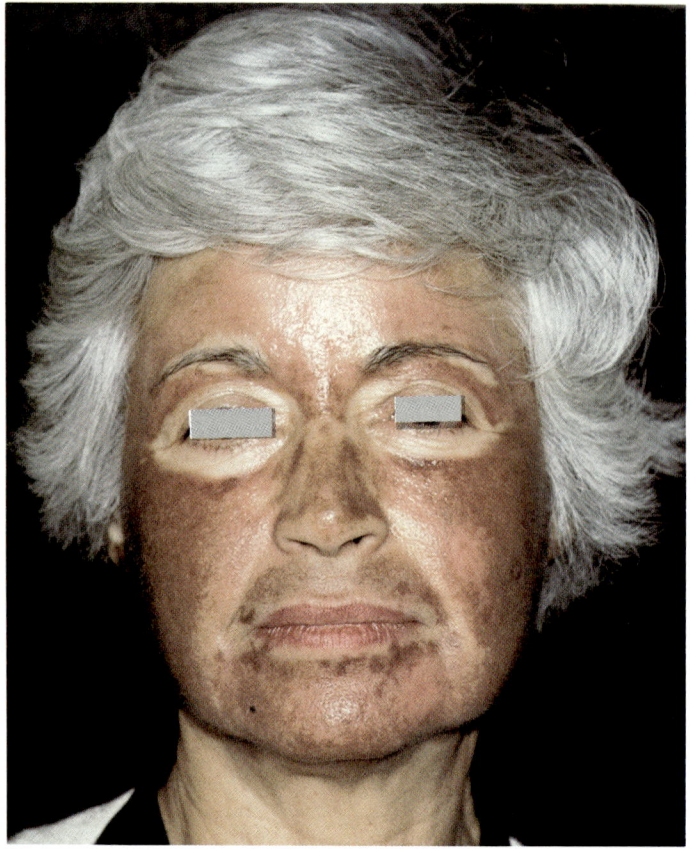

Postpeel hyperpigmentation. This unfortunate patient had a skin peel performed by a lay practitioner. Her undisclosed partial American Indian ancestry contributed to the poor result shown here.

One should be certain to ascertain the presence or absence of a history of reactive pigmentation to previous surgical procedures, including dermabrasion — the procedure that most closely mimics peeling in its effect on skin pigmentation. One should inspect surgical scars, if present. Likewise, one must always seek to examine unexposed skin — such as within the scalp — to determine the "true" baseline tone of the skin.

I would be loath to peel a patient who had a history of very large doses of radiation to the face or long-term topical steroid treatment that may have resulted in dermal atrophy. Wolfe[119] in 1982 described a case in which a skin peel was performed on the perioral area. That skin had been subjected to 6000 rad of therapeutic irradiation for treatment of a carcinoma of the floor of the mouth. Wolfe noted:

> "The peel was deeper than usual and slow to heal, but in this particular patient, the eventual result was satisfactory. Further experience will need to be obtained with chemical peeling in irradiated areas before the procedure can be considered safe, however, and until then, patients should be advised of the risk of a full thickness skin loss."

In his paper, it was interesting to note the description of the healing process:

"... and the crust that formed after the topical treatment with thymol iodide powder did not loosen for two weeks. The redness required a full three months to subside...."

In 1952 MacKee and Karp[74] stated:

"We're cautious with patients who have had x-ray treatment: the first treatment is mild. However, many of the patients had received a full course of x-ray treatments (75 R once weekly for 16 weeks), yet their skin tolerated applications of full strength."

Large areas of scar or any area where there is an absence of the dermal appendages should never be treated, as it is from these pilosebaceous units that new epidermal cells arise to resurface the skin. In these cases, healing occurs by granulation tissue with additional scarring and distortion.[32]

Current medications must be reviewed. Female hormones and contraceptive pills, through interplay of the pituitary gland and its control of a melanocytic stimulatory hormone, may influence postpeel pigmentation. Our practice is to ask the patient to withdraw the medication for 6 weeks before and several months after the skin peeling. Since retinoic acid alone is an exfoliative, use of the agent immediately prior to the peel may result in a deeper peel. It is recognized that retinoic acid thins the stratem corneum and influences fibrogenosis.[59] The wisdom of deliberately employing retinoic acid as a pretreatment to enhance the peeling procedure is discussed later in this chapter.

Recently, there have been reports of postpeel scarring possibly associated with the prepeel or postpeel use of isotretinoin (Accutane).*[27] Since practitioners reporting observation of this complication indicate many variables in the patient's collective histories, including intervals between isotretinoin treatment and peeling, peeling solution, number of peeling processes, and so forth, further investigation is necessary to determine if there is a cause and effect relationship.*

PATCH TESTING

In the borderline patient, a hedge against the uncertainty of pigmentary response can be provided by a "patch" or sample test, usually conducted at a concealed site such as the frontal hairline. This test area should be observed for 10 to 12 weeks. In the patient who is having surgical face lifting or other surgical rejuvenative procedure, it is convenient and appropriate to perform the peel patch test at that session since the interval of several months during which the patch must be observed is parallel with the period of surgical healing.

---

*Roche Laboratories, Nutley, NJ.
*Personal communication, Harold Brody, M.D.

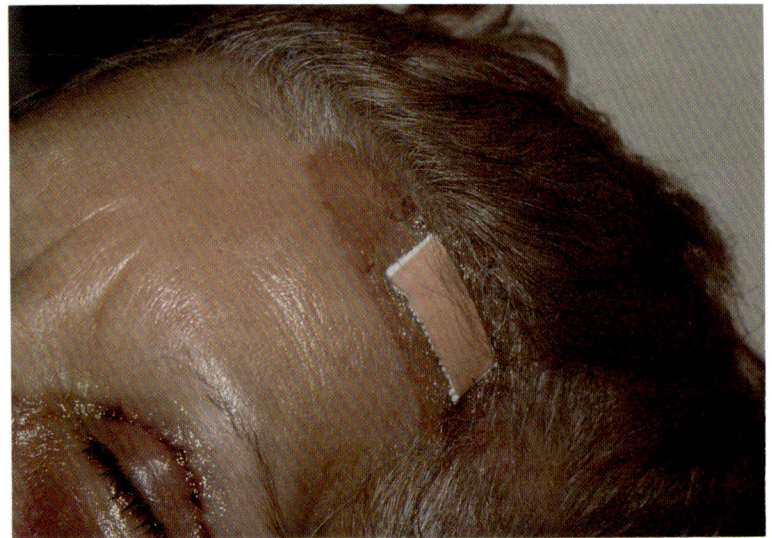
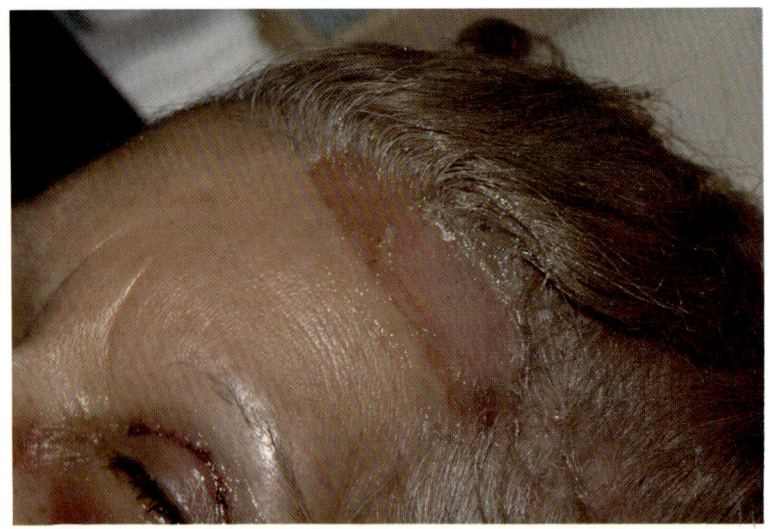
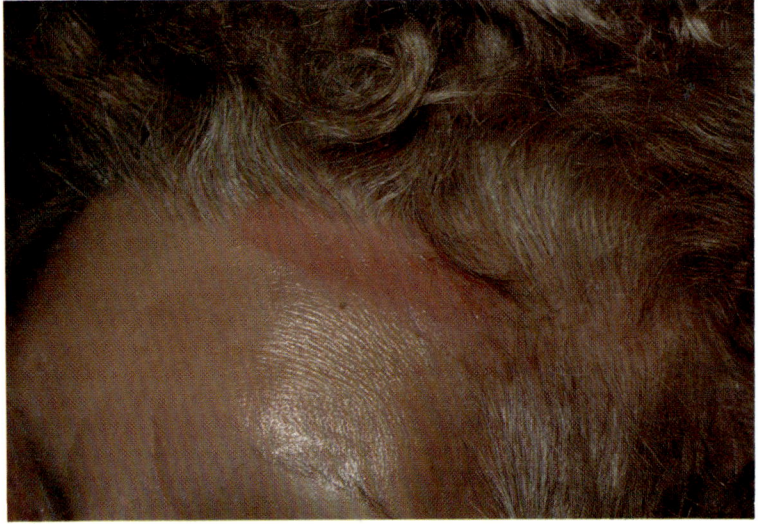

Patch testing. This patient's dark hair and complexion and Hispanic background make her a less than ideal candidate for chemical skin peeling. A patch test was therefore performed at the time of her blepharoplasty and face lift surgery. The timing took advantage of the 3-month interval (before a peel could be done) to evaluate the potential for postpeel discoloration. Close-up view of patch-tested area 2 days after application of Baker phenol solution shows a portion of the test area that was deliberately left unoccluded. The tape removed and tidying is performed. The appearance of the area after 30 days is satisfactory.

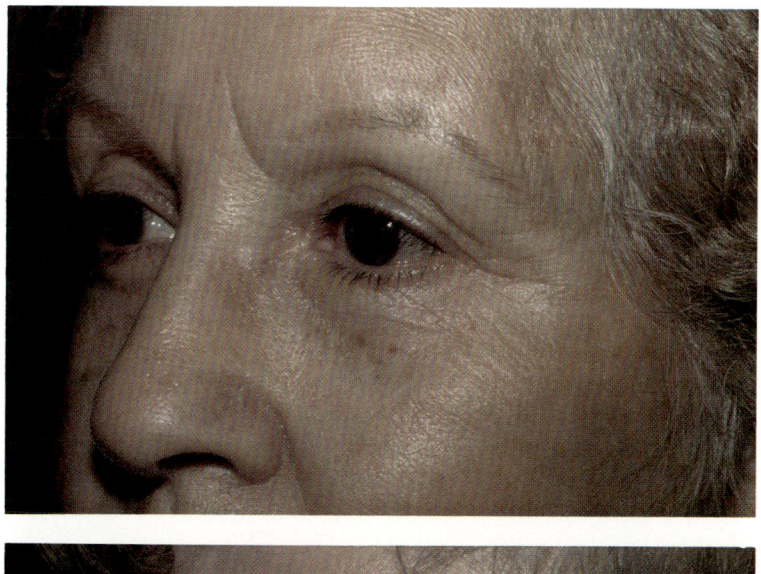

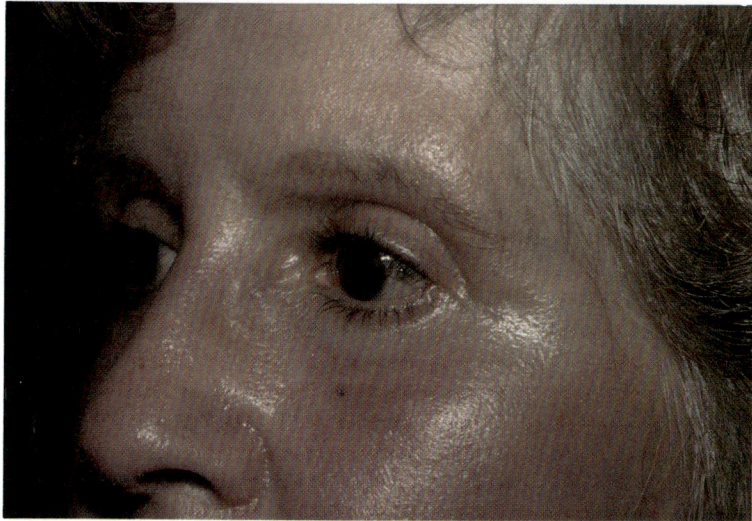

Final result: upper and lower blepharoplasty and face lift combined with chemical peel. Because the patient's patch test at the time of facial surgery yielded a favorable result, she was accepted as a candidate for a chemical face peel. The patient had an excellent result with an occluded Baker formula phenol peel; however, her postpeel redness took nearly 6 months to subside.

Patients may be disqualified from having the chemical skin peel for medical reasons (see box on p. 80). For example, since phenol, the most frequently employed major agent, requires conjugation by the kidneys, obviously those with borderline or poor kidney function are not candidates. Likewise, patients with cardiac and hepatic insufficiency are not candidates, in deference to the well-recognized potential cardiotoxic effect of phenol and detoxification of anesthetic agents by the liver.

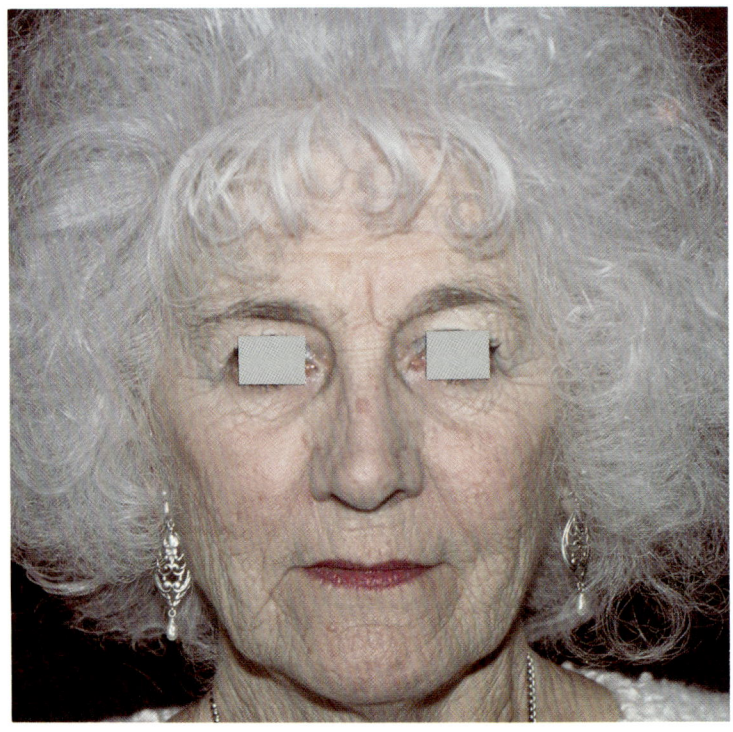

Patient selection. An ideal candidate with respect to skin color, blue eye color, and indications for chemical skin peeling, this patient nevertheless was disqualified for the procedure because of her unsuitable cardiac status.

RELATIVE CONTRAINDICATIONS

1. Inadequate photo protection
2. Skin types IV through VI
3. Keloid-prone individuals
4. History of herpes simplex
5. Unrealistic patient expectations
6. History of cardiac disease
7. History of hepatorenal disease
8. History of previous facial irradiation
9. Ehlers-Danlos syndrome
10. Recent isotretinoin treatment
11. HIV positive disease

From Brody HJ: Complications of chemical peeling, *J Dermatol Surg Oncol* 15(9):1010-1019, Sept 1989.

PRETREATMENT USE OF RETINOIC ACID

As retinoic acid has become an important member of the skin peeler's armamentarium, its role in enhancing the effect of chemical skin peeling has been raised. Collins[34] stated that prior application of retinoic acid will enhance the penetrance and thus the effectiveness of TCA by decreasing the debris and scales present on the epidermis. He noted that such peeling should be done with caution because of the potential enhancement of acid penetration. One could extrapolate the same conclusion with respect to the use of retinoic acid before peeling with phenol. Baker noted that he does not pretreat with retinoic acid if the patient is going to have a phenol peel but will if TCA will be used.*

Stegman[108] and associates noted that "patients who are pretreated with medicines that will correct the actinically damaged epidermis, such as Retin-A or the alpha-hydroxy acids, will absorb the agent better. This must be considered in order to dose the patient properly."

In our practice, many patients have used retinoic acid for some period of time. We factor this into the decision when determining the technique to be employed, but we caution the patient to inform us accurately as to the utilization. Signs of retinoic acid overuse call for cessation for at least 6 weeks prior to the procedure.

Some investigators favor the use of retinoic acid following chemical skin peeling. Stagnone[102] favors regular usage of retinoic acid beginning 2 weeks after dermabrasion or peeling "after resolution of any significant inflammation."

CONSULTATION AND INFORMED CONSENT

At initial consultation or reconsultation, the prospective patient is shown before and after examples of typical results. As indicated, the candidate is shown photographs of patients demonstrating uncamouflaged color differences between the treated face and untreated neck. This is an important part of the patient's informed consent to the procedure since it demonstrates the permanence of the color disparity and, pending the patient's personal makeup habits, the need for a long-term camouflage. Unless specifically requested, I do not show patients photographs of their appearance during the 1-week "healing" exfoliative process.

Photographs are taken in views that we have standardized for the practice. Consistency of photographic technique is important for the following reasons.

1. An unequivocal base-line medical record is established.
2. The photos must be consulted during the procedure when the patient is supine. In the supine position, in some anatomic zones, wrinkling will be less than in the erect position; conceivably, without the ability to reference accurate preoperative photographs, one could undertreat some areas.

---

*Personal communication.

3. Photos with standardized framing, camera exposure ("F-stop"), shutter speed, and lighting technique will allow consistency for the practitioner's quality control program.
4. Good quality "before" pictures are a practitioner's best response to an unappreciative, short-memoried patient. And, of course, it is the best resource when answering an inappropriate medical malpractice lawsuit.

The routine views employed in our practice are:

	Distance
Frontal face and neck	5 feet
Frontal face only	4 feet
Close-up frontal forehead	2 feet
Close-up frontal orbital	2 feet
Close-up oblique (face turned 45 degrees) of each orbital/ malar area	2 feet
Close-up frontal mid-face	2 feet
Close-up frontal lip and chin	2 feet
Close-up oblique (head turned 45 degrees) of each cheek	2 feet

As clinically indicated, other views may be taken. Scars — surgical or traumatic — and unusual skin abrasions should be recorded.

If the patient has had previous peels or dermabrasions and the "zone of transition" between treated and untreated skin exists, I would suggest recording the area photographically.

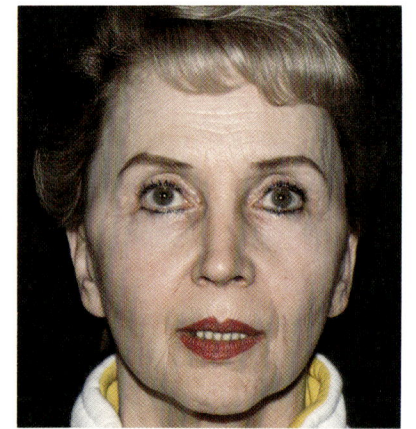 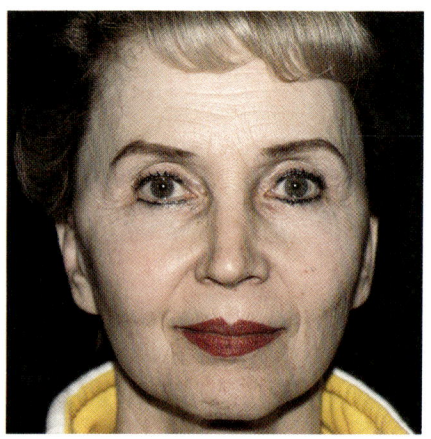

Photo technique. The standard photographic views employed in our practice are illustrated here. **A,** Frontal face and neck, 5 feet distance; **B,** frontal face only, 4 feet; **C,** close-up frontal forehead, 2 feet; **D,** close-up frontal orbital area, 2 feet; **E and F,** close-up oblique orbitomalar area, 2 feet; **G,** close-up frontal midface, 2 feet; **H,** close-up frontal lip and chin, 2 feet; **I,** close-up oblique left cheek, 2 feet; **J,** close-up oblique right cheek, 2 feet.

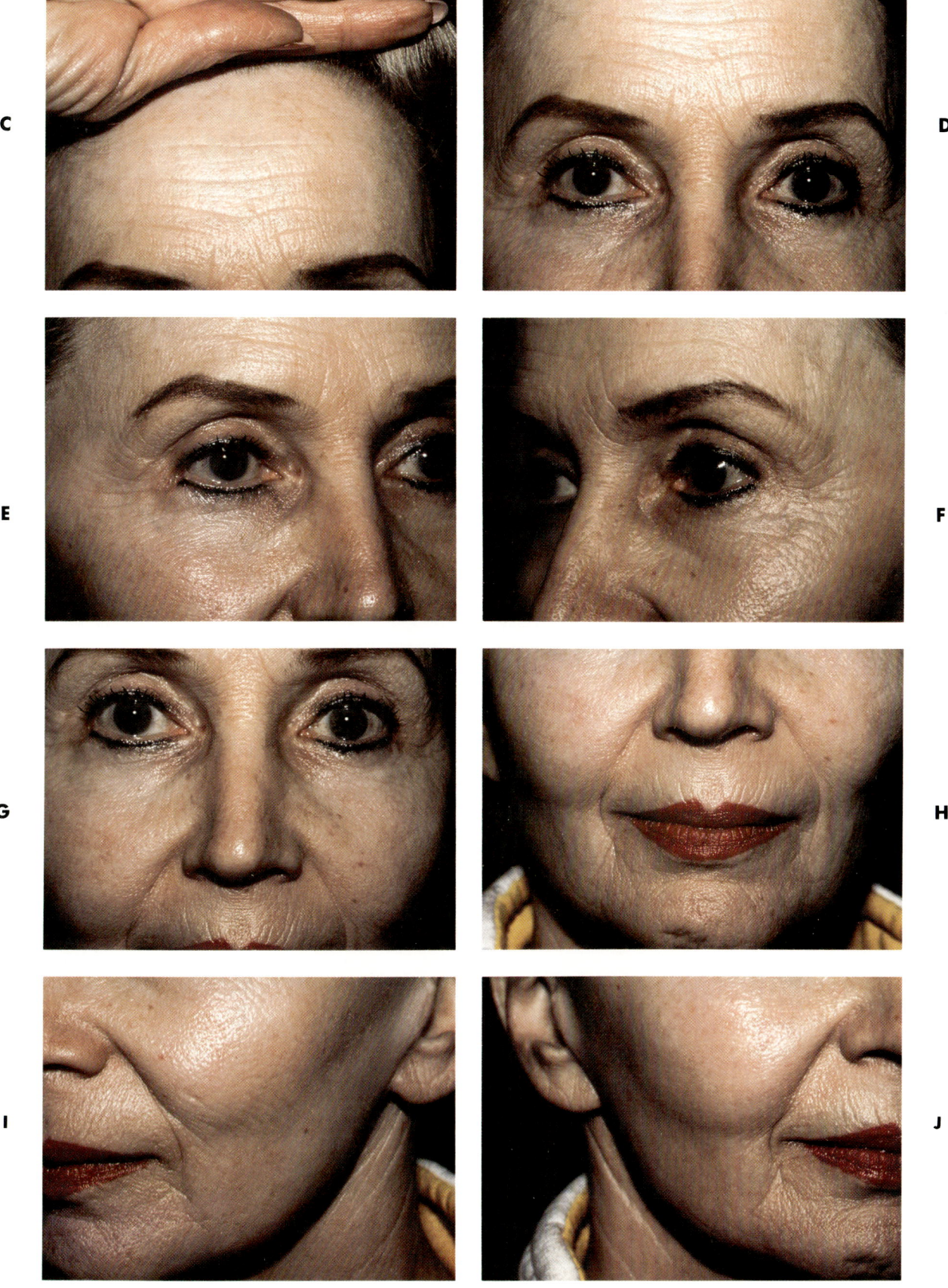

After answering questions posed by the patient, we provide an illustrated booklet about the procedure in addition to a "Face Fact" sheet that outlines the timetable for the first week following the procedure. The prospective patient is encouraged to record any further questions and present them at the time of the future preoperative visit, generally conducted 2 weeks before the procedure. Following consultation and just prior to the preoperative visit, the patient should have a preoperative medical consultation and clearance by the personal physician. This examination should include, minimally, a basic history and physical examination, complete blood count, urinalysis, and serum creatinine level. We prefer to have a baseline cardiogram provided as well. A chest x-ray examination is optional, at the discretion of the consulting physician, as is the matter of a chemistry panel, including liver function tests. Certainly, any history of alcoholism, hepatitis, etc., mandates a full liver function panel. For the examining physician's convenience, our office provides a "checklist" form for completion.

At the preoperative visit, the sequence of events of the precedure day is explained in detail to the patient. Consents are signed. The patient is given a prescription for pHisoHex to be used as the exclusive facial soap and shampoo for 5 days prior to the procedure. The patient is advised that nothing should be eaten or drunk after the midnight before the procedure and that the anesthesiologist will call the patient the evening before the procedure to obtain a history and discuss the anesthetic.

INTRODUCTION

This booklet describes one of modern medicine's most significant and truly astonishing accomplishments: the reversal of the skin's signs of aging through a medical—not surgical—process.

While perpetually youthful appearing skin has always been one of man and woman's most ancient desires, until the past several decades the goal was unattainable. The ancient Egyptians and other great civilizations sought means of smoothing wrinkled skin through applications of substances such as honey and milk and even practiced a rather crude method of mechanical sanding using alabaster stone (undoubtedly the forerunner of today's dermabrasion or mechanical sanding). Obviously none of these techniques ever achieved any level of success.

In Europe, in this century, there developed techniques of facial rejuvenation that were practiced by nonphysicians known as aestheticians. Akin to today's cosmetologists, these lay people prepared combinations of lotions and chemicals that could indeed remove the outer, worn layer of skin. With such a process, not only were age spots, brown spots and other blemishes removed, but the skin became smoother, less wrinkled, and remarkably younger appearing. Eventually, some of these lay-practitioners brought their techniques to the United States but were limited in their abilities to provide this process to the public, since there are more stringent laws controlling the dispensing of drugs and administration of anesthetics. As a few physicians developed an interest in performing the process, it became a practical, safe, and comfortable procedure. Through the rapid progress made in medical science and particularly anesthesia, it was practical to shorten the performance and recovery time of such a facial rejuvenation from weeks to days.

MY PERSONAL EXPERIENCE WITH REJUVENATION

In the late 1960s, when I was a surgeon-in-training in Chicago, I was astonished when I first saw the results of facial rejuvenation as performed by one of my teachers. This particular doctor—who was one of the first surgeons in Chicago to have become highly specialized in cosmetic facial surgery in its early days—took me under his wing so to speak and shared with me his knowledge and experience. For over ten years, I studied the process—both here and in Europe—and conducted my own research on the subject.

Fortunate was I that I had the opportunity to receive that training, for I had realized that surgery alone was incapable of making old skin look younger. In fact, it seemed to me that those surgeons who pulled the facial skin too tightly, in a vain attempt to pull out the wrinkles, did their patient a great disservice because these patients invariably wore a plastic or mask-like expression after surgery that hardly complimented them or their surgeon. It became apparent that unless a cosmetic facial surgeon could remove wrinkles, both he and his patient would be dissatisfied regardless of the quality of the surgery performed.

The extra time and effort expended in acquiring the skills to perform this procedure has brought a great sense of satisfaction and enjoyment to this physician. When the patient returns to the office one week after the procedure with the new, smooth, fresh pink skin and says "I still cannot believe it. The wrinkles are really gone!" I am as thrilled as I was when I started performing these procedures.

From brochure used in the practice of Robert Kotler, M.D. Copyright © Robert Kotler. *Continued.*

HOW FACIAL REJUVENATION IS PERFORMED
The Need for Anesthesia

Although chemical rejuvenation involves absolutely no surgery—the skin is never touched by a scalpel—it must be performed under an anesthetic administered by a specialist in anesthesia. There are several reasons for this:

- The anesthetic ensures that the process will not be uncomfortable.
- Bodily functions such as blood pressure, pulse, and respiration can be accurately monitored, since the medicines applied to the skin are absorbed into the body and can affect these functions.

Because rejuvenation is performed under anesthesia, and because one's general health should be good as for any medical procedure, a physical examination by a family physician or internal medicine specialist is required. Although such an exam need be only a basic type examination, it will also be accompanied by several appropriate blood and urine tests.

An Office Procedure

In keeping with today's trend to perform relatively noncomplex procedures outside the hospital setting, for economy, efficiency, and pleasantness, chemical facial rejuvenation is very appropriately performed in an office such as ours, which is equipped and staffed as is a hospital. Regarding comfort and safety, the standards for this process are no less than those for facial surgical procedures done in the office, such as cosmetic nasal and eyelid surgery and face and neck lifting.

One of our staff anesthesia specialists will call you the evening prior to the procedure to introduce himself and explain the anesthetic. When you arrive at the office surgical facility the following day, you will be greeted by our staff and the anesthetist will induce sleep intravenously.

The skin of the face is then cleansed thoroughly and the process of applying the prescription of medicines to the skin begins. Since each patient has unique skin properties, such as color, thickness, oiliness, and variations in the amount and depth of wrinkling, each patient's treatment is a unique process. But the basic principle is that any or all areas of the face are treated with gentle application of the prescriptions used for at least one hour (for an entire face). Additional time may be required to apply special protective dressings that stay in place from one to two days. At the end of the session, which lasts several hours in total, the patient awakens from the anesthetic but remains sleepy for the remainder of the day.

BEGINNING THE DAY AFTER

The rejuvenation process of going from "old" to "new" skin actually takes several days, and during this time a special high protein liquid diet is prescribed and one must refrain from excess speaking. For this reason, we recommend staying in our "recovery hideaway"—a retreat which is described later. A minimal stay of two days there is recommended, for this will ensure proper professional attention that is important in achieving the best possible result for you.

The hideaway's limousine will bring you to our office for a brief check-up for each of the first two days after the process was performed. On the third day, a

From brochure used in the practice of Robert Kotler, M.D. Copyright © Robert Kotler.

brief dressing change will take place painlessly under a very brief anesthetic delivered by the anesthetist. The following day—depending on the individual—you may be seen again in the office. By this time, you will be at home and able to participate in normal home duties, but you probably will not be ready to face the rest of the world because you will be treating your fresh new skin with our program of special powders and creams. These home treatments create somewhat of a mud-pack coating which washes off in the shower quite easily on a prescribed day.

By six days after the initial application, your skin is smooth and wrinkle-free; the blemishes, age spots, brown spots, and even freckles (if you ever had them) will also be gone. This new skin is quite bright pink in color—resembling a wind- or sunburn—but this begins to fade as you adhere to our "Skin Care After Rejuvenation" program. We will prescribe medications which will hasten the disappearance of the pink color. While this may take several weeks to achieve, the color is easily camouflaged by cosmetics. We shall also teach you how to perform cover-ups using allergy-free make up products.

GETTING BACK TO ACTION

Most of our patients are able to resume normal work and social functions about ten days after the start of the process. At that point, the most common complaint is dryness of the skin and perhaps some itching. We shall provide medications to correct this as this is temporary and due to the inactivity of the skin's own oil glands.

Under our direction, you will be able to care for your new skin and to keep it fresh and youthful appearing. We shall recommend specific lotions and moisturizers and shall anticipate your skin's needs during the first few months after the procedure. Generally, the pink color has faded completely by six to eight weeks. During that period, there are minimal restrictions on sunbathing, exercise, etc. that will vary with the individual. Contrary to some old wives' tales, you need not be a recluse, nor fear "ever going out in the sun again." You will be able to return to your previous lifestyle without major change.

Having been through the process with so many people, we are sensitive to your needs and have dealt with nearly every question or uncertainty that you could have. Your facial rejuvenation is your investment in a healthier, younger appearance and we shall do everything we can to keep you that way, since, as stated by one of our patients, your face is our reputation!

SUMMARY

Chemical facial rejuvenation is a modern, medical process to permanently (depending on age, of course) remove wrinkles and other outward signs of an aging skin. For safety and comfort, it is performed under anesthesia and requires seven days spent away from normal activities—two or three days in a professionally supervised recovery facility and the remaining time at home. Excepting the need for some cosmetics, women patients generally return to work and social functions within ten days, men possibly sooner.

From brochure used in the practice of Robert Kotler, M.D. Copyright © Robert Kotler. *Continued.*

YOUR QUESTIONS ANSWERED

Q. Could you describe this "hideaway"?
A. Recovery hideaways are literally "halfway houses" exclusively for post–cosmetic facial surgery or nonsurgery patients. They are not hospitals and not nursing homes but rather are unique retreats where your special dietary and medical needs are provided around the clock by registered and practical nurses who are specialized, as we are, in care of the face only. In addition to the professional care, the hideaway provides all the amenities of a fine hotel, with all private rooms, full meal service, and transportation to and from our office and the airport.

Your family and friends need not miss time from work nor concern themselves with being a nurse, and you are free from the nuisances of the curious or otherwise inquiring.

The facility is described in its own brochure, which accompanies our educational materials.

Q. Is everyone a candidate for the process?
A. No, regardless of anything else, if you have significant heart, lung, kidney, or liver problems, you cannot have the procedure any more than you could have any other elective surgical procedure. Second, candidacy depends on skin color, texture, and your skin's health history, which include previous treatments with x-rays or various potent medicines that were applied to the skin. Black or dark brown skin is not amenable to this process.

Q. Can cosmetic facial surgery be done at the same time?
A. That depends on how much of your face is treated.

Q. Does that imply that not everyone has the entire face treated?
A. Yes, depending on various factors, but particularly how fair the complexion is. Areas such as upper lip, or eyelids and crow's feet around the eyes, can be treated independently.

Q. If only the face is treated, will its color ultimately be different than the neck or other untreated parts of the body?
A. Depending on the shade of your skin (very fair skin is best) there may or may not be a slight difference in skin tone. By hiding the "line of demarcation" under the jaw line, the problem is usually obviated. For some, makeup may be necessary to conceal that transition zone. For the rare patient, the neck can be treated for the purpose of color match.

From brochure used in the practice of Robert Kotler, M.D. Copyright © Robert Kotler.

Q. Can blotchiness occur? If so, what can be done?
A. Your skin history and our examination can usually predict whose skin might become "blotchy" (slight differences in pigmentation or color in varying areas of the face). If we are particularly suspicious that this may occur, we shall perform a "patch test." We treat a small area of skin in a hidden area with a sample prescription and observe the skin's reaction for at least three months to see if any blotchiness may occur.

In any event, should any blotchiness occur, even if unexpected, there are now available prescriptions that can permanantly lighten the darker areas.

Q. What patient or what type of skin is generally considered the best candidate for chemical facial rejuvenation?
A. Fair-skinned people with blonde or red hair and green or blue eyes are invariably the best candidates and achieve the best results. Obviously, your ancestry helps to determine this, and for this reason, those of Central and Northern European ancestry, such as German, Austrian, French, English, and Scandinavian, are generally excellent candidates. Those whose ancestors come from southern Europe, such as southern Greece or Italy, or Central or South America, tend to have darker skin and may not be satisfactory candidates.

The latter group may take some comfort in knowing, however, that their skin generally does not become as wrinkled as the more fair skinned, since the darker skin with its more prevalent pigmentation acts as a natural sunscreen and helps prevent the sun's damaging rays from inducing the wrinkling and age-related changes of the skin.

Q. Is it true that smoking, excess drinking, and other poor health habits are detrimental to the skin and cause premature aging?
A. Yes.

Q. Is it better to have the procedure done at a relatively young age, such as in the forties, or wait until the wrinkles are "really bad" in the sixties and seventies?
A. My personal feeling is that when you see the wrinkles and find them unsatisfactory, that is the time to consider having the process performed.

From a technical standpoint, it is a bit easier for us to achieve a greater success when the wrinkles are not as deep as they may become at a more advanced age. Obviously, most people tend to be a bit healthier in middle age than they may be at an older age and will want to take advantage of their good health so that they may have the procedure performed safely.

You will enjoy many more years of younger and wrinkle-free skin if you have the process performed at a relatively earlier point in your life.

From brochure used in the practice of Robert Kotler, M.D. Copyright © Robert Kotler.

Face Facts
CHEMICAL REJUVENATION

OBJECTIVE: To recreate more youthful skin through a medical and hence non-surgical process that removes age spots and wrinkles and tightens the skin.

ANESTHESIA: Heavy sedation or light general anesthesia administered by a physician-anesthesiologist specializing in facial procedures. Under our anesthesia, there is no pain and no awareness. An intravenous infusion is started and you "drift off to sleep."

TIME: Approximately 2 hours in our surgical suite.

RECOVERY ROOM: Usually 2 to 3 hours in our fully monitored, computerized recovery room. Your care is supervised by a registered nurse further specialized in recovery and critical care.

CONVALESCENCE: One or several nights at the "hideaway retreat" or in a hospital or under the care of a professional experienced registered nurse in your home may be appropriate. We shall recommend according to the nature of your procedure. If dressings were applied to the facial skin, they will be removed without discomfort in our office under a very brief anesthetic 1 or 2 days after the procedure has been performed.

RETURN TO WORK, NORMAL ACTIVITIES, ETC. 7 to 10 days. During the first 7 days, your face is covered with either dressings or the "mud pack." No later than day seven, the mud pack will have been washed off revealing the fresh, smooth, reddish-pink skin (akin to a sunburn). Within 1 or 2 days, make-up can be applied. We provide appropriate skin care products such as cleansing lotion (instead of soap), softening oils, and sunscreens. Instructions on make-up techniques are also provided.

THE FIRST SEVERAL MONTHS AFTER: The reddish pink color fades naturally and the lightening process is accelerated by medications that we provide. The pink color is usually gone by 6 to 8 weeks after performance. Regardless of how long the natural fading takes, the ruddy color can be concealed with cosmetics. In some people, during the first several months, the skin tends to be dry (due to inactive oil glands) but this is easily corrected by the use of the products provided to you.

WHAT ABOUT GOING BACK INTO THE SUN? Generally, once the pink color has faded, the new skin may be slightly lighter than it was before and less apt to tan. Since suntanning may have been one of the factors that caused the skin to age prematurely, you will want to reduce the chance of burning and tanning anyway. Therefore, we will advise you on the proper sunscreens which will reduce the chance of burning and help keep your skin from becoming aged again.

From brochure used in the practice of Robert Kotler, M.D. Copyright © Robert Kotler.

PREOPERATIVE CONSULTATION REPORT

Patient's name: _____ Date of exam: _____

Proposed procedure(s) _____

History

   Significant abnormal medical or surgical history: _____
_____

   Significant family history: _____
_____

   Allergies:

     Drug: _____

     Other: _____

   Current medications (prescription and/or nonprescription):
_____

   Smoking: _____   Caffeine: _____   Alcohol: _____

Examination

   Blood pressure   Pulse   Temperature   Resp/minute

Heart:

Lungs:

Abdomen:

Neuro:

Patient is medically fit for proposed procedure   [ ] yes   no [ ].

Please include copies of lab results,   Consulting physician's signature
ECG, chest x-ray (reports only)

                                                     ( ) _____
                                                     Telephone number

                                                     Address

                                                     City, state, zip

From brochure used in the practice of Robert Kotler, M.D. Copyright © Robert Kotler.

Dear Doctor:

RE: _____
(patient)

Thank you for seeing our patient in preoperative consultation. Our required laboratory tests are to be done within 2 weeks of surgery date: _____

- CBC
- Platelet count
- Pregnancy test
- Urinalysis
- Creatinine (for chemical skin peel/rejuvenation only)

The following tests are valid for 3 months:

- Electrocardiogram (if patient is over age 40—or if indicated)
- Chest x-ray, two views (if patient is over age 40—or if indicated)

We **must** receive the completed physical forms and copies of laboratory studies, including the ECG tracing and chest x-ray report, 3 days prior to surgery (by _____.)

Please perform any other medical exams/tests that you feel are indicated to clear the patient for the planned procedure(s).

A self-addressed envelope is provided for your convenience.

Yours very truly,

Enclosures

From brochure used in the practice of Robert Kotler, M.D. Copyright © Robert Kotler.

CONSENT TO TREATMENT FOR COSMETIC PURPOSES FACIAL REJUVENATION

1. I hereby request and authorize Robert Kotler, M.D., to treat me on or about the _____ day of _____ , 19 ___ for the purpose of attempting to improve my appearance.
2. The effect and nature of the treatment to be given, as well as possible alternative methods of treatment, have been fully explained to me.
3. It has been explained that well qualified and trained personnel will assist Dr. Kotler with certain portions of the treatment under his supervision.
4. I also authorize Dr. Kotler to perform any other procedure which he may deem necessary or advisable in attempting to improve my appearance, or any unforeseen or unhealthy condition that he may encounter during the treatment.
5. I hereby authorize Dr. Kotler to administer such treatment to me, and agree to hold him free and harmless for any claims or suits for damages or injury or complications whatever for any result from conditions beyond the Doctor's control.
6. I know that the practice of medicine and surgery is not an exact science and that, therefore, reputable practitioners cannot properly guarantee results.
7. I acknowledge that no guarantee or assurance has been made to me by anyone regarding the treatment which I have herein requested and authorized.
8. I am advised that though good results are expected, they cannot be and are not guaranteed; nor can there be any guarantee against untoward results.
9. I acknowledge that no guarantee has been given me as to the number of years I may appear younger following treatment.
10. I acknowledge that no guarantee has been given me as to the condition of the complexion or size of the skin pores following treatment.
11. I acknowledge that no guarantee has been given me as to the amount of percentage of improvement expected following treatment.
12. I acknowledge that no guarantee has been given me as to the painlessness of the procedure. Some individuals, because of emotional makeup or low pain threshold, may experience severe pain. Heavy premedication is given to make the procedure as comfortable for the patient as possible.
13. I have been advised that the following conditions may arise after treatment. These conditions are uncommon and usually not serious, but may appear at any time because of circumstances beyond the Doctor's control.
    a. A darkening of the skin or blotchiness may occur at any time up to 3 months following treatment. This is usually due to excess sun or heat exposure. Special medication may be prescribed for this and will usually clear the condition completely. Occasionally further treatment may be required, consisting of a second procedure. Persons with dark complexions undergoing treatment are advised that a blotchy complexion may arise which will usually even out over a period of 3 to 6 months.

From brochure used in the practice of Robert Kotler, M.D. Copyright © Robert Kotler. *Continued.*

CONSENT TO TREATMENT FOR COSMETIC PURPOSES FACIAL REJUVENATION—cont'd

    b. The skin may be red for a 6 to 8 week period or possibly longer. The redness is due to increased blood supply to the new skin. The redness usually disappears over the 3 to 6 month period and the final complexion is somewhat lighter than the original complexion.

    c. On occasion, small areas of the neck and chin may show thickening for a variable period of time following treatment. These areas are buildups of underlying collagen and scar tissue and are usually easily controlled by periodic injections of medication.

    d. Every Facial Rejuvenation procedure is accompanied by swelling of the tissue of the face and neck. This is usually only temporary and will usually disappear within a short period of time. On occasion, the swelling may be persistent and will require further medication.

14. I have been advised that exposure to sun and excess heat must be avoided at all costs for a period of 6 months. No sunbathing is permitted for 6 months. To do so would encourage blotchy skin pigmentation requiring further treatment.

The operation has been explained to me and I fully understand the nature of the procedure and the risks involved. I acknowledge and understand that no expressed or implied warranty has been given to me.

Date _____ Signature _____

Witness _____ (If minor, signature of guardian)

_____

If patient is a minor, complete the following:

Patient is a minor _____ years of age, and we, the undersigned, are the parents or guardian of the patient and do hereby consent for the patient.

Witness _____ _____
(parent or legal guardian)

From brochure used in the practice of Robert Kotler, M.D. Copyright © Robert Kotler.

PREOPERATIVE INSTRUCTIONS

Patient: _____

Surgery date: _____ Time: _____

TRANSPORTATION: Make arrangements to have someone drive you to and from the office on your surgical day. **You will not be allowed to drive yourself home. Someone must accompany you home after surgery and stay with you the first night.** This person may wait for you in the waiting room or may be called after surgery. Please make sure that we have his/her phone number.

FOOD RESTRICTIONS: **No solid foods or liquids are to be consumed after 11:00 PM the night before surgery, and nothing the morning of surgery, unless approved by the anesthesiologist.** You may take heart and blood pressure medicine with a very small sip of water in the morning.

CLOTHING: Please wear comfortable underclothing the morning of surgery. Do not wear any clothes with small neck openings or high-heeled shoes. A night gown and robe or sweat pants and shirt are preferred. *Please leave all jewelry and valuables at home.*

FACIAL CLEANSING: Please use the prescription provided to obtain pHisoHex Soap. Wash your face using this soap twice daily, beginning five (5) days before your surgery. Your skin may become dry and moisturizers can be used up until the night before your surgery. Please also wash your hair with pHisoHex the night before your surgery, and refrain from using any shampoos, cream rinses, or conditioners. The morning of surgery, wash your face with pHisoHex.

MEDICATIONS: *Do not take any aspirin or aspirin-containing products at least two weeks prior to surgery. If you find it necessary to take something for pain, please* **use Tylenol instead.** Make sure that the office is aware of any medications that you are presently taking. Begin taking Zovirax the day before surgery.

ANESTHESIA: Our anesthesiologist will be calling you the evening before your procedure to discuss your anesthesia. If you will be staying elsewhere that evening, please make sure the office has this phone number. In case you miss his call, he will speak to you the morning of your scheduled procedure(s).

NOTE: If you should develop any pimples, rashes, or outbreaks on your face or develop a cold any time before your surgery, please **notify our office immediately.** Your surgery may be postponed if your symptoms do not subside and it may be necessary to obtain medical treatment preoperatively.

If you have any questions regarding your surgery, please do not hesitate to call our office. Our hours are from 9:00 AM to 5:00 PM Monday through Fridays.

From brochure used in the practice of Robert Kotler, M.D. Copyright © Robert Kotler.

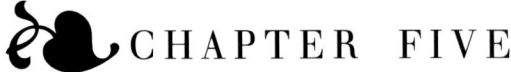CHAPTER FIVE

Anesthesia

Until 3 years ago, in our practice, chemical face peels were performed with the patient under intravenous sedation. A small number of arrhythmias occurred, none of which proved difficult to control. Since converting to general endotracheal anesthesia with full monitoring devices, such as electrocardiograph, pulse oximetry, and end-tidal CO_2 monitoring, we have seen a marked decrease in the incidence of arrhythmias. We attribute this to general anesthesia, more efficient exchange of oxygen and carbon dioxide, and less dependence on narcotic analgesics. We hypothesized that cardiac arrhythmia is more likely to occur under intravenous sedation than under general endotracheal anesthesia with assisted ventilation for the following reasons:

1. Sedatives, particularly barbiturates and benzodiazepines, tend to depress respiration, leading to hypoxia and hypercapnia. Both predispose to arrhythmia.
2. Narcotic analgesics likewise depress respiration, with the same potential ventilatory and cardiac consequences.
3. A sedated, but not unconscious, patient who is stimulated by the painful application of the chemical solution will become restless, agitated, and uninhibited—particularly under the influence of the sedatives. This uncooperative behavior can overlap with hypoxic restlessness and can be indistinguishable from it.
4. Painful stimuli promote endogenous catecholamine release. Such elevated levels of catecholamines in the presence of the aforementioned hypercapnia and hypoxia makes all the necessary ingredients for cardiac irritability, arrhythmia, and hypertension.

Certainly, the analgesic and anesthetic circumstances under which the procedure is done span a wide spectrum. Some practitioners find it very satisfactory to premedicate patients with narcotics and sedatives and then continue the procedure with the addition of similar medications as needed. Whether one wishes to employ the services of a nurse anesthetist or anesthesiologist is an individual consideration. Certainly, the patient should not be restless or combative during the procedure, for this can compromise the result and introduce additional risk factors. Nor should the patient have recollection of an unpleasant or trying experience in the operating room. By using whatever technique is effective for the patient and comfortable for the practitioner, the experience should not be a burden for either.

Some practitioners use a field block anesthesia for the entire face. A variety of agents, including longer acting anesthetics such as bupivacaine hydrochloride (Marcaine), can create a pain-free area for several hours, including the critical first 4 to 6 hours after the procedure. It is during that time that patients complain most of the "burning" sensation. Following that interval, the pain reduces significantly, perhaps because of the temporarily toxic effect of the phenol on the nerve endings (phenol is a well-recognized anesthetic, such as in over-the-counter sore throat preparations).

Stegman and associates[108] describe the following technique for local anesthesia face block:

> "Block the forehead with a ring block just above the eyebrows which hits the supraorbital, supratrochlear, and temporofacial nerves. The infraorbital and mental nerves are each blocked separately. The temporozygomatic nerves are blocked by entering the skin with a long spinal needle just preauricularly and sweeping over the entire lateral cheek. The nose is blocked by injecting the bridge at the bony cartilagenous junction, in each alar groove, and at the base of the columella."

But regardless of the technique of anesthesia, a cardiac monitor is imperative when a phenol solution is being applied to the full face. Changes in cardiac rhythm can be recognized before consequences occur. Should any abnormality be observed, further applications of phenol are obviously postponed until a normal rhythm is restored. For the same reasons of prudence, an intravenous line should be in place and appropriate medicines readily at hand.

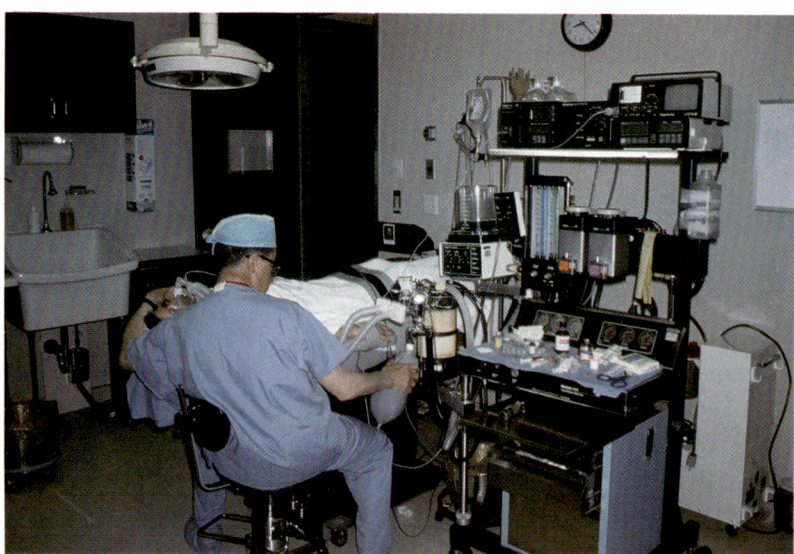

Operating room equipped to perform chemical skin peeling under general anesthesia. The anesthesiologist or nurse anesthetist must be supplied with all monitoring and resuscitation equipment necessary for the practice of his or her specialty.

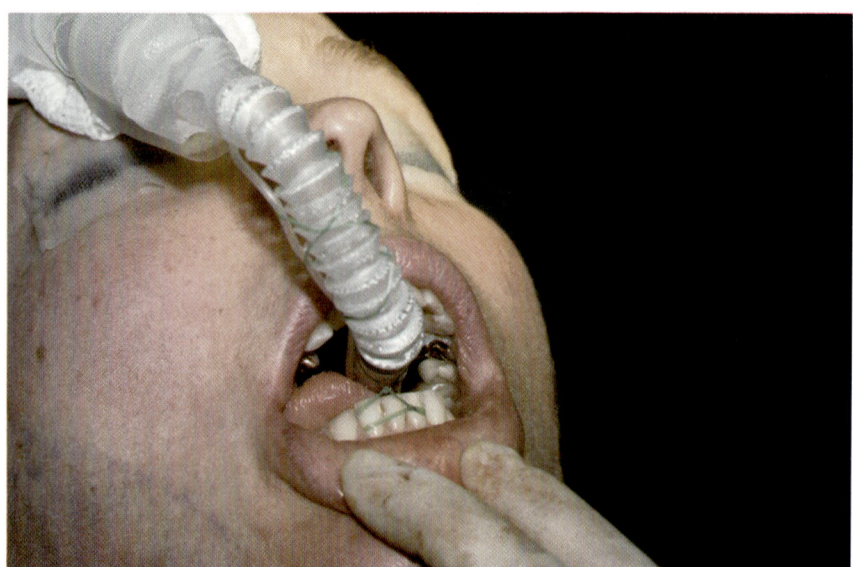

Anesthesia technique. The use of dental floss to secure the endotrachal tube reduces the chance of dislodgement. (Technique courtesy Juan Minelli, M.D.)

ANESTHESIA 99

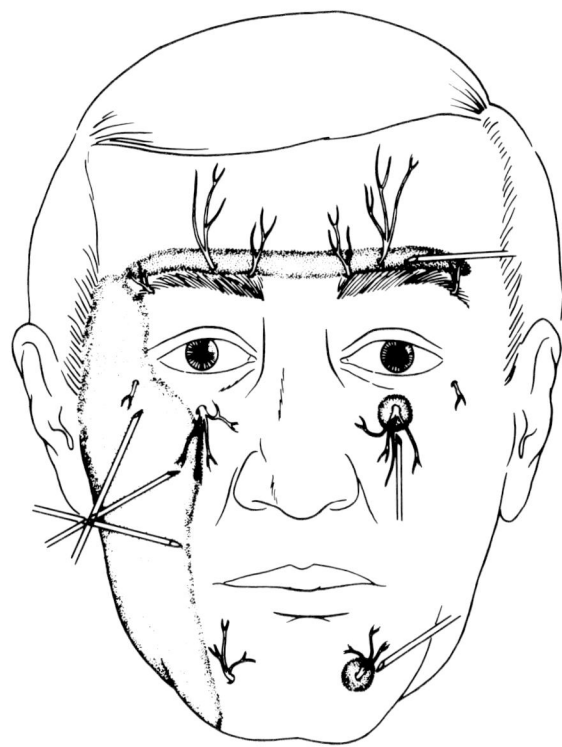

Sites for local anesthesia face block.
(From Stegman SJ, Tromovitch TA, and Glogau RG: *Cosmetic Dermatologic Surgery,* ed 2, St Louis, 1990, Mosby–Year Book.)

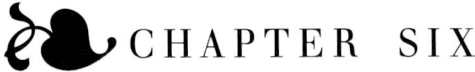 CHAPTER SIX

The Procedure

PREOPERATIVE PREPARATION

A surgical nurse receives the patient, reviews the history and physical examination, and confirms that the patient has had nothing to eat or drink since the prior midnight. A careful evaluation of the area to be treated is performed to detect signs of infection.

The patient is taken to the preoperative holding area where the hair is best placed into braids with rubber bands. An intravenous infusion of 5% dextrose and balanced salt solution is started by the surgical nurse or anesthesiologist. The patient is then brought to the operating suite and moved onto the operating table. Using a surgical marking pen, I delineate the inferior limit of the procedure (see p. 101). Such marking *must be done with the patient in the sitting position;* otherwise, normal anatomic landmarks may be misconstrued. Ideally, the procedure should end just beneath the inferior mandibular margin within the inframandibular shadow. Should a color demarcation between the treated face and untreated neck develop, it would be best concealed in this shadowed area. Patients of lean habitus with prominent mandibles afford the ideal circumstances for such concealing of this "zone of transition."

The patient then reclines into the supine position. Electrocardiographic leads and pulse oximeter are attached. The anesthesiologist then induces general endotracheal anesthesia. The surgical nurse cleanses the face with surgical soap, rinses it carefully, and uses acetone to remove residual oils from the skin. *Such oil removal is critical since failure to uniformly remove the oils may result in uneven penetration and, hence, inadequate peeling.*

Vigorous degreasing with acetone, soap, alcohol, or any combination of these injures or destroys the epidermal barrier, which allows more penetration of the peeling agent.[109] All these variables may have

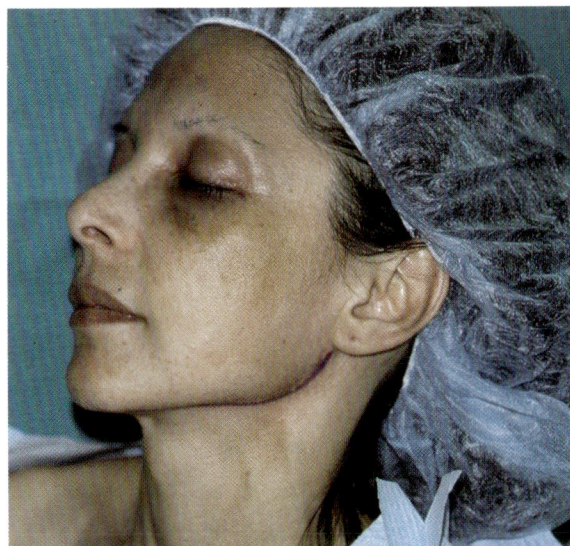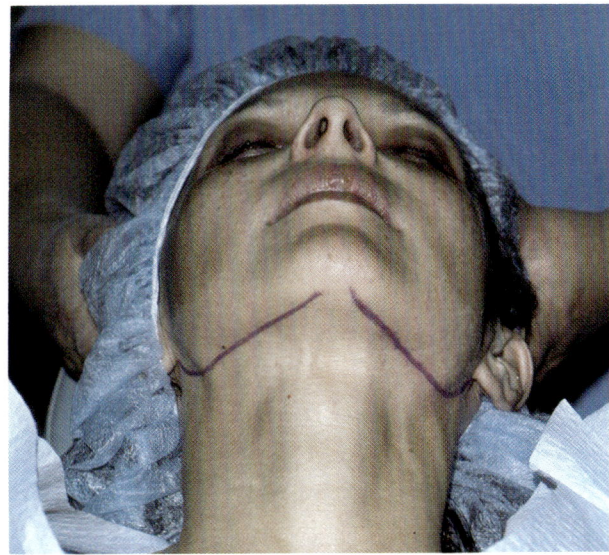

Line of demarcation. The inferior end point of the procedure should be within the inframandibular shadow. This should be delineated with a marking pen, with the patient in the sitting position before the procedure. It should be examined for symmetry by inspecting from the caudal perspective.

an effect on the end result of the peel. Stegman and associates cited "cases where the physician changed only the degreasing step of his routine and the patient subsequently developed a much deeper wound that progressed to scarring. Thus, more complete and rapid absorption of the agent can produce a deeper wound, and if phenol is used, there is a greater risk of cardiac toxicity."[109]

Stegman and others[108] reported a case whereby a "patient's face was vigorously cleansed with acetone, followed with a 35% TCA peel, and the patient developed some hypertrophic scarring. This type of situation is rare but it illustrates the point that the degreasing step, if carried to the point of breaking down the epidermal barrier, must be considered to be one more way to affect the depth of the wound, just the same as if more escharotic agent or occlusion were added."

Stegman also showed that an actinically damaged epidermis has impaired barrier function. Therefore patients with severe sun damage, the most common indication for phenol peel, will require more or stronger agents to penetrate the epidermis than will patients with minimal sun damage who might be peeled for other indications.

CHEMICAL APPLICATION

For extremely deep, craggy lines of the glabella and nasolabial creases of the cheeks or forehead, a pretreatment with 50% trichloroacetic acid to these specific lines appears to enhance the phenol peel. Whether the peeling effect of the pretreatment with TCA and then with phenol is

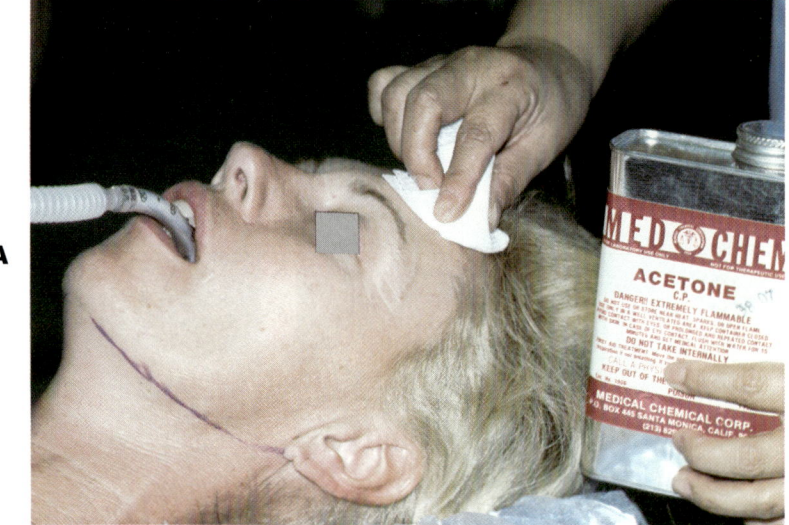

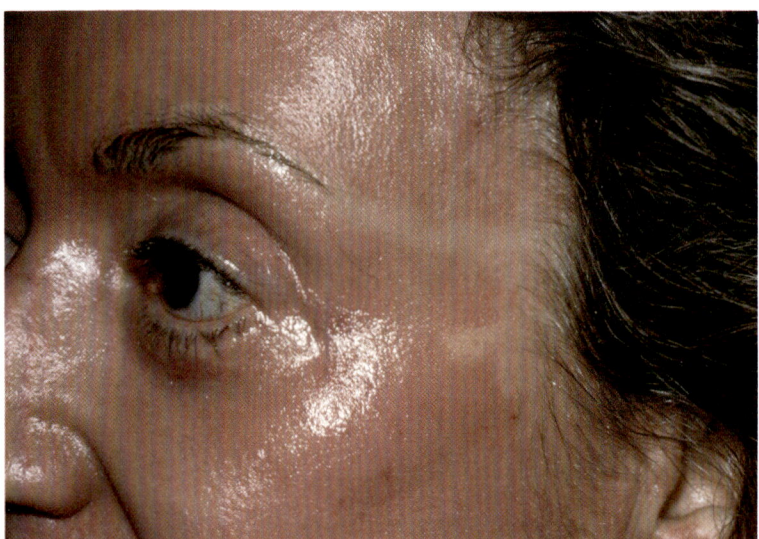

Degreasing with acetone to prevent "skip" areas. The face is degreased with acetone while the patient is under general anesthesia and in a supine position. Note the line demarcating the inferior limit of the procedure within the inframandibular shadow. The "skip" areas in the temporal area shown here appeared 7 days after peel and may have been due to inadequate removal of facial oils before the application of peeling solution. These areas can be spot-peeled later as needed.

additive or whether the pretreatment—through creation of edema that effaces the deeper creases and, hence, makes the phenol absorption more likely—is uncertain. Having been very pleased with the effects of this "dual treatment," we are currently evaluating whether a similar excellent result can be achieved without the TCA pretreatment, substituting or not substituting different skin preparation techniques, including more vigorous degreasing with acetone. That itself may provide a superficial abrasion that would more effectively clear the skin of keratin and enhance the exfoliative process by the acid.[35]

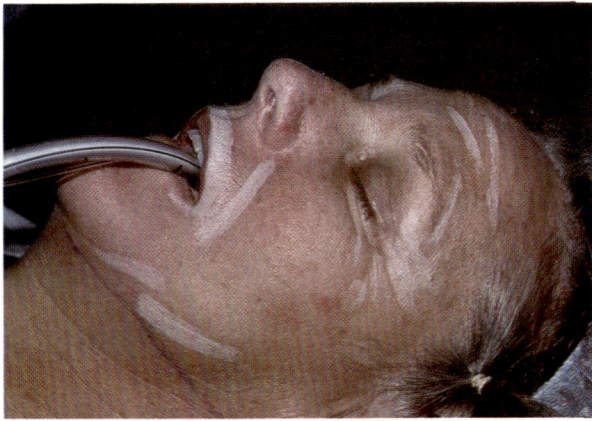 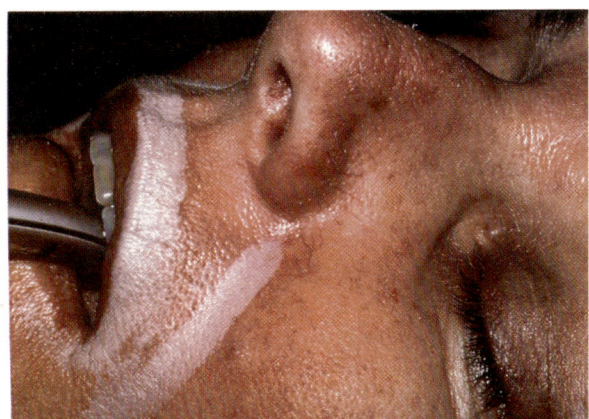

Pretreatment with trichloroacetic acid (TCA). The areas of deep wrinkling are pretreated with 50% TCA. Recall that the "frost" takes longer to develop with 50% TCA than with Baker's formula phenol solution; therefore the operator is advised to apply one and two streaks of 50% TCA and then wait 3 to 5 minutes for maximum frosting to become apparent.

Pretreatment TCA is applied with one or two strokes, waiting 3 to 5 minutes to allow the white "frost" to develop. TCA is reapplied only if no frost develops. Extreme caution against overapplication is advised. In the very thick-skinned patient, overapplication of TCA can result in overthinning of the stratum corneum in those areas pretreated with TCA. This could manifest as a contour discrepancy that cannot be concealed.

The phenol solution is prepared in the classic manner described by Baker and Gordon.[16]

> "The solution used for a chemical peel must be mixed so that it is fresh each time it is used. Four separate, carefully labled bottles contain the individual ingredients. First, 3 ml of USP phenol, solution #1, is drawn into a regular hypodermic syringe and transferred to a medicine glass. Using the same syringe, 2 ml of water, solution #2, is then added. Eight drops of solution #3, Septisol, that is, a liquid soap, is next. Finally, 3 drops of croton oil, solution #4, is transferred. The sequence is always the same and the bottles are clearly labeled to prevent any errors. The resulting mixture is a suspension because of the immiscibility of the combined ingredients. The oils lie above, separated by the aqueous components beneath. When the combination is mixed with a Q-tip, the mixture becomes white, as it is converted into a suspension. It is very important that it be mixed freshly each time is it used.

> "Each time the applicator is inserted into the mixture, it is used to agitate and thus resuspend the ingredients. As it is withdrawn, the Q-tip is compressed to remove excess agent, as it should be semi-dry before contacting the skin. After application of the agent, the skin quickly assumes a frosty appearance...

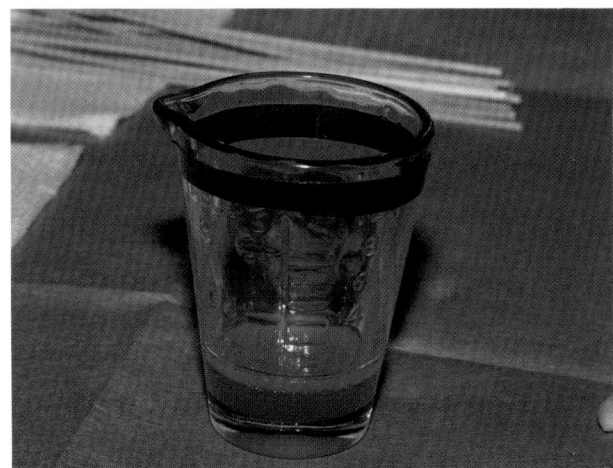 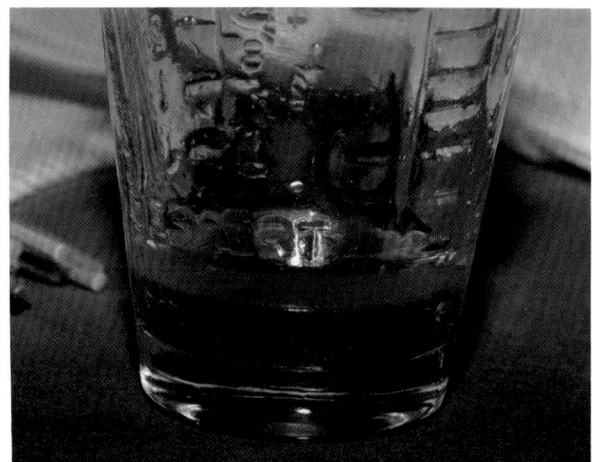

The Baker formula phenol peeling solution. The Baker formula is not a true solution but an emulsion. Consequently the liquid should be stirred well before each application.

"The solution is always kept on the Mayo stand. The cotton-tipped applicator is dipped into the solution, the solution is stirred vigorously, and then the applicator is pressed against the sides of the cup so that no dripping can occur. The Q-tip is then carried to the face to perform the applications. The Mayo stand itself is kept several feet away from the patient, reducing any chance of spillage onto the face. And, of course, the cup is never carried by the physician lest inadvertent and catastrophic spillage on the face occur."

I agree with Dr. Baker's admonition that "it is safer, also, for the surgeon to prepare the mixture personally rather than depend on a nurse, technician, or pharmacist, since a mistake here could have tragic consequences."

I prefer to perform the procedure in stages with given aesthetic zones being treated sequentially. The forehead zone is treated first, beginning with the glabella and inferior forehead. The application continues in a cephalic direction until the hairline is reached. Great care must be taken to apply the solution well beyond the first rows of hair to avoid a visible strip of untreated scalp at the hairline. As classically described, the end point of chemical application is when the skin develops a chalk-white color, the so-called "frost." Fewer applications or applications using an applicator that is too dry will result in a less profound white "frost," indicating less dense penetration and portending a "weaker" peel. One should strive for uniformity of application as judged by the uniformity of the white color. The white color gradually disappears over a period of 5 to 10 minutes; the skin appears pinker, shows signs of early edema, and has a waxen appearance. The face changes to a dark, red color because of the inflammatory response from the second degree burn. If the patient is responsive — not under general anesthesia or very heavy sedation — as the cauterant touches the skin, the patient experiences

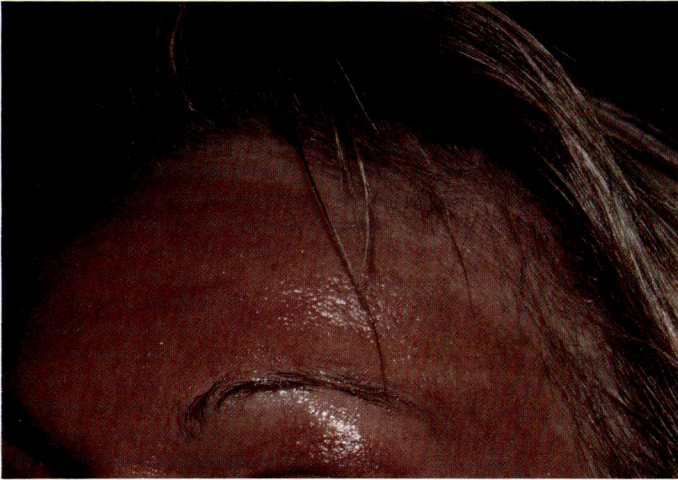

Failure to carry peeling into the forehead hairline. Failure to peel the hairline generally will not be visible if the patient's hair style conceals it. If it is visible, the unpeeled area may be peeled without anesthesia at a later date as an office procedure.

an immediate stinging that gives way to a throbbing, burning sensation. Depending on the patient's pain threshold, thus may linger 30 minutes to 1 hour.[5]

Between each aesthetic zone treatment, a "rest break" is taken for 10 or more minutes. This diminishes the clearance load to the excretory organs; phenol toxicity is related to blood level, the latter being a function of the application dose, time, and size of area treated.[40]

The next zone treated is the nose and orbital area. We begin with the eyebrow and infrabrow skin. (There is no untoward effect on hair follicles.) The application is carried inferiorly from the brow to the supratarsal crease. The eyelid skin below the crease is usually not peeled, since it is usually not wrinkled.

The lower eyelid skin application must avoid inadvertent application to the globe. To minimize the chance of such a maloccurrence, we recommend the following precautions.

1. Advise everyone in the room "not to move" to avoid accidentally bumping into the operator during application.
2. Advise the anesthesiologist or anesthetist that you are about to begin the application so that he/she can be certain of satisfactory anesthetic state.
3. Retract the cheek downward, allowing the lower lid to retract from the globe. Simultaneous elevation of the upper lid by an assistant gains additional exposure.
4. Always begin the application at the lower portion of the eyelid, away from the margin, so that even if there is movement by the patient during the application, the risk to the globe is minimal. Beginning application away from the lid establishes the pain

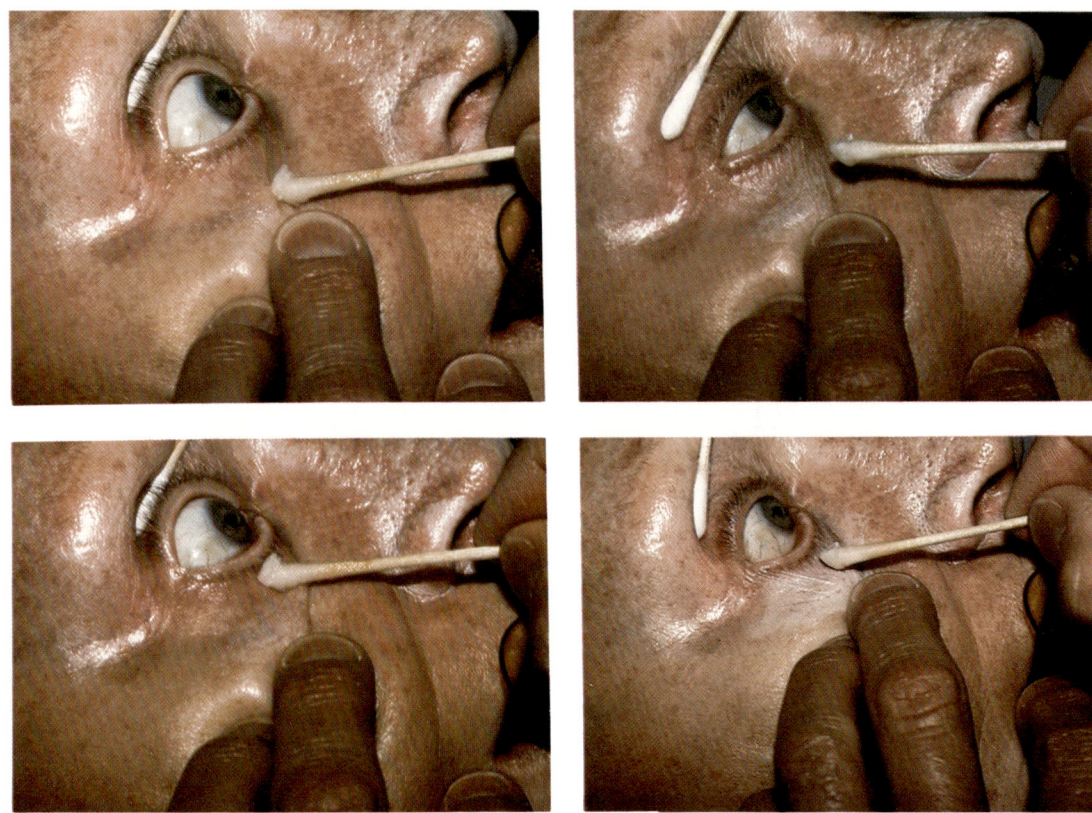

Lower eyelid peeling technique. The first application of peeling solution to the lower eyelid is begun over the malar eminence and away from the lid margin. The development of "frost" shows adequate penetration. As the applicator tip approaches the lashes, it is critical that the lower eyelid be retracted by the operator's hand so that the lid is withdrawn from the globe. The lid continues to be retracted downward and away from the globe as the final application is made to the lash margin.

threshold for possible reaction to the stimulus of peel solution application. This is in contrast to beginning the application near the lid margin whereby any movement by the patient could be critical.
5. Proceed cephalically with the application of the peel solution up to the lash margin, always retracting the lower lid away from the globe.

The identical procedure is then performed on the opposite side.

To ensure against "skip" on untreated areas, the chemical solution application onto a given zone should overlap onto the adjacent, previously treated zone. Untreated areas noted after completion of the application procedure may be treated immediately.

Following treatment of the nose and both periorbital areas, the forehead will have lost its frostlike appearance. An efficient use of the "break time" between chemical application is to apply dressings to a previously treated zone, if needed. Dressing application is discussed separately.

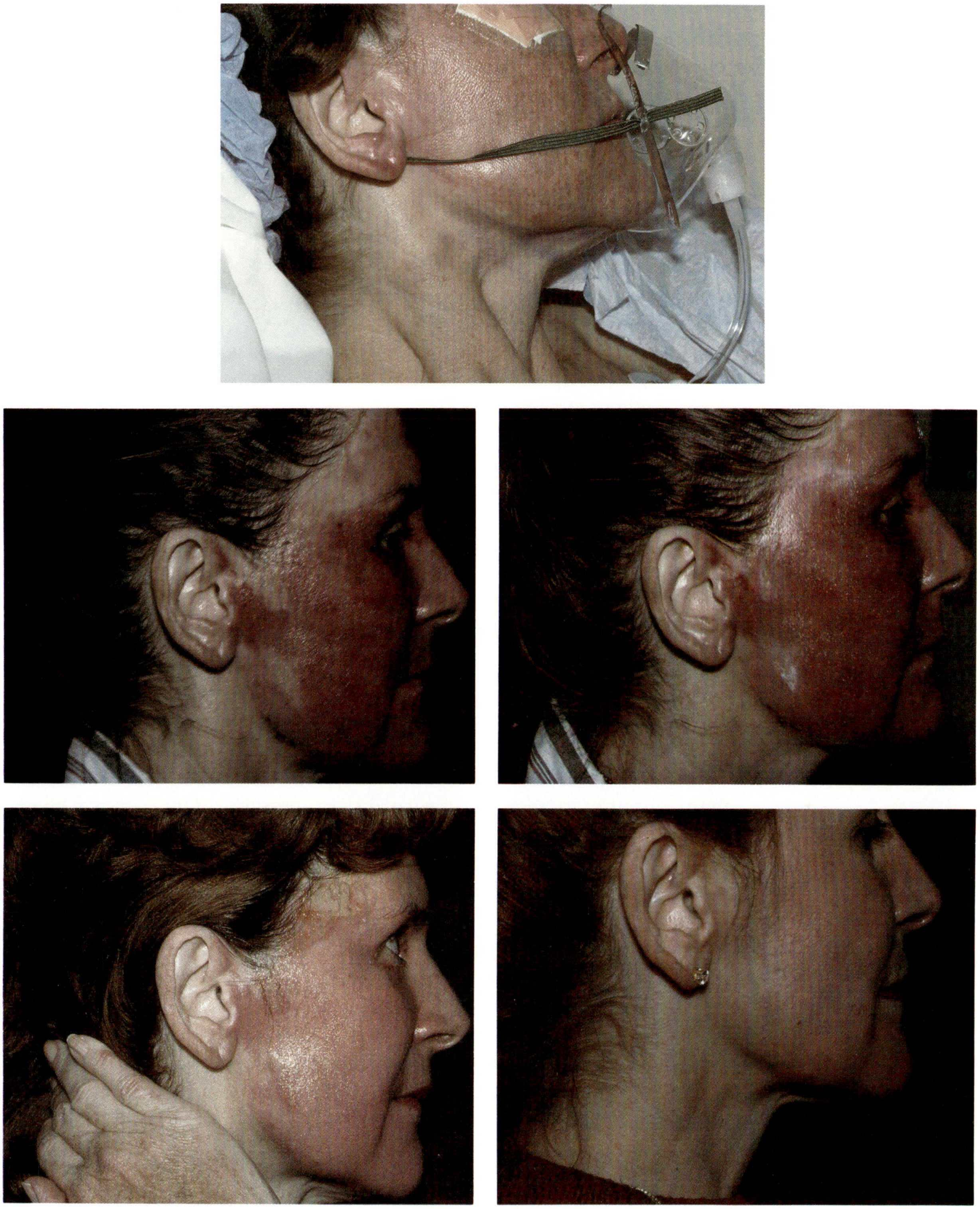

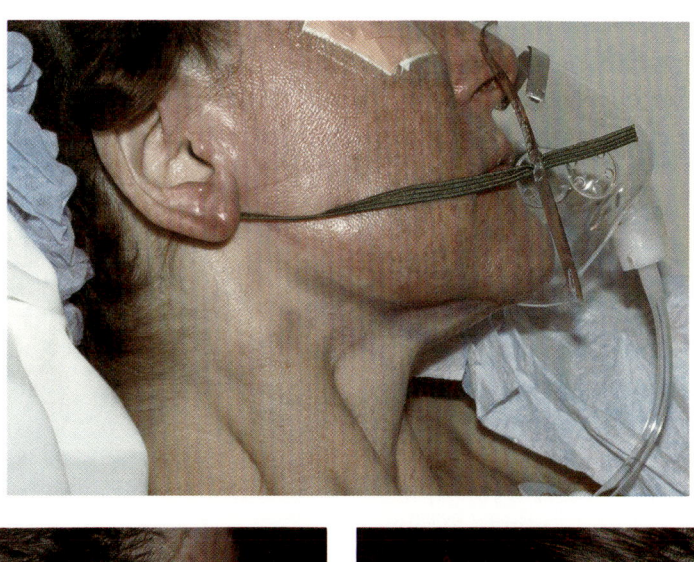

Skip areas. A skip area in the right posterior mandibular region was noticed while this patient was in the recovery room, and 50% TCA was applied at that time. At the 6 day postpeel visit the skip area that was treated in the recovery room looks satisfactory, but just above it in the temporal hairline are two others that were previously unrecognized. These areas were spot peeled with Baker formula and observed 2 days later. At 6 weeks after peel the areas show some irregularity of coloration.

The next zone to be treated is the left cheek, extending medially to the nasolabial crease. After the usual 10-minute pause, the right cheek zone receives the peel solution. The tragus and earlobe are treated. The final zone is the upper and lower lip and chin areas.

Our technique allows a minimum of 1 hour for application to the entire face. Since faces come in various sizes, of course, one might expect to take longer and to apply more solution to the patient with the larger facial surface area. Total "operative" time, including anesthesia induction and emergence and dressing application, may be 1½ to 2 hours. The anesthesiologist administers 1 liter of fluid over a 2 to 3 hour period for an average-size patient of 60 to 70 kg.

Asken[7] emphasized the following:

"1. The skin should be thoroughly degreased.
2. A fresh applicator should be used each time the solution is applied.
3. The solution should be thoroughly stirred before each application.
4. The wet applicator should never be moved over the patient's eyes.
5. The wet applicator should be rolled on a dry gauze before treating the eyelids.
6. Fifteen minutes should elapse between applications and the monitor watched for cardiac arrhythmias throughout the procedure. Should this occur, and if warranted, the anesthetist can usually treat it with lidocaine intravenously. I have never seen such arrhythmia occur during 15 years' experience with this procedure."

The beginning practitioner of this technique is advised to use every means possible to accurately record the technique. The use of a "work card" or sheet of some type will facilitate later recall of specifics of the procedure (see pp. 110-111). While relatively simple in concept, skin peeling calls for many judgments to be made at the operating table, and without such a record details are quickly forgotten. I would also urge the use of a Polaroid camera as well as permanent slides or prints to record the details of tape occlusion. All this provides an excellent record to aid in a "quality control program."

Brody[29] also urges the practitioner to develop a standardized qualitative and quantitative approach to peeling to provide a better analysis of results. He included a very handy worksheet he uses during the procedure (see p. 113).

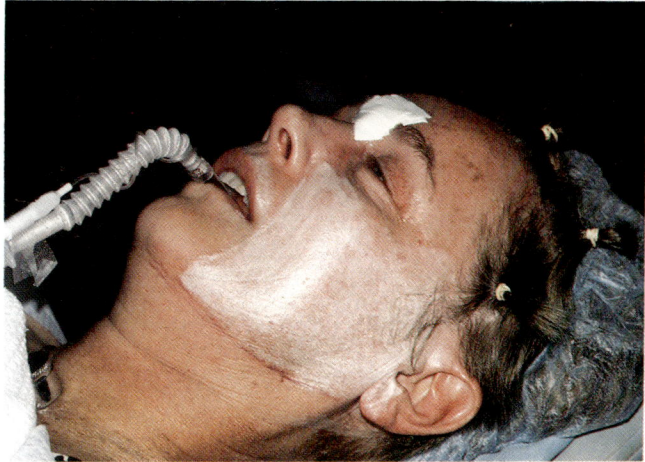

Peeling technique. The patient is shown here after a standard application of Baker formula phenol solution to the cheek, tragus, and ear lobe.

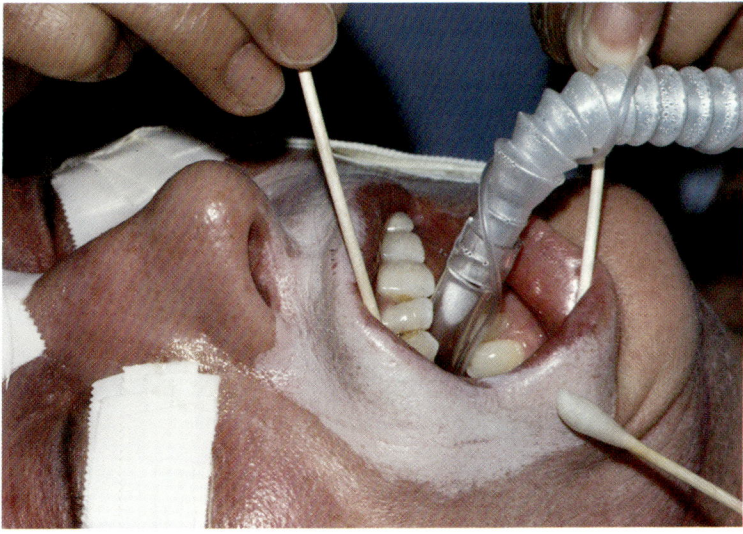

Perioral peeling technique. To ensure penetration of the peeling solution into the fine lines around the mouth, the lips are placed on traction by means of applicators as the operator works the solution into the crevices and grooves found in this area.

REJUVENATION

Name _____ Date _____

Formula _____

1. Full Face _____
2. Neck _____
3. Upper half of face _____
4. Lower half of face _____
5. Eyelids _____
6. Mouth _____
7. Forehead _____
8. Cheeks _____

Tape

1. _____
2. _____
3. _____

Adhesive _____

Powder _____

Remarks:

Day 1 _____
    2 _____
    3 _____
    4 _____
    5 _____
    6 _____
    7 _____

REJUVENATION—cont'd
Remarks: _____

Day 1. _____

Day 2. _____

Day 3. _____

Day 4. _____

Day 5. _____

Day 6. _____

Day 7. _____

112 CHEMICAL REJUVENATION OF THE FACE

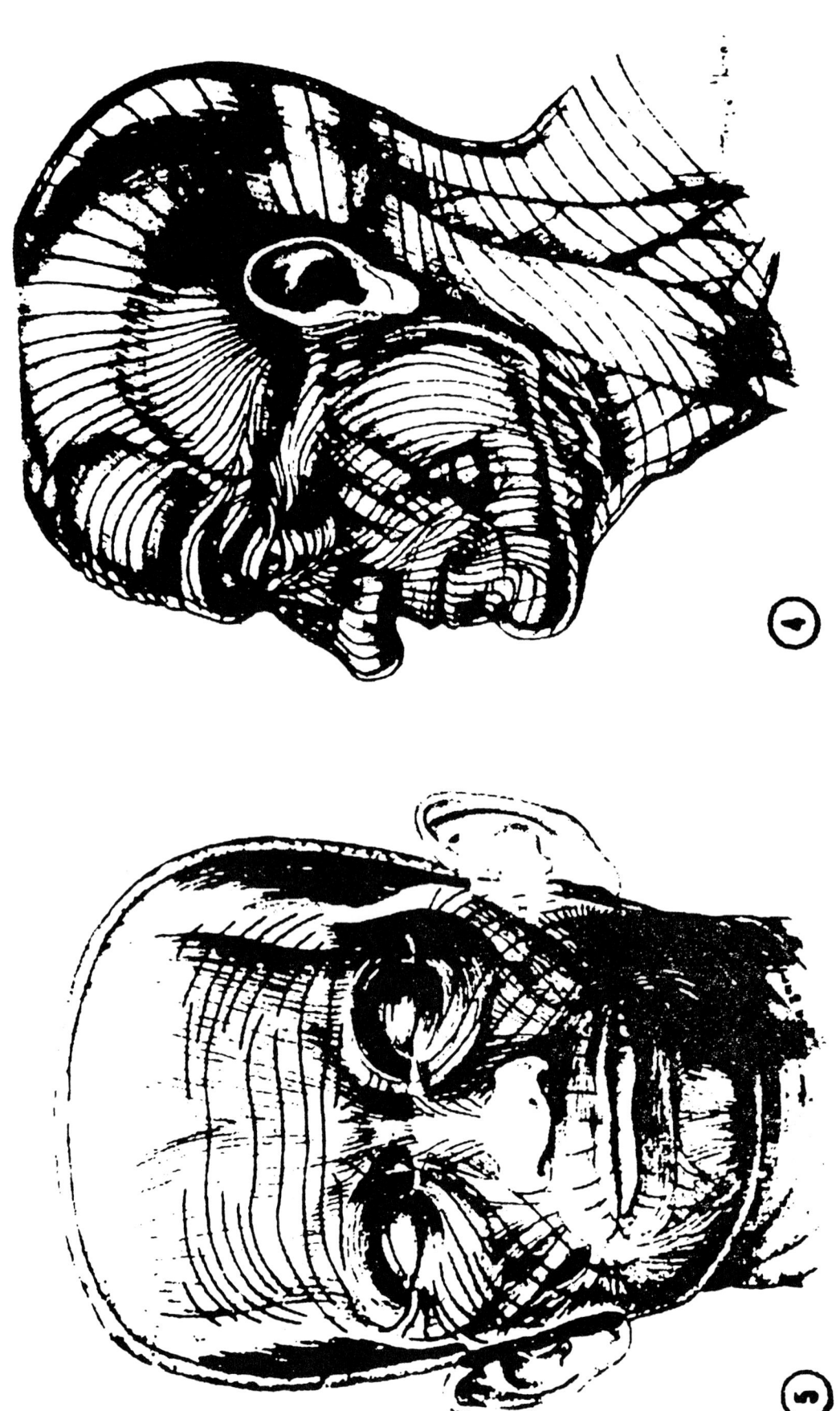

CHEMICAL PEELING

Date: _____

Patient name: _____

Age: _____

Clinical skin description:

   Diagnosis _____

   Skin type _____

   Actinic degree _____

   Sebaceous degree _____

   Photographs taken _____

Size of area peeled: _____

Location (Diagram):

Preoperative skin preparation and degreasing:

_____

_____

_____

Preoperative analgesia: _____

_____

Anesthesia: _____

_____

Chemical agents and mode of application:

_____

_____

_____

Area   Time applied

_____

_____

_____

Keloid former? _____

Operative time: _____

Postoperative condition (dressings, medication) _____

_____

_____

_____

Attending physician: _____

OCCLUSIVE DRESSING APPLICATION

It is axiomatic in chemical skin peeling that should deeper penetration of the chemexfoliative agent be desired to create a deeper peel, the primary technique is to occlude the peeled surface. Whether or not occlusion should be performed is a factor of the clinician's judgment, although occlusion is but one of several techniques that deepen the peeling. Mechanical and chemical breakdown of the epidermal barrier by vigorous preparation with ether or acetone or the application of agents such as carbon dioxide (dry ice) or exfoliating solutions such as Jessner's solution may also promote the same result (see Chapter 3).

The question of occlusion and its importance as one of the variables in the scheme of peeling has been raised by authors when discussing the possibility of imitating the deep peel that results from tape occlusion by nontape techniques. Beeson and McCollough[21] cited Stegman's[105] studies, which noted that the more phenol applied, the greater the penetration. They also noted that the nontape technique may feature greater application of phenol to perhaps compensate for the lack of taping. The degree of mechanical, active preparation of the skin with acetone or other degreasing agents may also affect penetration.[21] With the introduction of retinoic acid into the practitioner's armamentarium, some have sought to enhance the process by both pre- and postoperative application of retinoic acid. Whether absence of tape occlusion can be compensated for by retinoic acid's further exfoliation is a subject of study.[103]

Classic concepts of occlusion have been modified recently to exclude covering with adhesive tapes. Some veteran practitioners have been satisfied with petrolatum or vegetable shortening coating instead of tape.[21,110] Such a technique avoids the need for a separate dressing removal session. Stuzin, Baker, and Gordon[112] in 1988 reported to the American Society for Aesthetic Plastic Surgery that:

> "For the last 18 months, we have abandoned tape occlusion following phenol peel and have substituted an occlusive dressing using a thick layer of petroleum jelly (Vaseline). The occlusiveness provided by the petroleum jelly has proved to be almost as effective as the standard tape mask, and the results using this technique parallel those with the tape mask. The advantages of Vaseline occlusive dressing include greater patient comfort, the ability to evaluate the wound beneath the petroleum jelly and the prevention of streaking, which can occur from uneven tape application. Eschar formation and cross separations are avoided after the peel by the constant use of facial lubricants...."

Later in the same paper they noted[112]:

> "Some clinical situations require a deep peel to produce significant improvement, and it is our impression that tape occlusion produces more profound results in these problem patients. Patients with deeply lined faces that appear weather-beaten who

have sustained significant actinic damage merit tape occlusion. In contrast to fine facial wrinkling, the improved appearance of patients with deep wrinkles and sun-damaged skin following chemical peel is greater with the use of tape occlusion as compared with the results using Vaseline occlusive dressings. We reserve tape occlusion only for those difficult types of clinical problems."

Alt[2] states:

"My personal experience has shown that untaped phenol peels do not achieve the depth of penetration that is possible with the taped variety. The therapeutic and cosmetic results are diminished when compared with the taped method."

My observations cause me to concur with these comments. We also are comparing this nontaping technique to the classic technique. Traditionally, our preference has been to use white waterproof tape in four layers to all such areas that are deemed in need of moderately aggressive peeling. Frequently, significant portions of the face may not require such an aggressive technique. Therefore, the dressing is customized for each patient. In our experience with a quite sun-damaged population, 20% of patients will require dressings to the entire face.

This issue of "to tape or not to tape" has challenged many investigator/practitioners. Stegman,[106] in a letter to the editors, responding to an article by Beeson and McCollough in the *Journal of Dermatologic Surgery and Oncology* entitled "Chemical Face Peeling Without Taping,"[21] raised the issue of other factors besides occlusion that may intensify the skin peel process.

"I have had the opportunity to observe at meetings and by videotapes and to see in person the excellent results obtained by the technique described in the paper, 'Chemical Face Peeling Without Taping' by Beeson and McCollough. The paper is presented as an advantageous technique because 'It eliminates the need for repeated anesthetics and postoperative visits and provides an atmosphere for accelerated wound healing.' My letter has two purposes: I want to add histologic support to the contentions made by the authors as to why their technique is effective, and I want to question whether or not the technique is truly meritorious.

"The contention is made by Beeson and McCollough that having the patient wash multiple times with soap and water plus vigorous scrubbing with acetone so damages the stratum corneum that the phenol penetrates deeper, thus creating a wound as deep as the tape-occluded technique. Their evidence for this is some work I had published in 1980 comparing the various depths of wounding produced by different escharotics and occlusion versus nonocclusion. (This work has been further proven in humans.)

"Some years ago, I heard Dr. McCollough present this technique at a meeting in Birmingham, Alabama. I was so intrigued by the fact that he obtained excellent results (as also shown in this paper) without occlusion that I tried to understand better the mechanism of action. I felt it was clinically obvious that there was more penetration of the phenol when the patients were prepared by the washing and acetone technique, because on the videotapes and live demonstrations some patients developed cardiac arrhythmias—fortunately mild, benign ones which were easily controlled by the anesthesiologist present.

"Conversely, I have had only one instance of cardiac arrhythmia in all of the years I have been performing phenol peels. (Fortunately this, too, was easily controlled.) Deductive reasoning would suggest that at least more phenol is absorbed or the phenol is absorbed more rapidly by the McCollough-Beeson method. The critical question is: Does the increased penetration or the increased speed of penetration effect the wound depth? Wound depth is the primary factor to determine the efficacy of chemical peels.

"Therefore, when I had my next opportunity to work with a pig, I set up a small portion of the study whereby I would peel two 1 cm areas of the pig's back with Baker's formula without occlusion. One area had been prepared with Hibiclens* only, and the other with Hibiclens followed by extensive rubbing with acetone. Thirty days later biopsies were taken from these sites and the depth of the ongoing healing reaction compared. The 30-day posttreatment biopsy at a site prepared by Hibiclens only revealed an epidermis of normal thickness with rete pegs. The skin appeared fairly well healed with the exception of a slight lymphocytic infiltrate and some new collagen formation in the papillary dermis. On the other hand, the specimen taken after Hibiclens and acetone showed an epidermis that was still hyperplastic with no rete pegs. This would indicate that the epidermis was not as completely healed as the other specimen. Also, inflammation and interstitial edema extended into the dermis at least three times deeper and the lymphocytic infiltrate was thicker and more pervasive. My conclusion is that the second wound was not as completely healed as the first. I extrapolate this to mean that the acetone-cleansed area was much deeper. This small animal study would support the contentions by Beeson and McCollough that the washing in acetone causes enough damage to the epidermal barrier, so that the ensuing wound by phenol is deeper than when the barrier is not destroyed.

"The second portion of my comments, however, concerns the question of creating a deeper wound by greater or faster absorption of phenol. I should prefer that we try to develop techniques which would use less phenol, since this is a toxic and potentially

*Stuart Pharmaceuticals, Wilmington, DE.

fatal agent. Thus, enhancing the effect of smaller doses of phenol with occlusion might be a safer technique. When one compares the small inconvenience of returning to the office to remove the tape versus the potential toxicity of phenol, it is not difficult to choose the former path.

"In addition, in 15 years of performing chemical peels, I have never administered anesthesia of any type in order to remove the tape. About half of my patients remove the tape themselves at home and call me, as instructed, to report that everything is all right. These patients usually do not come back to the office for 7 to 10 days. Others who prefer to come to the office for tape removal are there only a few minutes, because it seldom takes me more than 30 seconds to remove the tape. They sigh in relief and head home to the shower.

"The other observation by the authors is that the moist postoperative care accelerates wound healing. I am not sure about the speed of wound healing, but I am very sure about the comfort of the patients. After observing the technique of Beeson and McCollough, all of my postoperative peel and dermabrasion patients now have the luxury of immediately going to the shower which makes them infinitely more comfortable. They wash their face twice a day (why the authors have their patients wash five times a day I will never understand) with a soap of their own choice, followed by a thin, smooth application of an antibacterial ointment. Crisco works, as suggested by the authors, but I think there are many more elegant preparations available which can be washed off easier and contain antibacterial agents and antirancid agents superior to those used in Crisco vegetable shortening.

"We must all be cautious, however, about extrapolating too much information from what we observe clinically. Surely the moist technique as presented by the authors and which I have adopted leads to healing with a great deal more comfort and maybe even quicker healing. The new semipermeable and semipermeable/gel dressings also provide more comfort to postoperative dermabrasion patients and I think have been proven to measurably speed epithelialization after a peel or a dermabrasion is valuable.

"The epidermis plays a very small role, if any, in the cosmetic appearance of final healing. Some of the ugliest scars have a normal epidermis. It is the dermal healing which determines the cosmetic quality of the skin. In chemical peeling, it is the replacement of the elastotic dermis with a new and thick papillary dermis and a mid-dermal partial fibrotic replacement which seems to produce the salutary results. One could even theorize that rapid epithelialization decreases the amount of dermal replacement and thus would be detrimental to the desired goals."

118 CHEMICAL REJUVENATION OF THE FACE

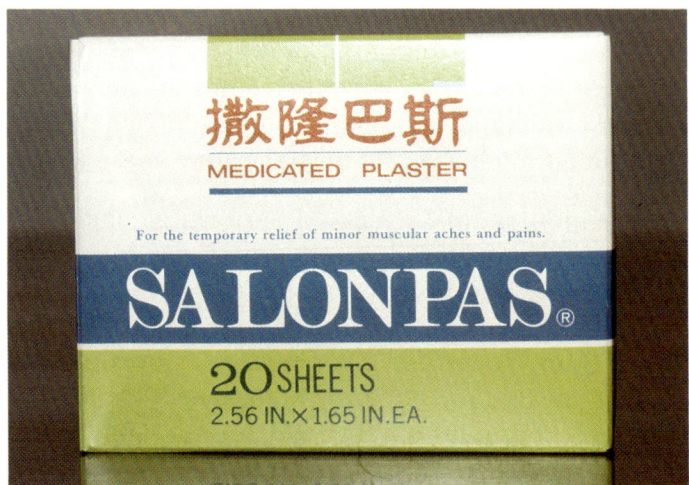

Technique: tape occlusion. Salonpas, a medicated plaster tape found in most Oriental food stores, often is used as the first layer of a tape mask to intensify the effects of the peeling solution in deeply wrinkled areas.

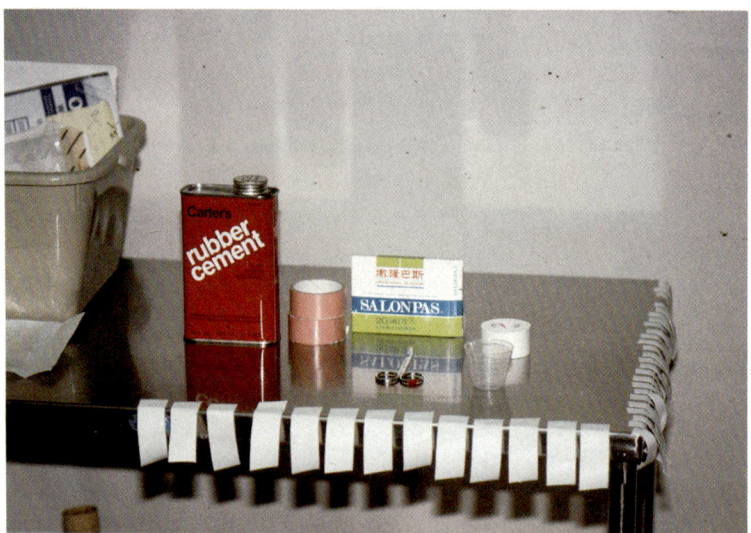

Technique: tape application. This view of the taping table shows tapes that have been precut for efficiency in mask application.

Alt[2] favors a film of petrolatum being applied to the surgical site and then a layer of plastic film (Saran Wrap) being applied over the petrolatum to prevent desiccation. Vaseline and Saran Wrap are applied until all the surgical sites reepithelialize.

For the patients in whom there are profoundly deep wrinkles in the glabellar, periorbital, or perioral area, it has been our experience that a more potent taping technique is needed to produce a superior result in those zones. The use of a medicated plaster tape containing methylsalicylate, menthol, camphor, and glycol salicylate apparently yields better results by causing additional irritation and maceration of the skin. This becomes the "first layer" of tape over the deepest wrinkles and is then covered by the standard white, waterproof tape mask. It must be emphasized that while the rewards and satisfaction of removing nearly all the wrinkles become greater, the attendant potential for scarring also increases. However, this remains a proven technique for eliminating the deepest wrinkles otherwise not removable. This tape, marketed under the trade name Salonpas,* is made in Japan and is generally available in Oriental food stores, where it is sold for "temporary relief of minor muscular aches and pains." The active ingredients in Salonpas are:

> Methylsalicylate
> Menthol
> Camphor
> Glycol salicylate
> Thymol
> Tocopherol acetate

Tapes may be applied in the same "zone" manner used for application of the chemical peeling solution. If one chooses to use an adhesive, various adhesives are appropriate, including the aerosol spray adhesives frequently used to apply Elastoplast† dressings or commercial grade rubber cement. After the application of the waterproof tape layers, an additional two layers of pink Hi-Tape‡ may be applied. This plastic tape is an excellent outer layer since it resists staining and may be easily washed.

To achieve maximum chemexfoliation, drying of the skin surface must be avoided and taping must be meticulously done. Careful overlapping of the edges provides the most effective airtight seal that helps ensure against an uneven result.

---

*Hisamitsu Pharmaceutical Co., Inc.
†Biersdorf, Inc.
‡Hi-Tape Surgical Products.

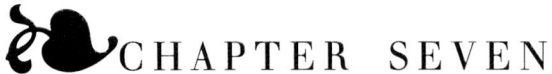
CHAPTER SEVEN

Dressing Removal and Aftercare

FIRST 48 HOURS

Our policy is usually to remove tape dressings 48 hours after application. It may be appropriate to remove the dressings after 24 hours; previously peeled skin or very thin atrophic skin requires greater caution and hence a more conservative taping approach. Certainly, it is technically easier to remove the dressing at 48 hours, by which time there has been liquefication of the chemexfoliated skin, allowing the dressing to spontaneously loosen from the face.

Our preference has been to treat the patient with intravenous sedation for the 5 to 10 minutes that it takes to remove the dressing, cleanse the skin of the desquamated and necrotic epithelium, and perform general tidying about the face and neck. Our practice is to have our anesthesiologist perform the intravenous sedation, although with proper monitoring equipment and experience the operator may choose to perform the procedure independently.

Very rarely spot peeling and retaping may be done if the skin appears underpeeled, particularly where the wrinkles have been very deep (for example, in the glabella, orbital, and lip areas). I have spot peeled with the Baker solution in all these areas. White waterproof tapes have been reapplied to the glabella, forehead, and orbital area using commercial rubber cement. I do not retape with Salonpas. These tapes are removed the following day without sedation. I have not had success attempting to retape around the mouth, mainly because the tapes almost immediately loosen, perhaps because of more active movement in these sites.

Upon initial dressing removal a serous exudate covers the face. The weeping is stopped by blowing the face with a hair dryer. Routine culture of the exudate from both occluded and unoccluded areas shows the presence of a variety of common bacteria (see p. 126). Infection is rarely a complication of the peeling procedure; however we routinely apply Bactoban, a newer broad-spectrum antibiotic ointment with specific antistaphylococcal properties, at this point.

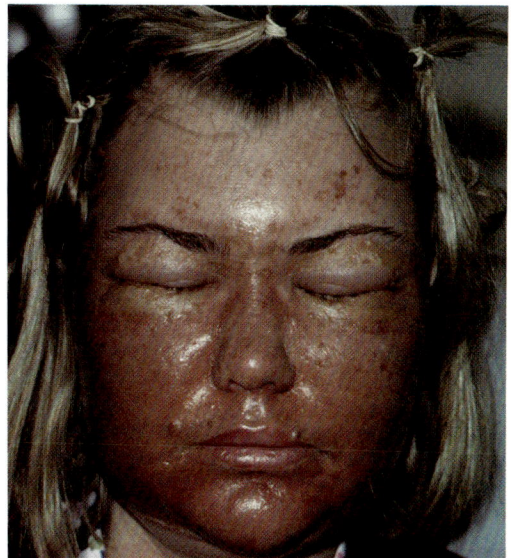 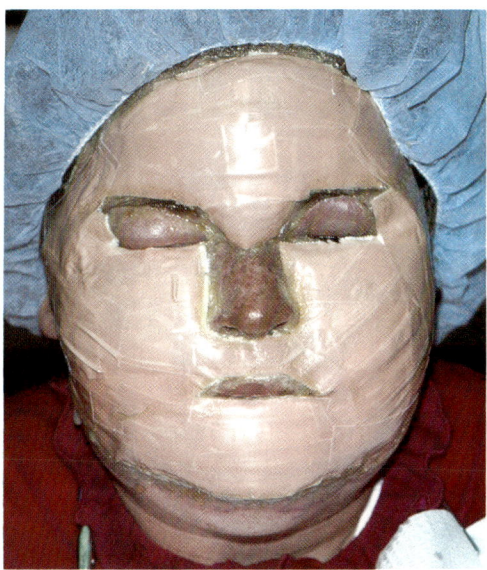

Appearance 24 hours after peel. Both patients have had Baker formula phenol peels, one unoccluded and the other with mask occlusion covering all areas but the nose, upper eyelids, and infrabrow. There is less swelling in the face and neck without occlusion; however, the eyes will swell shut in either case. The eyelids should be opened at this time to examine for ocular function.

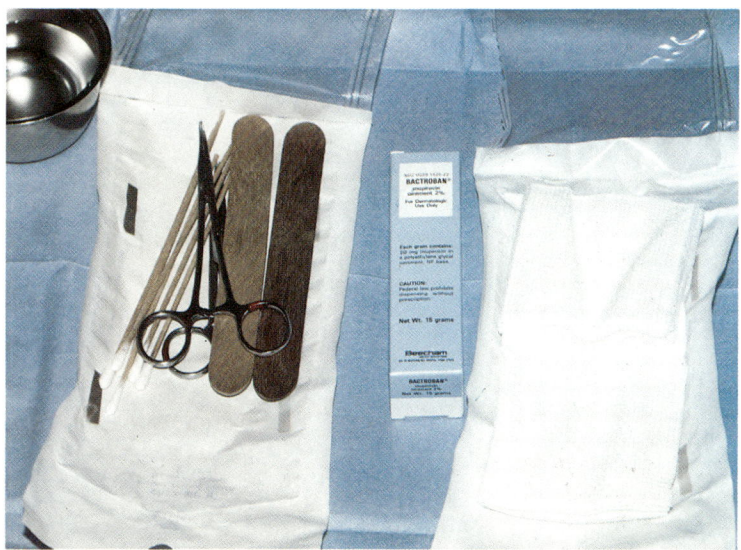

Supplies and equipment for mask removal. A sterile basin contains sterile saline. All instruments, tongue blades, applicators, and 4 × 4 gauze pads are sterile. Bactoban, a broad-spectrum antibiotic ointment, is used for the initial coating after mask removal.

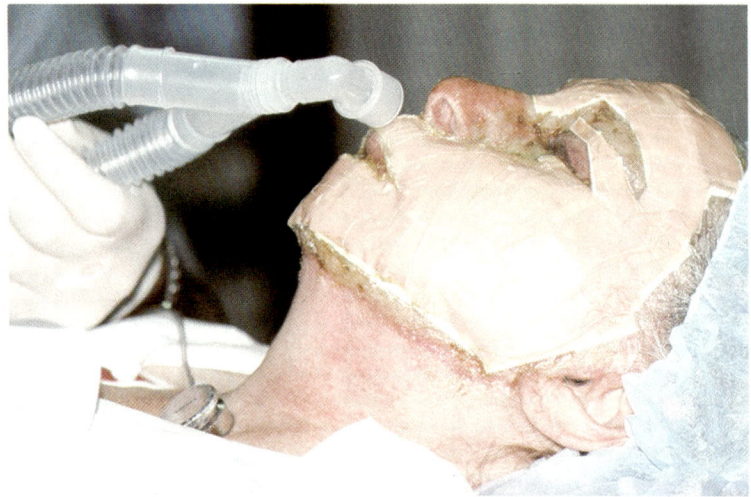

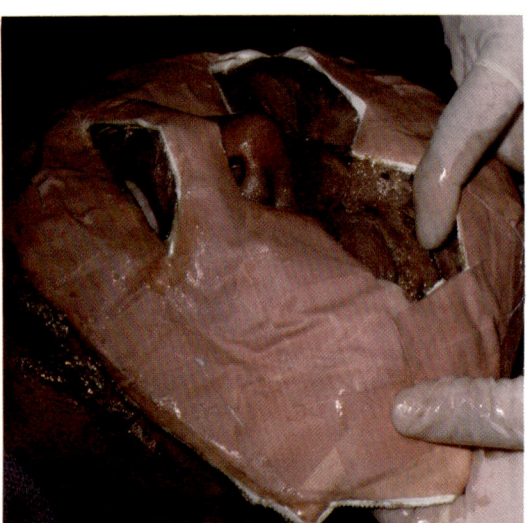

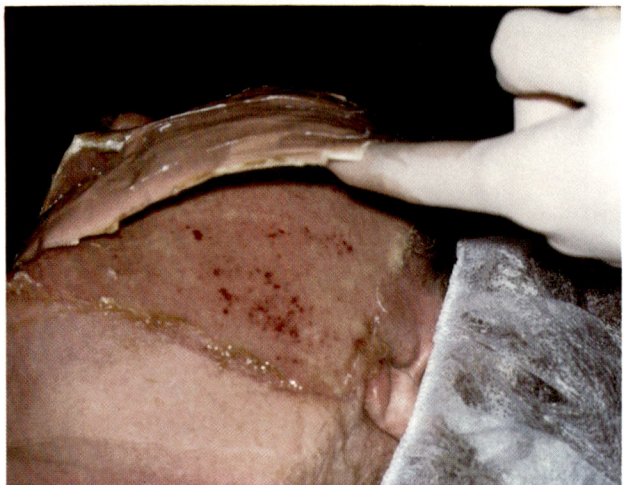

Mask removal. The mask is removed 48 hours after application of the chemical peeling agents. The patient is sedated and the anesthesiologist administers 100% oxygen to prepare for mask removal. Note that in removing the mask the operator gently dissects it from the eye area using an index finger to protect the eyebrow hairs from being inadvertently plucked as the mask is lifted off the face. Removal of the mask reveals a raw and unreepithelialized skin surface.

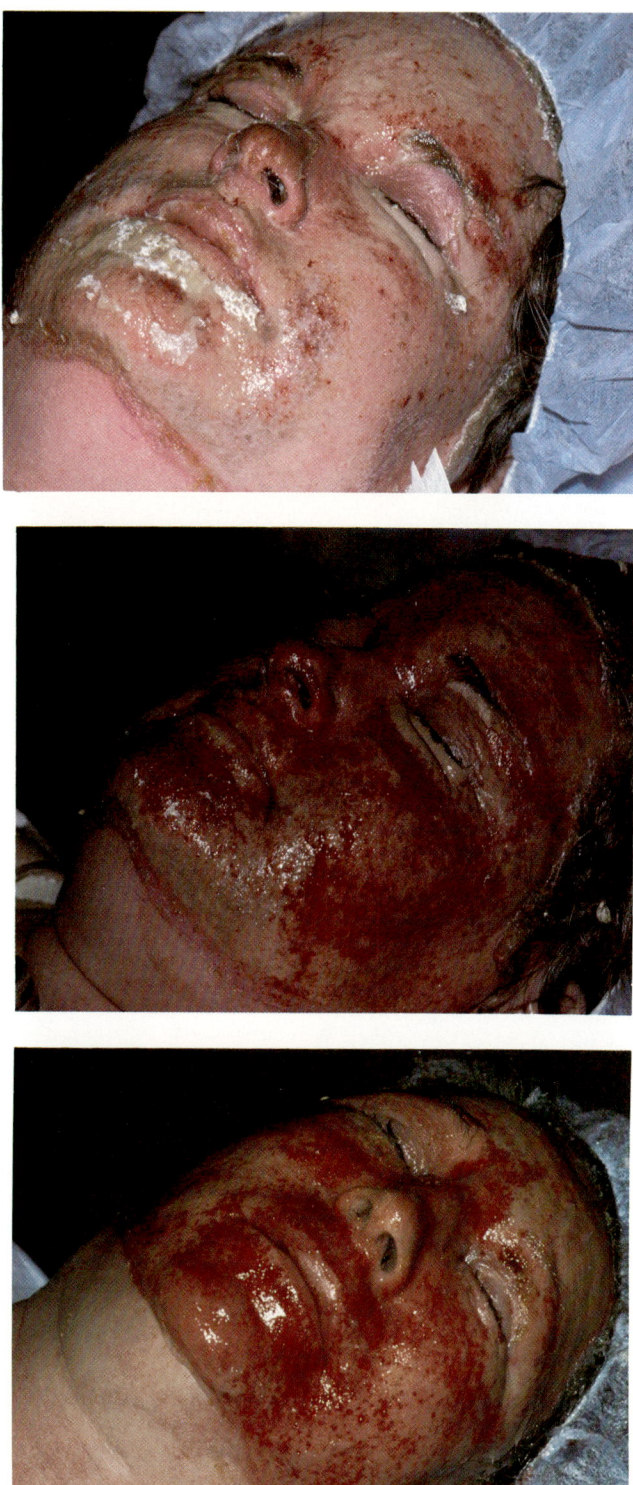

Immediately after mask removal. The significant amount of exudate seen here after mask removal is a sign of the "deep peel." Bits of adhesive that remain attached to the skin are removed and the skin is cleansed with use of 4 × 4 gauze pads. Note the appearance of the skin after overvigorous cleansing (middle). We have abandoned overly aggressive débridement in favor of gentle cleansing for fear of causing scarring. After cleansing, Bactoban ointment is applied.

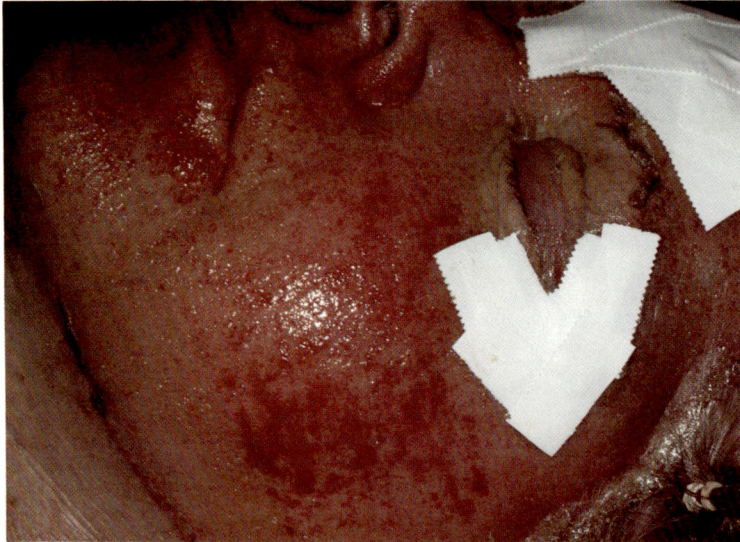

Tape reapplication. Retaping may be indicated for those patients in whom deep lines are still visible immediately after the 48-hour mask removal and cleansing. This typically involves lines in the crow's-feet and forehead areas. New tapes are secured with a rubber cement. It is nearly impossible to secure tapes around the mouth at this stage because of jaw movement.

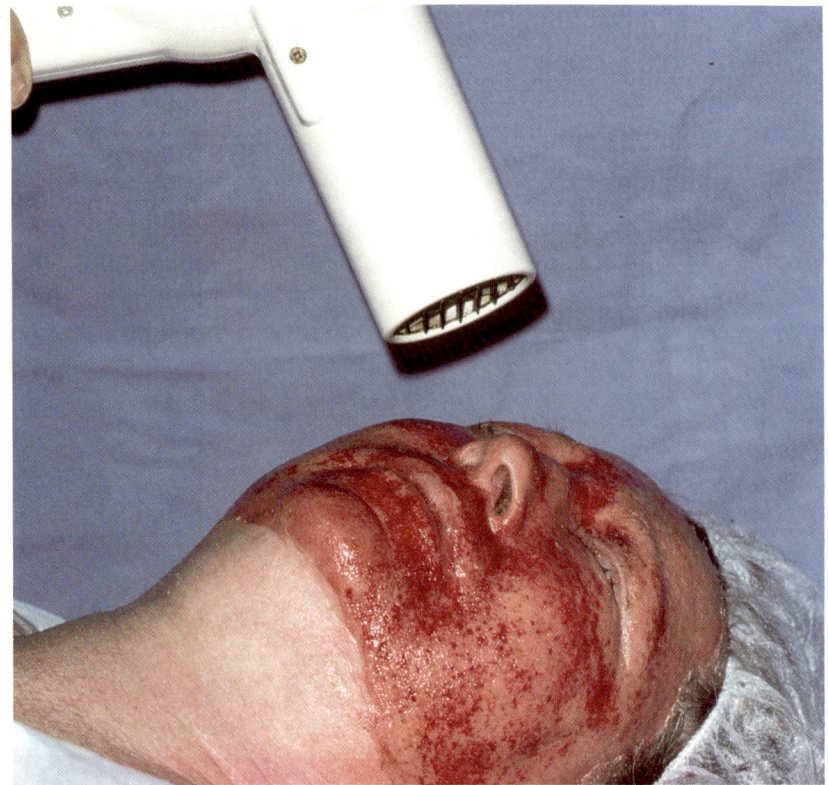

Drying the skin after mask removal. A hair dryer is used on the medium setting to gently dry the oozing skin. This promotes coagulation. After drying, antibiotic ointment is applied.

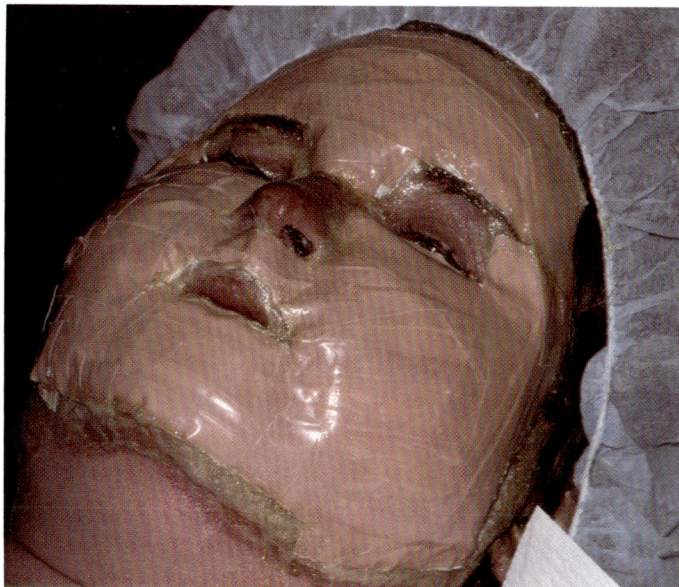

Neck swelling. The patient is shown here 48 hours after peel, ready for mask removal. Although there is profound swelling of the neck and upper portion of the chest there is no airway obstruction. Patients must be reassured that this is a normal occurrence and that it will abate very quickly.

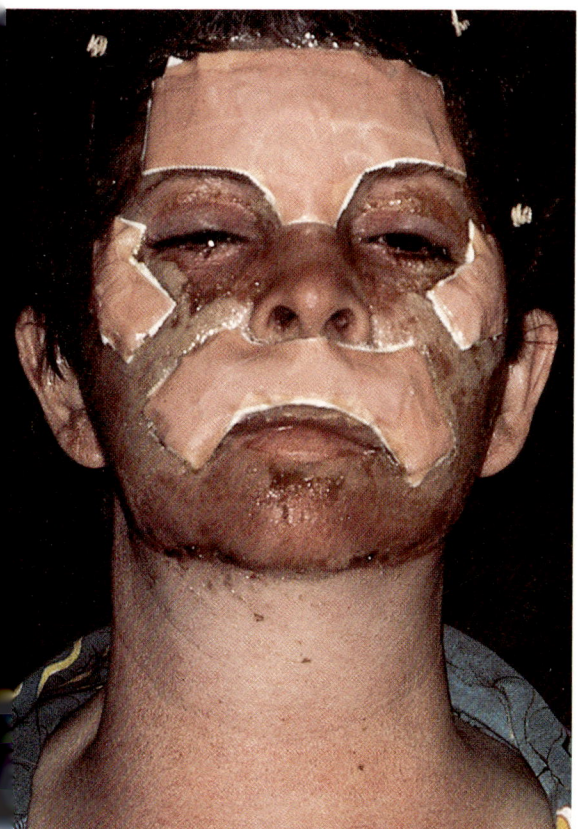

2 days post peel

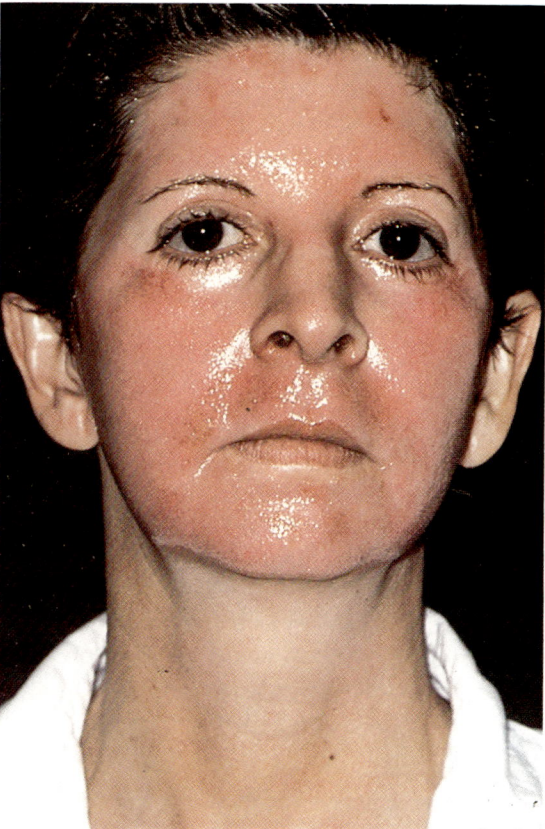

6 days post peel

Neck swelling. This patient also experienced swelling of the neck and upper portion of the chest following a maximum technique phenol peel. As seen here, however, the swelling has almost completely resolved by 6 days post peel.

NECK SWELLING

Neck swelling is expected after an aggressive peel. We have never witnessed airway obstruction as a consequence of this, but it has been reported in the literature.[68] The swelling typically resolves completely within 4 days following mask removal. Patients need to be reassured that this is a normal consequence of the peeling process and that it will resolve rapidly.

AFTERCARE FOR THE NEXT 4 DAYS

After the 48-hour dressing removal, patients recover in the office for an appropriate period of time and are then discharged to home with appropriate supplies and instructions.

We no longer routinely use thymol iodide powder, preferring to coat the skin with antibiotic ointment. This shortens the time between dressing removal and erasure of the "crust" that forms on the skin surface. Our timetable calls for 2 days of Polysporin antibiotic ointment coating, followed by 2 days of two facial cleansings per day using Ivory soap to remove the crust from the face. What crusting remains after these washings is retreated with the antibiotic ointment. Generally over 95% of the face is free of the crust within 48 hours of beginning the washing. Those areas most apt to remain crusted are the crow's feet, forehead, and mouth. Generally these areas will have been treated more aggressively, evoking a deeper peel process and hence development of a thicker crust. The patients are comfortable, do not require pain medication, and complain only of the sunburnlike sensation. This may be relieved with a mild antiinflammatory medication such as aspirin, acetaminophen, or a nonsteroidal antiinflammatory agent.

ROUTINE CULTURE OF EXUDATE 48 HOURS AFTER PEEL

Source: Upper lip under tape (pink)
  Staphylococcus, coagulase positive, isolated—heavy growth
  Alpha streptococci isolated—heavy growth
  Enterobacter species isolated—heavy growth
  Pseudomonas aeruginosa—moderate growth
  Diphtheroids isolated—few

Source: face—eyes uncovered
  Staphylococcus, coagulase positive, isolated—heavy growth
  Enterobacter species isolated—heavy growth
  Klebsiella species isolated—oxytoca, heavy growth
  Diphtheroids isolated—heavy growth

GENERAL INFORMATION

During the first several weeks and the first 7 days in particular, for your new skin's benefit, please heed the following advice:
1. Avoid excessive chewing and speaking.
2. Avoid direct sunlight.
3. Whatever swelling is present will disappear.
4. The initial redness will change to pinkness and fade.
5. The skin tends to be very dry initially; we shall tell you how to correct that.
6. Be sure to tell us about any new medications that you may be taking.
7. Smoking is not advised.
8. CALL US AT <u>ANY TIME</u> IF YOU HAVE <u>ANY</u> QUESTIONS.

FACIAL REJUVENATION POSTTREATMENT INSTRUCTIONS

Day 1 and Day 2	The dressings, if placed, stay on skin. Liquids per straw only. No chewing. Skin not covered by dressings turns dark and becomes dry. The face and neck are normally swollen.
Day 3	If your face has any dressings on it, you will have them removed in the office, usually under a brief anesthetic; DO NOT eat or drink anything after 11 pm the evening before coming to the office. Some areas may be re-dressed for another 24 hours. Today we begin covering the entire face with the antibiotic ointment. Swelling begins to subside. "Weeping" may still be present.
Day 4	Continue to apply the antibiotic ointment to the entire face. Ointment should be applied as often as necessary to keep the entire treated area covered at all times. This ointment helps to soften and remove the old skin.
Day 5	Begin to wash off remaining crust with Ivory soap and water. If some crust remains, keep applying ointment to soften. Wash several times during the day and apply ointment to keep skin from being dry. Continue this process until all the "crust" is off. This may take another day or so.
After Day 5	We shall set an appointment for you to be seen.

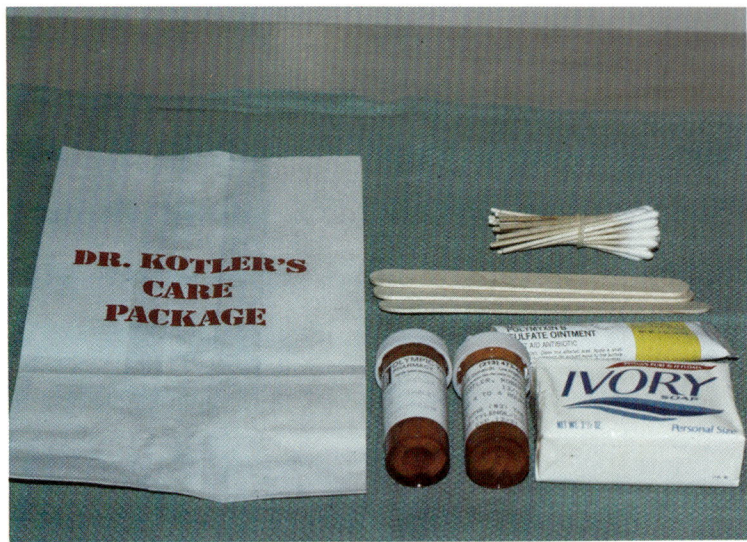

Postpeel take-home kit. Patients leave the office after the skin peel with a "care package" containing all the supplies needed for the next 5 days. While the mask is still in place during the first 48 hours, they will require only an oral antibiotic such as erythromycin and acetaminophen with codeine or methadone for pain. Ivory soap and Polysporin ointment are to be used in the "washing off" process, which generally begins on day 4 or 5. Patients are previously given a supply of acyclovir (Zovirax) to be used beginning the day before the peel to prevent herpes simplex.

"1 WEEK VISIT"

An appointment is always made for the patient to be seen 6 or 7 days after the "application day." By this time most or all of the face is now clear of the crust. It appears bright pink. The patient is told that at that point we will begin a program of "skin care after rejuvenation." Our center's pharmacy compounds 2.5% hydrocortisone in Aquaphor ointment. There are no additional ingredients such as alcohols or propylene glycol, which are frequently found in commercial preparations. The patient is advised to use this at least once a day. Those who will not be returning to work or venturing forth into the world may use the hydrocortisone ointment preparation continuously. This provides moisturization and some degree of antiinflammatory effect. Patients not infrequently complain of itching beginning 10 to 14 days after the procedure is performed. A prescription is given for Temaril 2.5 mg four times a day. We have recently added nonsteroidal antiinflammatory agents to the regimen and are evaluating the efficacy of this additional treatment. For those patients for whom itching becomes intolerable and who complain of the tightness and soreness of the skin, we have not infrequently resorted to a 6-day Medrol Dose Pak with excellent relief of symptoms. Neither steroidal nor nonsteroidal medication appears to compromise the cosmetic outcome.

Generally, the patient's most trying time will be in the second and

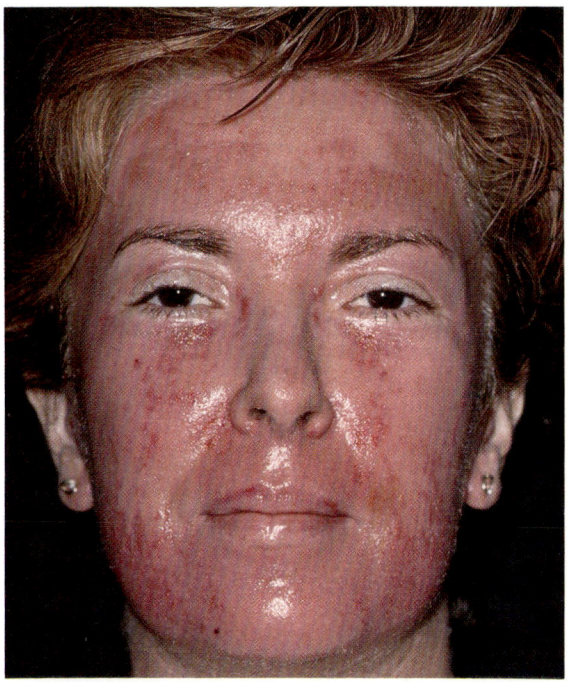

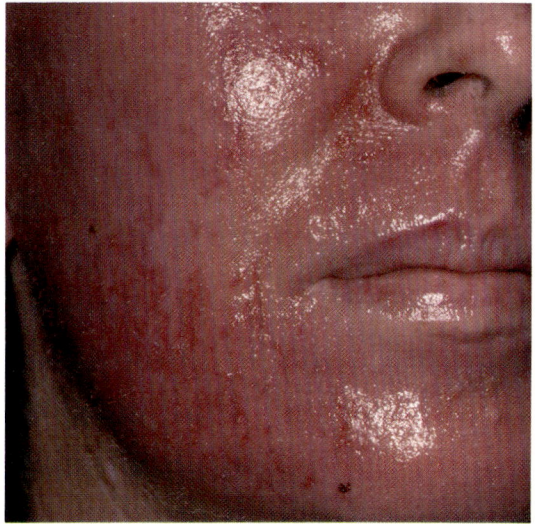

Appearance 1 week after peel. The patient is shown here at the 1-week visit after an occluded Baker formula phenol peel. The reddish areas seen in the close-up view of the cheeks are thought to be areas in which thickening of the epidermis has yet to occur. Within a matter of days, the skin will take on a more homogenous appearance.

third weeks of the process, when the skin is quite red, often itchy and dry, and when the patient is uncertain if this discomfort will last forever. The patient must be reassured that, indeed, the pink color will fade, the skin will become less sensitive, and the itching will disappear. Not infrequently we have had other patients who are "veterans" of the experience consult with the patient to provide support and rejuvenate morale.

SKIN CARE AFTER REJUVENATION; LONG-TERM MANAGEMENT

We believe that patients need education concerning the long-term optimal management of the skin following the procedure. For this reason, we provide them with a "starter kit" of products that are reliable, and not apt to cause sensitivity. This includes a non-PABA sunscreen, a hypoallergenic moisturizer, and—as needed—an emollient oil for those in whom dry skin has always been a problem. We advise against using soap, preferring lipophilic cleansing lotions. Patients are urged to apply the moisturizer during the day as an integral part of their makeup technique. Our office staff provides advice on cosmetic techniques, particularly those to obscure the red hue of the skin. Pamphlets concerning skin care are included in our starter kit.

The patient is seen at least twice in the first month. This gives us a chance to be aware of any problems, complications, or dissatisfactions. Our instruction sheet provides a list of the most common side effects or possible complications (for example, milia and pigment formation). The peak incidence for milia is generally in the sixth to eighth week after the process. Pigmentary problems have been observed as early as 2 to 3 weeks after the process, particularly in those who were obviously predisposed to such. The management of these is discussed in the following section. The patients are reminded that they can expect 8 to 12 weeks to elapse before the redness will disappear and that ultimately the skin color of their face may be lighter than that of their neck. We have photographic examples of patients with an obvious demarcation between the face and neck—with and without makeup—to share with the patients. Thus they can understand that this is not necessarily an insurmountable or unacceptable result of the procedure.

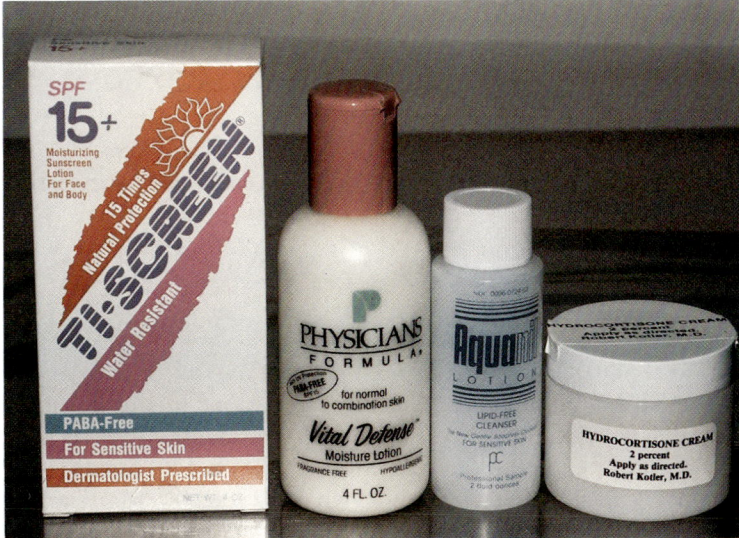

Postpeel skin care. The patient is supplied with 2.5% hydrocortisone ointment, a gentle skin cleanser, moisturizer, and a sunscreen preparation to care for her new skin after peel.

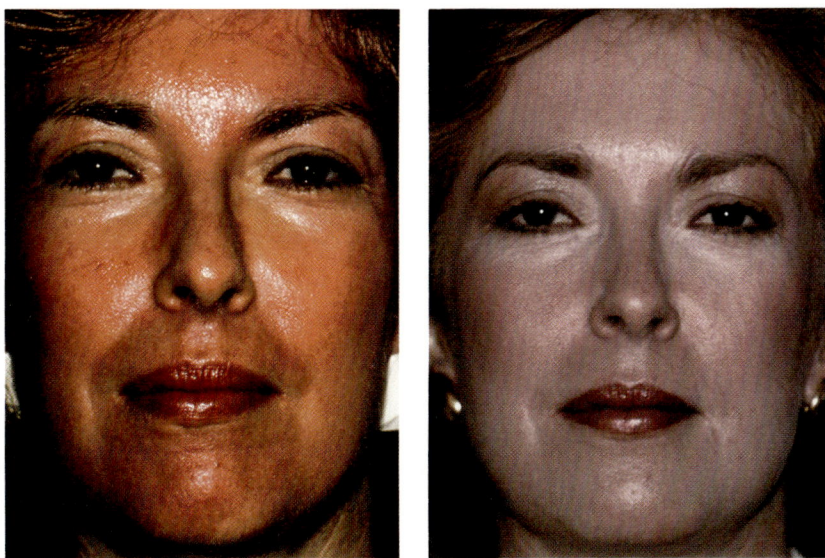

Makeup camouflage after peel. The patient seen on p. 129 is shown 1 week later. Without makeup *(left)*, the skin is still quite red; however, with makeup applied *(right)* there is a satisfactory contrast to the untreated neck.

❧ POSTOPERATIVE FACIAL SKIN CARE AND COSMETIC TIPS

This brochure will familiarize you with some basic facts about enhancing the results of your facial plastic surgery by following basic skin care, cosmetic and grooming tips. It will give you enough background to make you an "educated consumer." Your facial plastic surgeon will explain how these tips apply to individual conditions.

Common problems

After facial plastic surgery, it is not uncommon to have high expectations about the surgery and to be anxious to see the "new you." It is important to remember, however, that cosmetic surgery *is* major surgery and the healing process naturally takes time. Although actual pain is minimal, it is not uncommon to feel fatigued, tired, or just "run-down" for a day or two after surgery. Many people experience depression during the weeks or months it takes for final results to be visible, while surgical scars mature and shrink.

Some solutions

Fortunately, during and after the healing process, there are many skin care, cosmetic, and grooming procedures that will promote healing and enhance surgical results. Following these suggestions may help you maintain the positive attitude that is essential to looking your best.

Basic hygiene rules

After any kind of facial plastic surgery, proper hygiene is important to promote healing. Your surgeon will give you specific instructions to follow regarding the care of the affected area after your bandages are removed.

Gauze pads, or a clean, soft facial sponge, may be used to cleanse affected areas and to soften crusts. After washing, gently pat the area dry using a soft clean cloth or a gauze pad.

An antibiotic ointment or a vitamin preparation may be recommended to help prevent infection and speed healing. Sometimes hydrogen peroxide is used to soften and remove crusts. Moisturizing is important after dermabrasion or chemical peeling. You may be advised to apply a thin layer of bland vegetable oil shortening to the area, or your doctor may recommend a medicated ointment. Follow the specific instructions that you are given carefully.

Incision scars often seem to get worse as they heal, but this is normal. Incisions heal in three stages. The first stage, characterized by swelling and redness, lasts a few days to a week. Then scar tissue begins to form, causing the scar to look pink, lumpy and noticeable. This period can last up to six weeks, but it is followed by a period of shrinking and softening that can continue for up to a year. Eventually, for most scars, only a fine, white line remains.

Copyright © 1986 by the American Academy of Facial and Plastic Reconstructive Surgery.

POSTOPERATIVE FACIAL SKIN CARE AND COSMETIC TIPS—cont'd

Resumption of normal activities

Most people can resume normal activities after about two weeks, but care must be taken to protect incision sites and swollen or reddened areas. After surgery, sleep with your head elevated during the first two weeks and use cool compresses to help reduce swelling. Take care to protect the incision from being accidentally struck by children or bed-mates. Avoid foods that require strenuous chewing. Try not to get involved in any arguments or spirited discussions, since exaggerated facial movements may place a strain on the incisions. If you have had a facelift or neck surgery, avoid turning your neck vigorously from side to side.

After dermabrasion or chemical peeling, use warm compresses to soothe the affected area. It is essential to avoid exposure to the sun during the first six months, as this can cause blotchy pigmentation. Wear a wide-brimmed hat and sunglasses, stay in the shade if possible, and use a good sun-block (SPF 15 or higher) if you are going to be outside any length of time. Also avoid excessive exposure to heat, cold, and wind as well, as these can cause drying of the skin. Continue to use a moisturizer for at least several weeks.

Don't use aspirin or any aspirin-containing product from approximately two weeks prior to and two weeks after the procedure, as aspirin may increase your tendency to bleed. Avoid alcohol and smoking during this four week period as well. Don't do any bending, heavy lifting, or other activities that may elevate blood pressure or cause sweating.

If you have had surgery on your nose, glasses cannot be allowed to put pressure on the nasal bones for at least six weeks. If you need to wear glasses, ask your doctor about an eyeglass cradle. This clear plastic device is attached to the forehead with special tape and supports the nosebridge of the glasses.

If you wear contact lenses, you should be able to resume wearing them within two weeks. In some patients, however, eyelid surgery temporarily affects the eye fluid, causing the eyes to be drier than normal. It may be necessary to wait an extra week or two before using contact lenses if this occurs.

You should wait three to six weeks before resuming such activities as aerobics, tennis, weight-lifting, contact sports, and swimming or diving. Check with your doctor before going back to your athletic routine.

Copyright © 1986 by the American Academy of Facial and Plastic Reconstructive Surgery. *Continued.*

POSTOPERATIVE FACIAL SKIN CARE AND COSMETIC TIPS—cont'd

Cosmetic tips after surgery

Women can usually resume cosmetic use about one week after surgery and ten days after dermabrasion or chemical peeling. Careful use of makeup can help camouflage bruising and discoloration and can do wonders for your self-esteem during the healing period.

Water-based cosmetics are usually recommended during the first three weeks, since they can be easily washed off with water if irritation occurs. If your skin is particularly sensitive, you may want to use hypoallergenic makeups. Avoid products that contain fragrance or alcohol during the first few months.

Generally, you can return to your former makeup routine (including oil-based or perfumed cosmetics) about six weeks after surgery, but many women feel that this is an ideal time to reassess their beauty routine and perhaps make some changes. A consultation with a professional cosmetician can give a real boost.

Incision scars from many facial plastic surgery procedures are hidden and do not present a cosmetic problem. Scars in a noticeable location present problems because they tend to be a different color from surrounding skin, show a texture difference (such as a shiny surface), or they may be slightly raised or lowered.

The first two problems are dealt with by using a foundation makeup with good coverage. Surface irregularities are harder to camouflage because they create shadows that do not mask easily. Avoid trying to cover an irregular scar with makeup. Makeup tends to collect in slight depressions or along the edges of raised scars, making the blemish even more noticeable. Try using a sheer foundation and play up other features to draw the eye away from the scar. It may be possible to use dermabrasion at a later date to even out irregular facial scars.

If regular makeup does not adequately cover bruised or reddened areas, special corrective cosmetics are available. High-coverage makeups have been developed for use by both men and women after plastic, burn, or cancer surgery or to conceal port-wine stains and other severe birthmarks and scars. Such products are available in a variety of shades for all skin tones, including black. Special skin toners or "color block" products are also available in green, pink, and purple to neutralize skin discolorations. Corrective cosmetics and skin toners are available commercially and can be purchased at most department store cosmetic counters.

Copyright © 1986 by the American Academy of Facial and Plastic Reconstructive Surgery.

POSTOPERATIVE FACIAL SKIN CARE AND COSMETIC TIPS—cont'd

Makeup tips for a natural appearance

- Always select a foundation that is one shade lighter than your natural skin tone.
- Use a translucent powder after foundation for complete coverage with a soft, natural look.
- A concealer (stick or cream) may be applied under the eyes to mask bruises or dark circles. Apply it under your foundation, and use a shade slightly lighter than your base color.
- Use a green skin toner to balance excessive redness, pink to counteract a sallow complexion, and purple to mask yellow discoloration.
- Avoid brown or black eyeliner after eyelid surgery, as these colors tend to emphasize redness. Blue eyeliner, smudged along the lash line on both the upper and lower lids, helps to minimize redness and dark circles.
- Scars in the eyebrow area may leave brow hairs missing. Use a small, angled brush to shade the missing area using a flat shadow color close to your hair color. This looks more natural than shading with eyebrow pencil.
- A soft eyeshadow pencil in slate or taupe can be smudged toward the outer corner of the eye to correct any visible scars in this area.
- Avoid using metallic or iridescent eyeshadow or face makeup as these colors emphasize open pores, scars, and other skin flaws.
- After a facelift, choose a soft, face-framing hairdo. Hair that is too short around the face, and hair that is swept up off the forehead may reveal scars. Medium-length bangs, perhaps gently curled, can help to camouflage scars in the forehead area.
- If hairline and forehead scars are not a problem, a soft, full backswept hairstyle can promote a youthful appearance. Avoid severely pulled-back styles.
- If you have a reddened complexion or redness around the eyes, never wear fuschia, rose, red, or hot pink. Instead, choose soft shades of blue and green for both wardrobe and makeup.

Copyright © 1986 by the American Academy of Facial and Plastic Reconstructive Surgery.

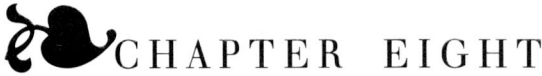

CHAPTER EIGHT

Complications

Since complications in cosmetic procedures are of the greatest concern to practitioner and patient, I urge the serious student of chemical skin peeling to study some of the classic papers on the subject. Spira, Gerow, and Hardy[100] wrote a superior paper on the subject in 1974. They wisely noted that "there is little place for the experimenter or innovator in employing this treatment, as the margin for error is too small."

COMBINING PEELING WITH SURGERY

On combining a face and neck lift with peeling, Asken[7] stated:

> "A phenol chemical peel should not be performed concomitantly with a rhytidectomy. The marked inflammatory reaction induced by the peel combined with the undermining of the skin can compromise the vasculature as well as the lymphatic drainage in that area. This can cause tissue sloughing with subsequent scarring. Instead, one should wait 2 to 3 months before performing a phenol peel on a patient who has recently had a face lift. The same interval should be applied to the periorbital peel following a blepharoplasty."

In 1986, Litton, Scachowicz, and Trinidad[68] reviewed nearly a quarter century of the experience practicing the technique. Their discussion of complications is excellent and is highlighted by discussion of whether to peel any skin that has been undermined for a surgical procedure. They recommended that "6 months elapse before chemosurgery is used as an adjunct to surgical blepharoplasty to avoid ectropion and possible scarring."[69] A somewhat contrary position had been taken by Ariagno and Briggs[3] in 1975 when they proposed a combination procedure whereby two different strengths of phenol were applied to the face following a face and neck lift. "A stronger solution (65% phenol) is applied to the T-

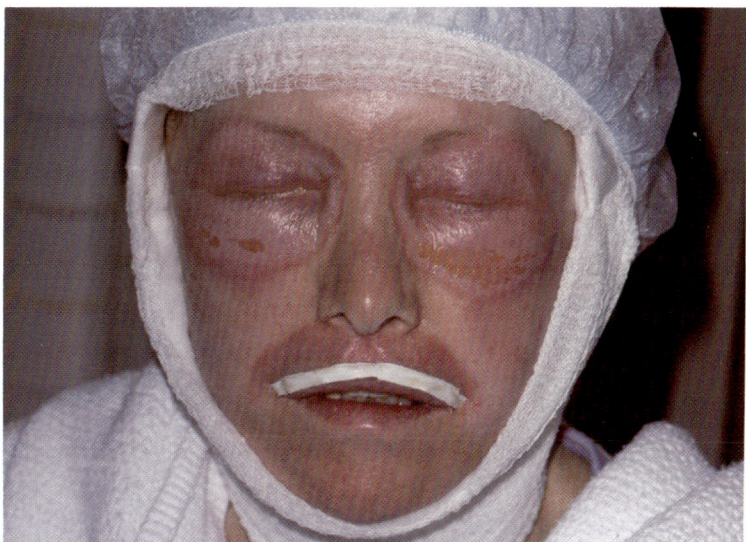

Combining chemical peeling with facial surgery. Areas that have not been undermined in the course of face and neck surgery may be chemically peeled. Here the patient has had a periorbital and upper lip peel performed at the same time as a face and neck lift. Note that the inferior edge of the lip is taped to promote deeper penetration at the vermillion border.

zone. The remainder of the face and neck is blended with a weaker (35% phenol) exfoliant. The undermined or blended areas may or may not be taped. If taped, the tape should be removed from this area within 24 hours." They noted the importance of not taping below the hyoid level citing "a relative paucity of adnexal structures in the reticular layer of the dermis in the neck skin, resulting in the possibility of delayed epithelialization hypertrophic scarring." However, their position stands as a distinct minority view as most current practitioners advise against peeling of skin that has been undermined. Based on several clinical cases that I have seen in consultation, I would strongly advise the novice practitioner not to perform concomitant peeling and either blepharoplasty, forehead and brow lifting, or face and neck lifting. In our practice, the standard interval between the surgery and peeling is 3 months. The consensus in the medical literature is that combining surgical procedures with chemical skin peeling is inadvisable. Spira, Jerow, and Hardy[100] admonished, "Never insult a skin by peeling and undermining the same area simultaneously. These two procedures should be separated by at least 6 to 8 weeks."

In one of the earliest papers on chemical skin peeling, Baker[13] favored an interval between surgery and peeling by stating, "This delay is necessary because the blood supply of the cheek flaps is already embarrassed and to further insult with the chemical burn would be dangerous."

CARDIAC ARRHYTHMIAS

Since phenol is a known cardiac irritant, the issue of potential cardiac arrhythmias must be understood by the practitioner. The proposed scenario under which arrhythmia may develop is discussed in the chapter on anesthesia.

In 1979, Truppman and Ellenby[114] reported that 23% of their patients developed an arrhythmia during peeling. They determined the positive correlation between arrhythmias and the size of the area treated and the duration of the procedure. The average lag time for the onset of arrhythmias was 17½ minutes, by which time over 50% of the area being treated had formula applied. The study included 43 patients. Ten out of 20 patients who had their peel completed in 30 minutes or less developed arrhythmias, including premature ventricular contractions, ventricular tachycardia, bigeminy, and premature atrial tachycardia. No patients in a subgroup of 23 in whom the total peel exceeded 60 minutes developed arrhythmias.

Gross, in his 1984 paper,[51] related the controversy that then arose in the literature. It appeared that the rise in use of cardiac monitoring was matched by a parallel curve of recognition of arrhythmias. A survey by Litton and Trinidad in 1981[69] showed that 13% of the respondents to their survey reported cardiac arrhythmias. Based on his study of 100 consecutive cases, Gross[51] concluded that "cardiac arrhythmia in phenol peeling can be reduced by dividing the face into several units and spacing the application of phenol to each 20 minutes apart." This would appear to confirm the consensus by most practitioners that it is an overload of phenol to the circulatory system manifesting in cardiac irritability that is responsible for the arrhythmias. However, other factors must be considered in terms of the overall physiology of the patient undergoing the procedure. Carbon dioxide levels, which are dependent on the ventilatory state, may also influence cardiac arrhythmia since hypercapnia is known to potentiate myocardial irritability.

To reduce the incidence of arrhythmia, Brody suggests peeling the face in five to eight sequential aesthetic units allowing 10 to 20 minutes between each unit.[27] He adequately hydrates the patient with at least 500 ml of lactated Ringer's solution prior to the procedure and 1000 ml during and after the peel to enhance phenol excretion, allowing 60 to 120 minutes for the entire procedure. He further recommends employing cardiac monitoring, blood pressure checks, and pulse checks with emergency cardiopulmonary resuscitation equipment available. The extent of cutaneous absorption depends more on the total area of skin exposed than on the concentration of solution applied. If arrhythmias occur, the application of phenol should be stopped until normal sinus rhythm has returned for 15 minutes. The procedure may be resumed, extending the peel intervals for an additional 15 minutes.

Here is a case history of the only case of arrhythmia that we have had in our practice in over 200 consecutive cases since converting to general endotracheal anesthesia:

> This patient was a 50-year-old female who weighed 140 pounds, obese, 5 feet 2 inches, heavy cigarette smoker. She had an otherwise normal physical examination except for increased cholesterol level and high triglycerides. During the phenol peel—specifically, during the application to the upper lip at 1 hour and 5 minutes following the initiation of the procedure—the patient developed classic ventricular bigeminy and was observed for approximately 60 seconds, during which time the Forane inhalant anesthetic was reduced. Following the 1 minute observation, the anesthesiologist administered lidocaine 100 mg intravenously, and the patient converted to normal sinus rhythm within 30 seconds. The remaining portion of the face—lower lip and chin area—was treated with the phenol solution in the usual manner with no change. Blood pressure remained stable throughout. This patient had a large face and required a larger amount of phenol solution than usual; at the end of the procedure, almost no solution remained in the treatment glass jar. Our feeling is that this patient may have had borderline cardiac competency and received a larger than usual volume of the phenol solution, although within a normal parameter of time. These two events together may have predisposed to the arrhythmia.

ATROPHY

Depending on the aggressiveness of the procedure (for example, strength of solution, application of occlusive dressings), there may be atrophy of the skin. Thus repeat skin peels are to be avoided or performed in a very conservative manner. Obviously, a thicker-skinned patient will offer greater latitude and will tolerate more procedures.

Brody states that "atrophy or loss of the normal skin markings in the absence of scarring may occur after multiple deep peelings with phenol but has not been seen usually after superficial or medium depth peeling involving multiple applications of trichloroacetic acid."[27]

SCARRING

Scarring remains the most feared complication of chemical skin peeling. Unquestionably, its development is related to the depth of dermal injury produced by the chemexfoliative process. As Ayres[8] stated, "There is no positive assurance in any case that scars will not occur, but by erring on the side of conservatism and reducing the concentration of cauterant used, the likelihood is minimized." Therefore, it is most likely to occur in areas where more potent solutions have been generously applied and where the skin has been occluded. Intercurrent infection, which deepens the level of tissue injury, will predispose to such scarring.

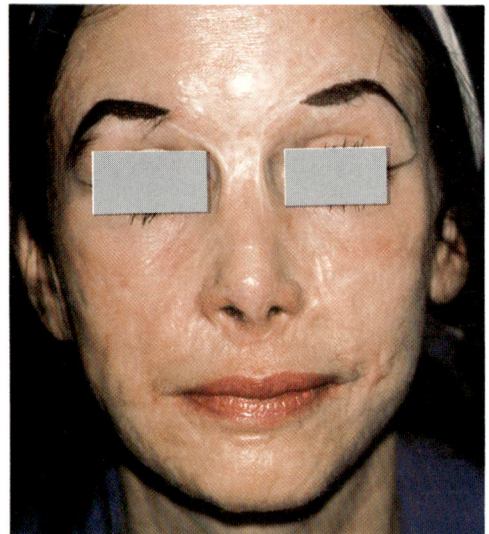 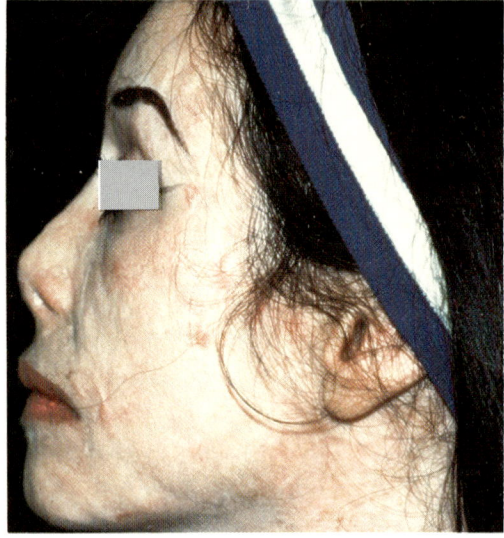

Scarring. This patient exhibits diffuse scarring subsequent to a chemical peel performed by a lay practitioner. The patient reported that occlusive dressings were left in place for 7 days after the procedure. The peeling agent is unknown.

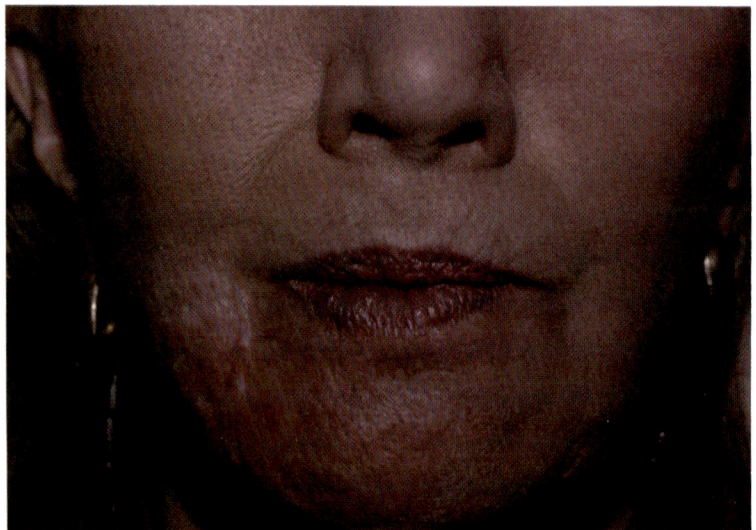

Scarring. This patient had several peels performed on the same area of the lip and chin within a short period of time by another physician, with resultant scarring. Whether infection intervened is uncertain, but the patient reported that the "right chin area had pus on it for a long period of time."

It has been observed by several experienced practitioners that scarring almost always occurs in the lower third of the face. When it does occur, it usually occurs in the perioral or mandibular region.[34] Perhaps this is related to the greater amount of tissue movement during eating and speaking. My observation has been that patients whose mouths habitually widen greatly during speaking or who gesticulate with very broad lip and mouth movements have more prolonged posttreatment perioral stiffness and edema. Lober[70] noted that "whether we elect trichloroacetic acid or phenol mixtures, there are certain complications inherent in chemexfoliation of the skin including hypertrophic scarring and keloid formation, particularly in the perioral area near the mandible." Ayres[8] noted that "the neck and beneath the chin are the areas most prone to this."

Brody[27] states that:

"Previous peels, previous dermabrasions, and previous isotretinoin (Accutane)* usage may be risk factors for scarring. Reasonable time intervals between repeat superficial, medium depth, and phenol peels are difficult to ascertain and are variable; superficial epidermal peeling is sometimes done on a weekly basis or certainly on a monthly basis without difficulty. Some feel that when postphenol erythema is clinically involved, peels can be performed again to achieve cumulative results.

"The interval between termination of isotretinoin treatment and dermabrasion is at least 6 months. With deeper peels, this interval would be warranted at minimum.

"The fact that some individuals scar while others do not may be the result of a mild variant of the Ehlers-Danlos syndrome, mitis form, which may have been overlooked in the patient and may be present in as high as 9% of the population. Scoring the patient based on joint hypermobility, increased skin extensibility, abnormal spreading scars, and easy bruisability may be helpful."

The incidence of hypertrophic scarring can be reduced to nearly zero if early warning signs such as persistent induration, edema, and redness of skin are aggressively treated, particularly with topical steroids. Lober[70] cited Gross and Maschek's[52] paper which stated, "Any area ... with a persistent erythema darker than the surrounding areas is considered suspect and is treated with topical corticosteroids and systemic antibiotics." A high potency topical steroid, Diprolene, is extremely effective in reversal of that persistent induration and edema that may predispose to scarring. The medication must be used twice daily for a period of 2 weeks, at which time the patient is reevaluated. I have used it "prophylactically" in those patients who appeared to be at higher risk for scarring, as manifested by persistent redness and induration of the tissues, as per Gross and Maschek's admonition. Whether or not any of

---

*Roche Laboratories, Nutley, NJ.

these patients would have necessarily gone on to develop hypertrophic scars is uncertain, but the treatment has been successful in early resolution of those prognostically unfavorable findings. Should such scarring actually manifest, intralesional steroids should immediately be injected and reinjected until the scar has disappeared. My preference is triamcinolone 20 mg/ml. Surgical excision and repair are less favorable modalities and should be reserved for circumstances that fail to respond to more conservative treatment.

Stegman, Tromovitch, and Glogau[109] concur in their approach:

> "We treat scars with time, support, and intralesional triamcinolone acetonide 5-20 mg/ml every three weeks. If, when we see patients three weeks post-operatively, we detect areas of slow healing or areas still scabbed, we will start them on strong topical steroids twice daily. Often this will prevent true scarring. If not, we switch to intralesional steroids at the first sign of true scar development. Early prevention and treatment greatly shorten the time it takes for the scar to mature and nearly dissolve. Most of the time, these scars will almost completely resorb. For these early scars, triamcinolone acetonide 40 mg/ml is too strong and may cause atrophy or will deposit out as small, milia-like droplets."

Asken[7] would appear to concur when he states that "persistent erythema may be a warning sign, and these areas should be treated with topical steroids or with Cordran* tape."

The two patients in my experience who developed perioral hypertrophic scars had both failed to report for routine posttreatment evaluation. Had they been seen as I would have preferred, perhaps early intervention could have prevented frank scar formation.

*3M, St. Paul, MN.

Case Presentations: Scarring

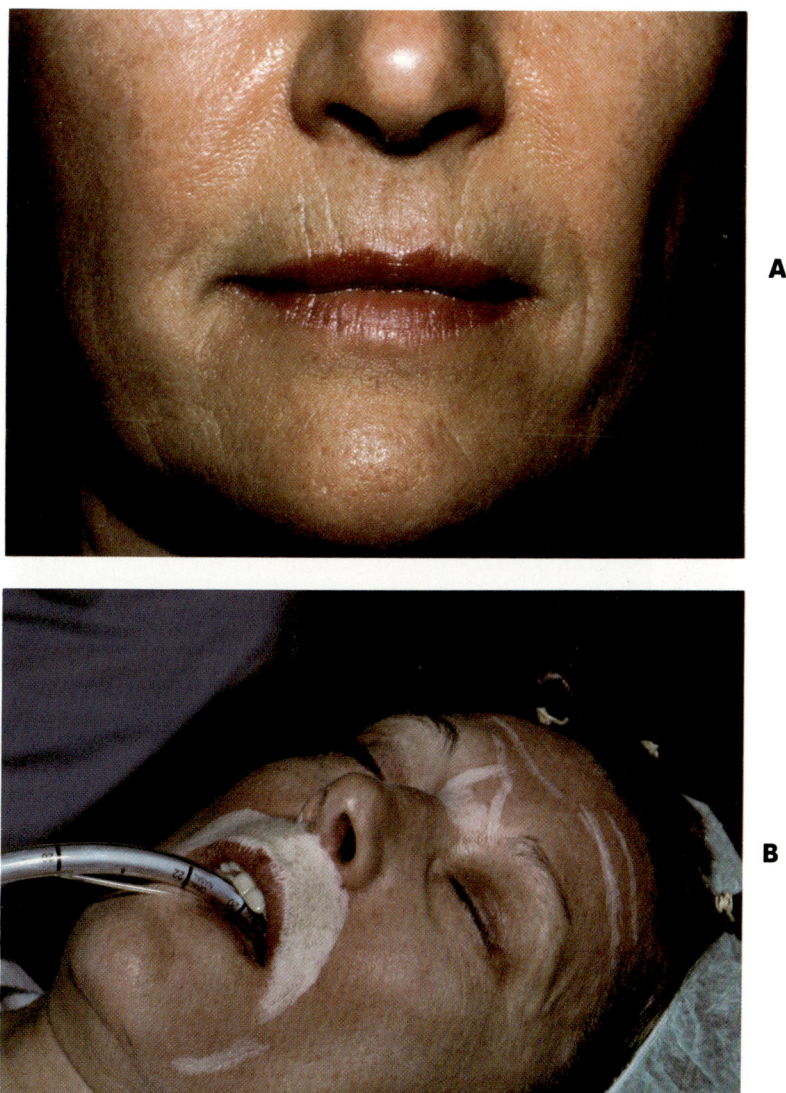

Case 1: Scarring of the upper lip. This patient received a standard full-face Baker formula phenol peel with pretreatment application of 50% TCA and occlusion to the upper lip. **A,** Pretreatment view. **B,** Application of 50% TCA to deepest wrinkles.

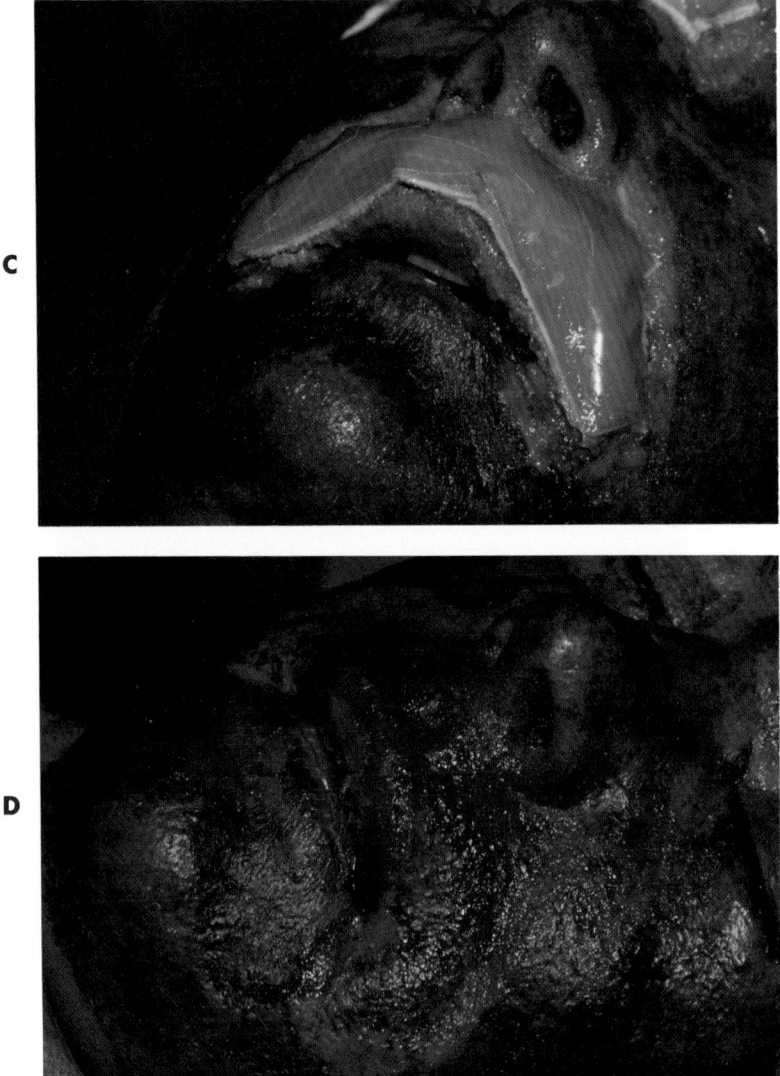

Case 1, cont'd. C and **D,** Two days after the peel procedure, the tapes were removed from the upper lip and the area was abraded with 4 × 4 sterile gauze pads to remove necrotic debris and conceivably enhance the effects of the peel. In retrospect, this probably represented overaggressive technique. **E,** Delayed healing of the upper lip contrasted with the surrounding face, a harbinger of difficulties to come. **F,** At 30 days after peel, persistent redness and induration to the touch suggested possible incipient hypertrophic scar formation, and betamethasone (Diprolene) topical steroid treatment was begun. **G,** At 45 days post peel, injection with triamcinolone, 20 mg/ml administered intralesionally, was initiated on a fortnightly basis. Patient is shown here 4 weeks after the first triamcinolone injection.

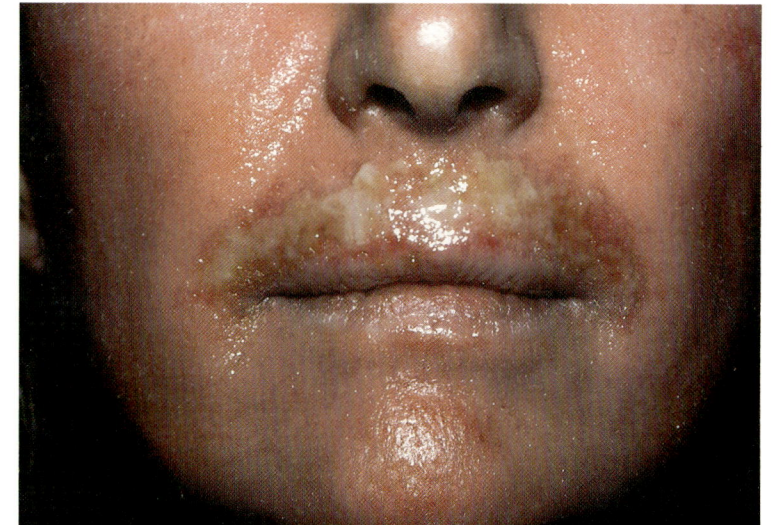

E

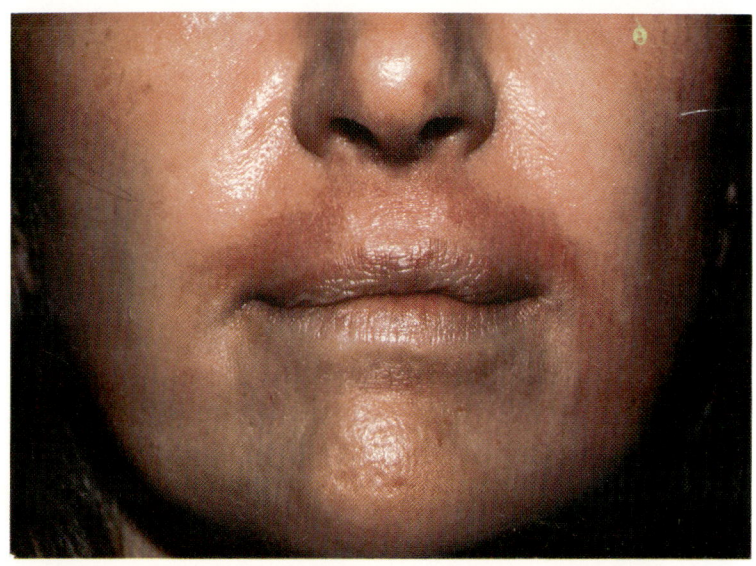

F

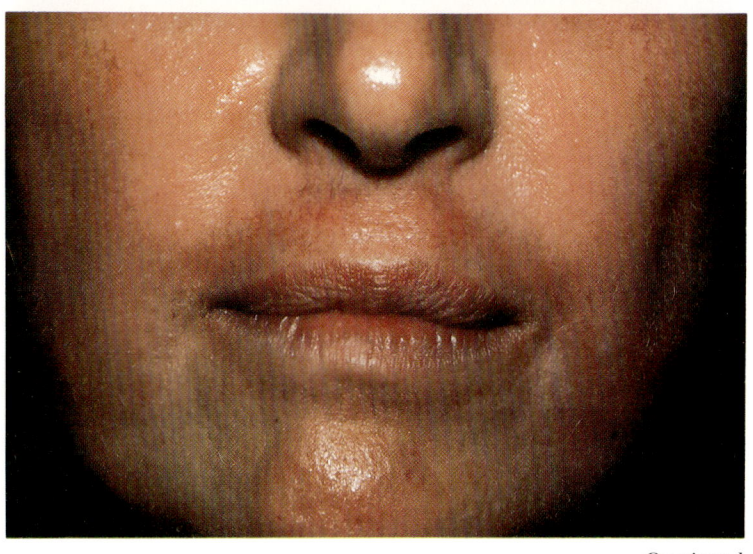

G

Continued.

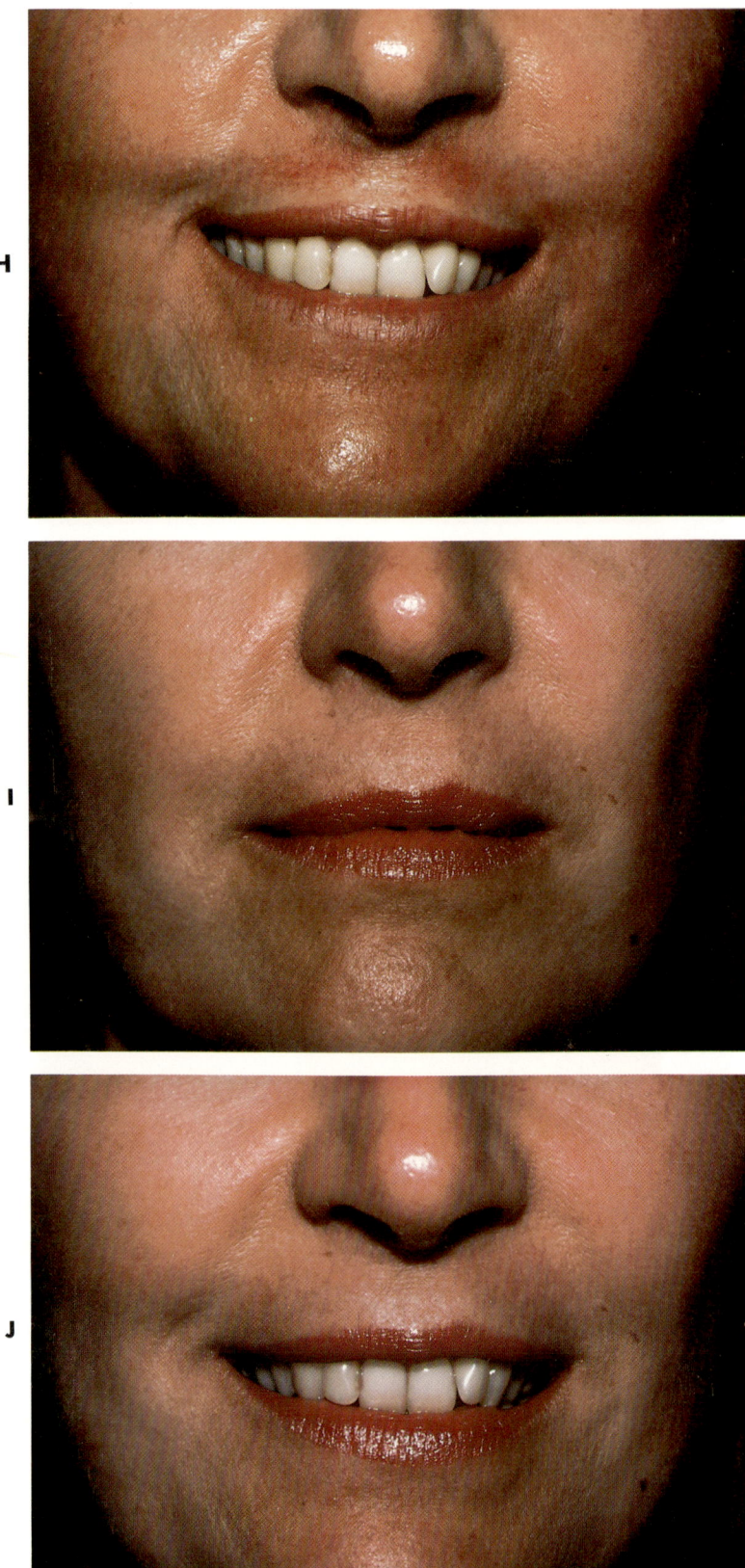

Case 1, cont'd. H, Note the "tight" appearance of the upper lip with smiling. **I** and **J,** Satisfactory resolution of the problem has been achieved. At 180 days after peel the area has taken on a normal appearance and the tightness of the upper lip upon smiling has abated.

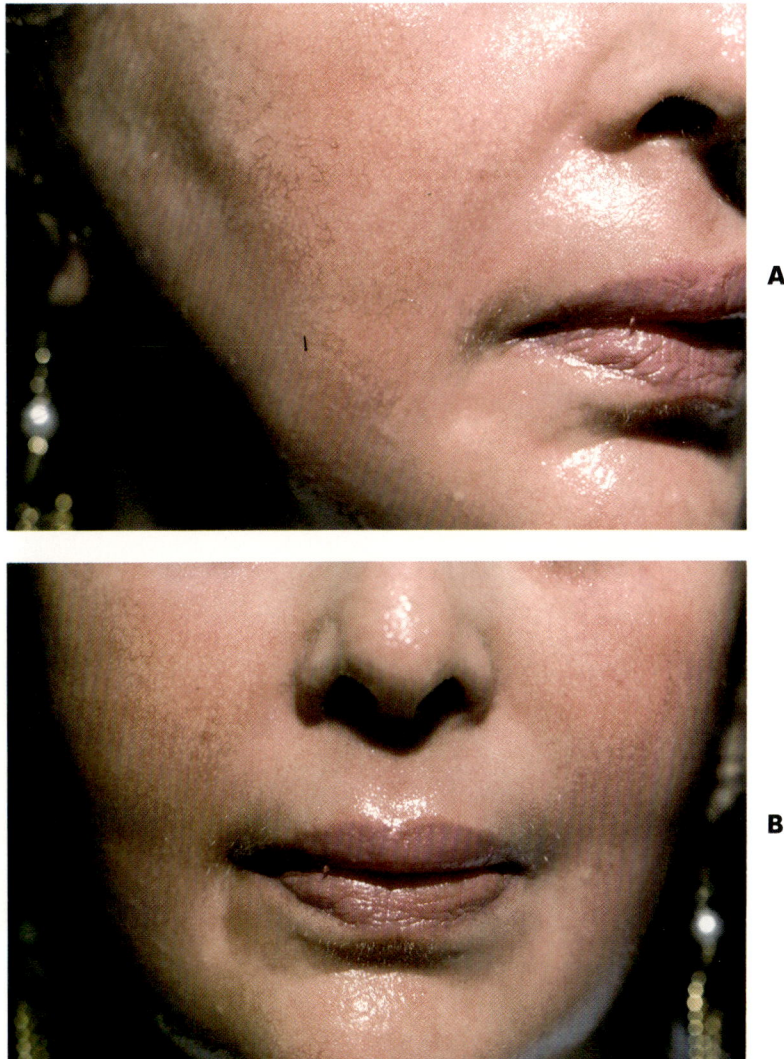

Case 2: Hypertrophic scarring. This patient was treated with a chemical peel, including an aggressive taping technique around the mouth. Immediately after the procedure there were no areas of distinction or particular concern, and the appearance of the taped area 21 days after peel shows no evidence of unusual erythema or any other predictors of problems. The patient lived in a distant community, however, and did not return for all routine follow-up care as recommended.

Continued.

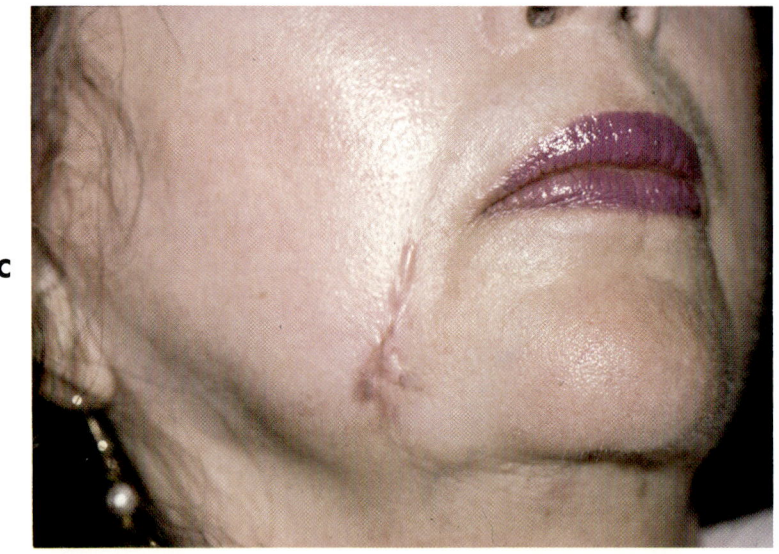

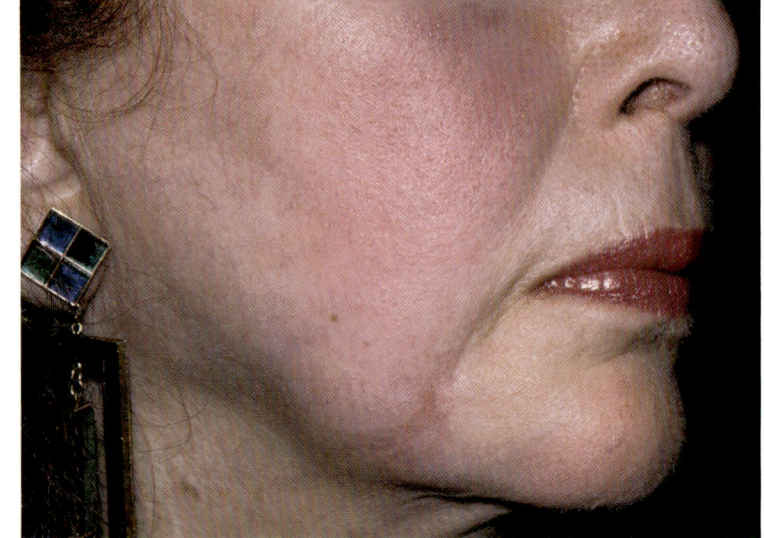

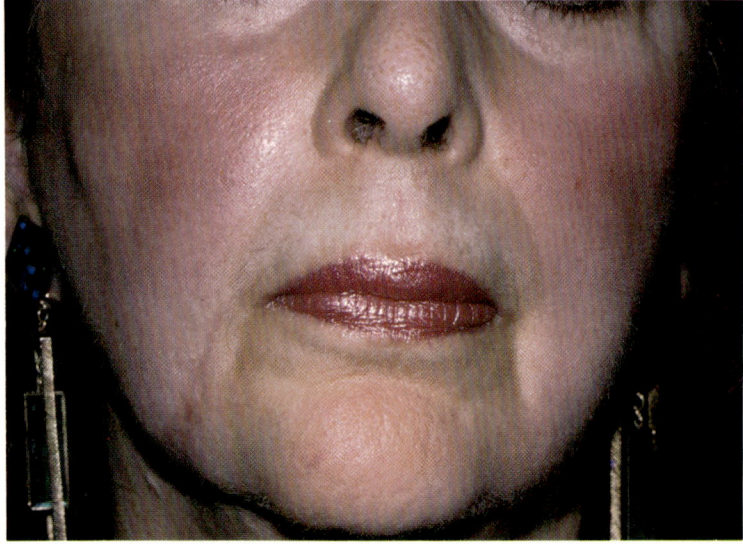

Case 2, cont'd. C, At 270 days after peel, hypertrophic scarring of the right mandibular and perioral area had developed. The upper portion of the scar was excised surgically and the lower portion treated with a series of steroid injections. **D and E,** At 300 days after peel the scar's appearance was considerably lessened and the area exhibited a pink color. The patient later reported that the color had abated, and the appearance of the area was very satisfactory, requiring no further treatment.

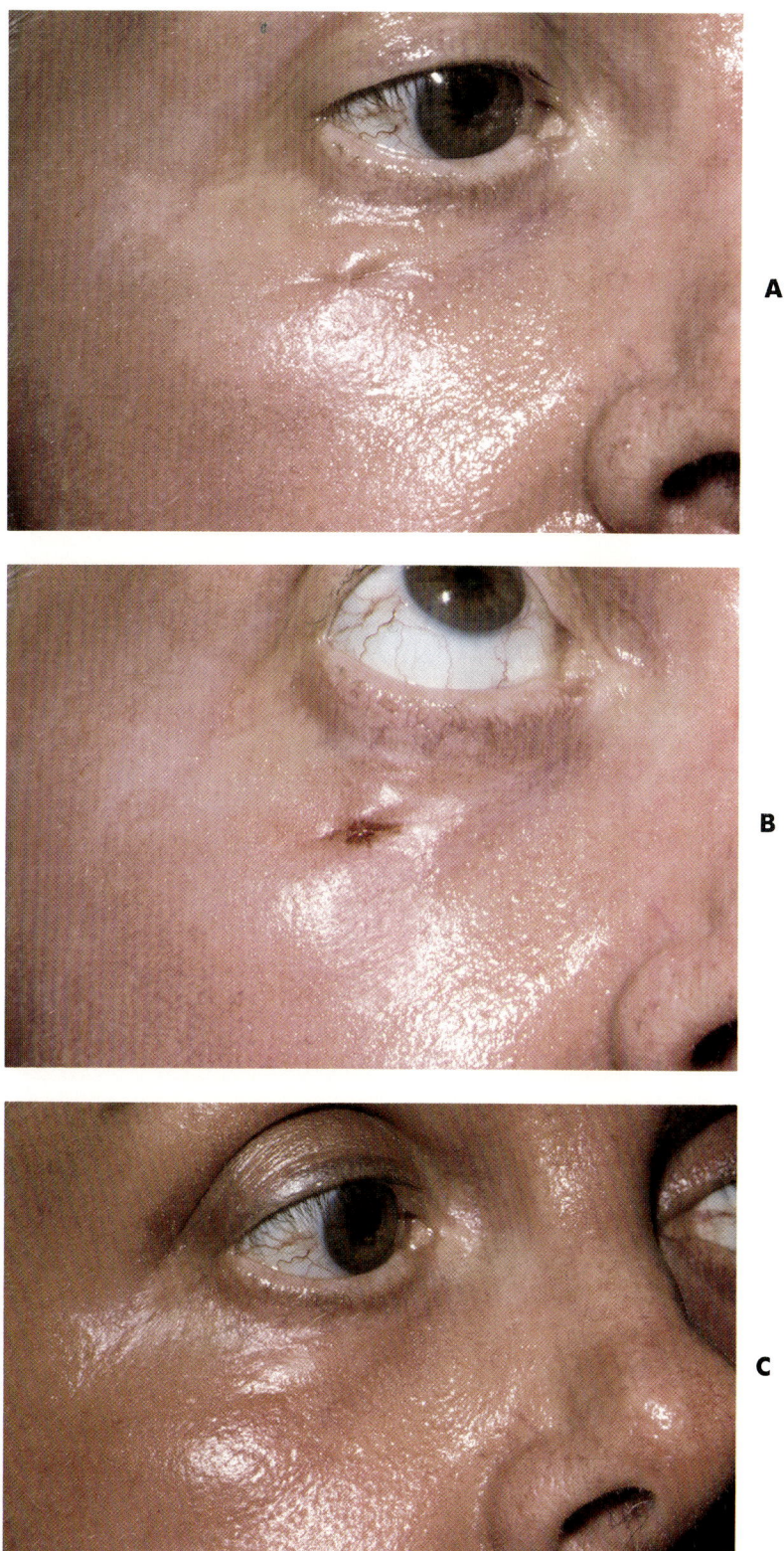

Case 3: Unusual scarring. A, An unusual pleatlike crease developed over the right malar eminence in this patient within the first 10 days after a Baker formula phenol chemical peel that included tape occlusion. It appeared that the tape had caused the skin to "roll over" on itself. **B,** The skin above the scar was retracted upward and the skin below retracted downward, undoing the pleat. **C,** The appearance 14 days later shows successful resolution of the problem.

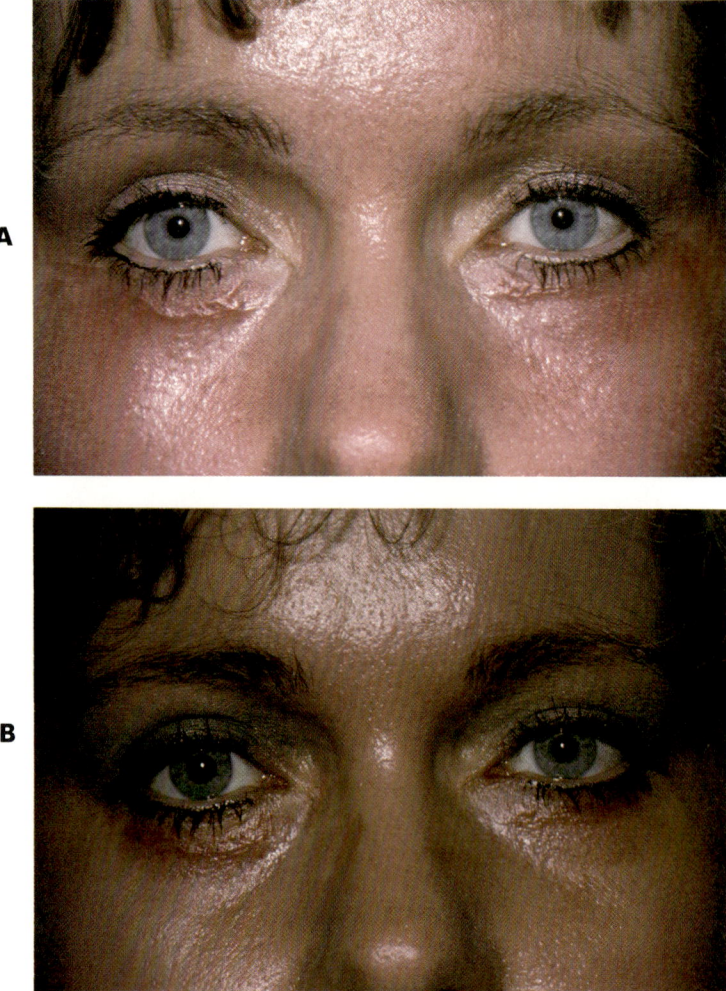

Case 4: Unanticipated hypertrophic scarring. A, Unanticipated hypertrophic scarring of the medial aspect of the lower lids developed in this patient. Although her Baker formula chemical peel included occlusive taping over the crow's-feet area, no tapes were applied to the area of the lower lids where these scars appeared. **B,** Topical steroid therapy with betamethasone (Diprolene) cream was begun upon first appearance of the scars, with improvement becoming evident after 30 days of treatment.

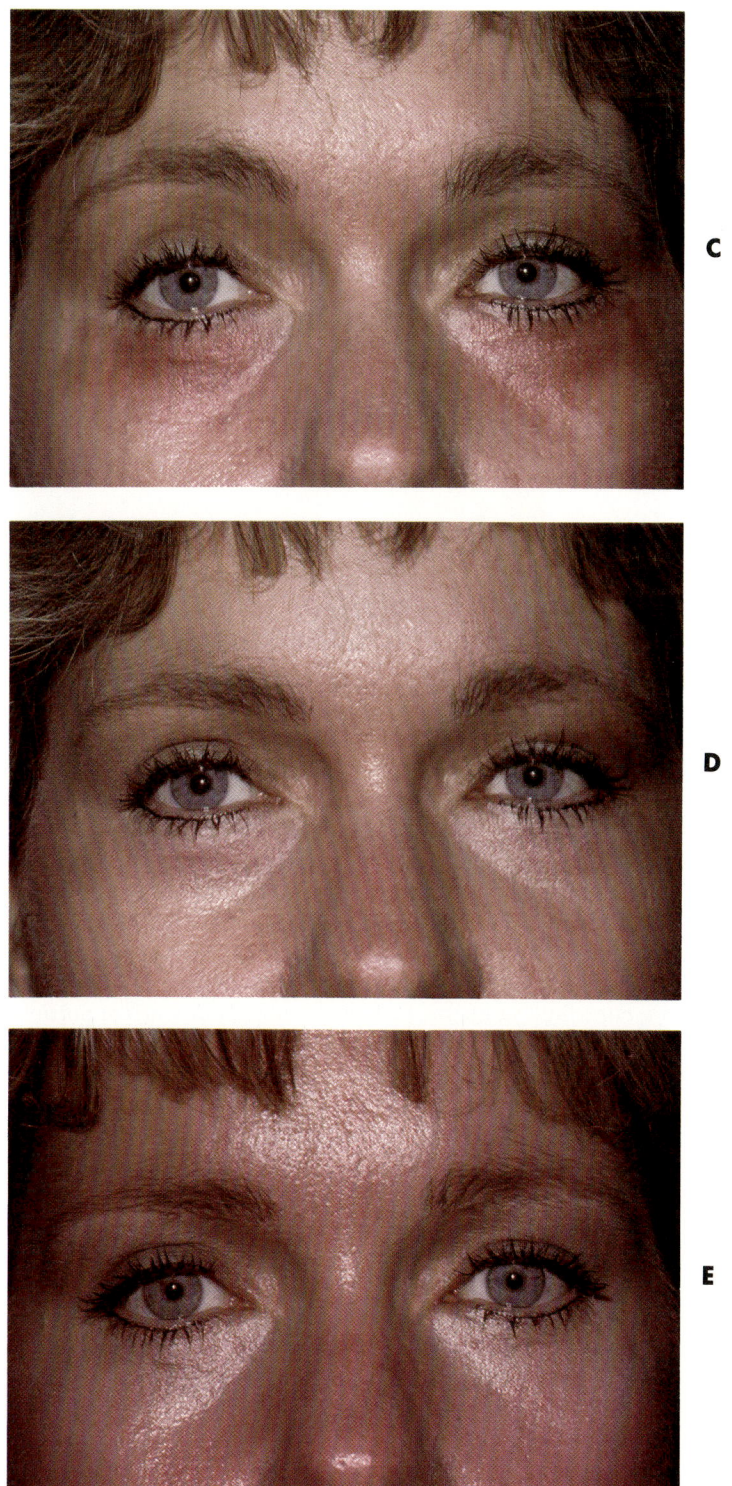

Case 4, cont'd. C and **D**, At 120 days after the development of the scars their appearance without makeup was satisfactory and with makeup excellent camouflage was achieved. (The ability to camouflage a problem is very important to bolster the patient's morale while the complication is being resolved.) **E**, The outcome 240 days after the development of the scars was excellent.

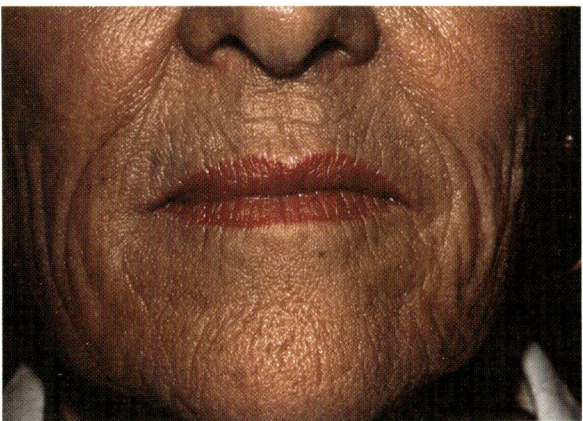

Case 5: Complications of an aggressive technique. This case illustrates the hazards the practitioner must accept in performing very aggressive peeling. Hypertrophic scarring developed in the perioral area, as well as temporary ectropion of the left lower lid. The latter resolved promptly without treatment, but the scars required treatment with steroid injections. The apparent predilection for scarring in the perioral area suggests movement of the lips, chin, and mandible as a possible cause. In my experience, this site appears to develop more problems than any other on the face. I would advise the beginning practitioner to be conservative, particularly with those patients who gesticulate actively while speaking. Because this particular patient did not live in our city, her postpeel follow-up care was not ideal, and the lack of frequent observation and early intervention must be considered a contributing factor. For this reason I am wary of performing very aggressive skin peels on patients who do not live in the area and who are unwilling to come for the standardized program of follow-up visits and regular observation. This patient underwent the most aggressive type of skin peel, which certainly must also be implicated as a potential cause of the resulting problems. The use of a phenol-based peeling solution with a Salonpas occlusive mask represents our most effective technique for treating the very deep and craggy wrinkles that this patient demonstrated; nonetheless, aggressive techniques always carry a higher risk of complications. Each practitioner must develop a comfort level with the procedures he or she performs. Through experience an "acceptable complication ratio" evolves that is unique to each practitioner. If one seeks to remove all wrinkles on the face, including the very deepest ones, then one must accept the increased risks. Of course, one must consider the issue of patient reliability and compliance, which I believe was a significant factor in the development of this particular patient's complications.

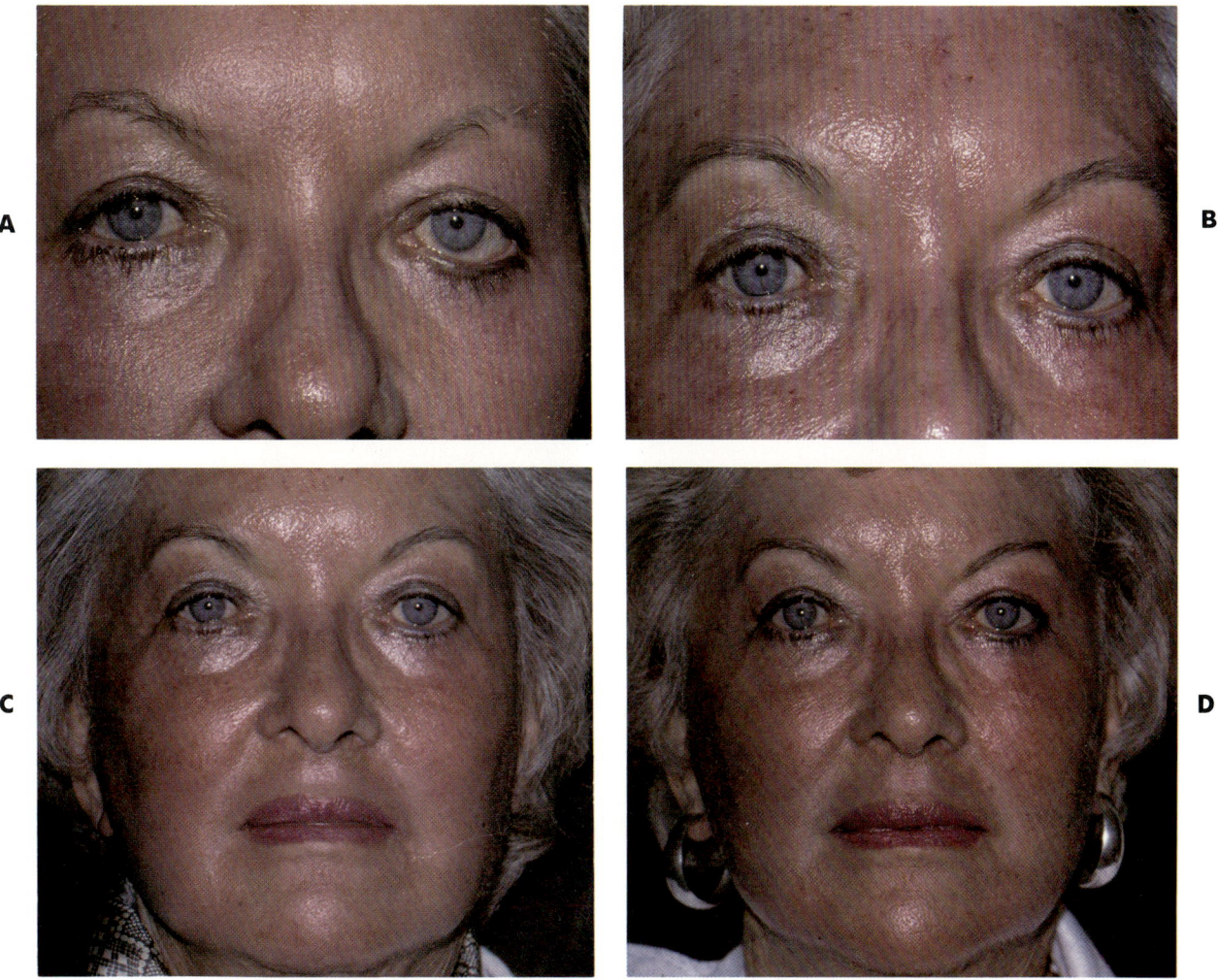

Case 5: cont'd. The patient is seen here 4 weeks after treatment with a maximum technique Baker formula phenol peel, including Salonpas tape occlusion of the upper and lower lip, chin, and anterior portion of the cheeks. **A,** Ectropion of the left lower lid developed despite the fact that no tape had been applied to the lower lids. Frequently this is related to edema of the tissues inasmuch as the ectropion disappears when the patient is in a supine position, and hence conservatism is advised. **B** and **C,** Two months after peel the condition had spontaneously improved and all looked well. **D,** At 4 months after peel persistent redness of the right anterior mandibular area became apparent. In retrospect, this was a harbinger of problems to come.

Continued.

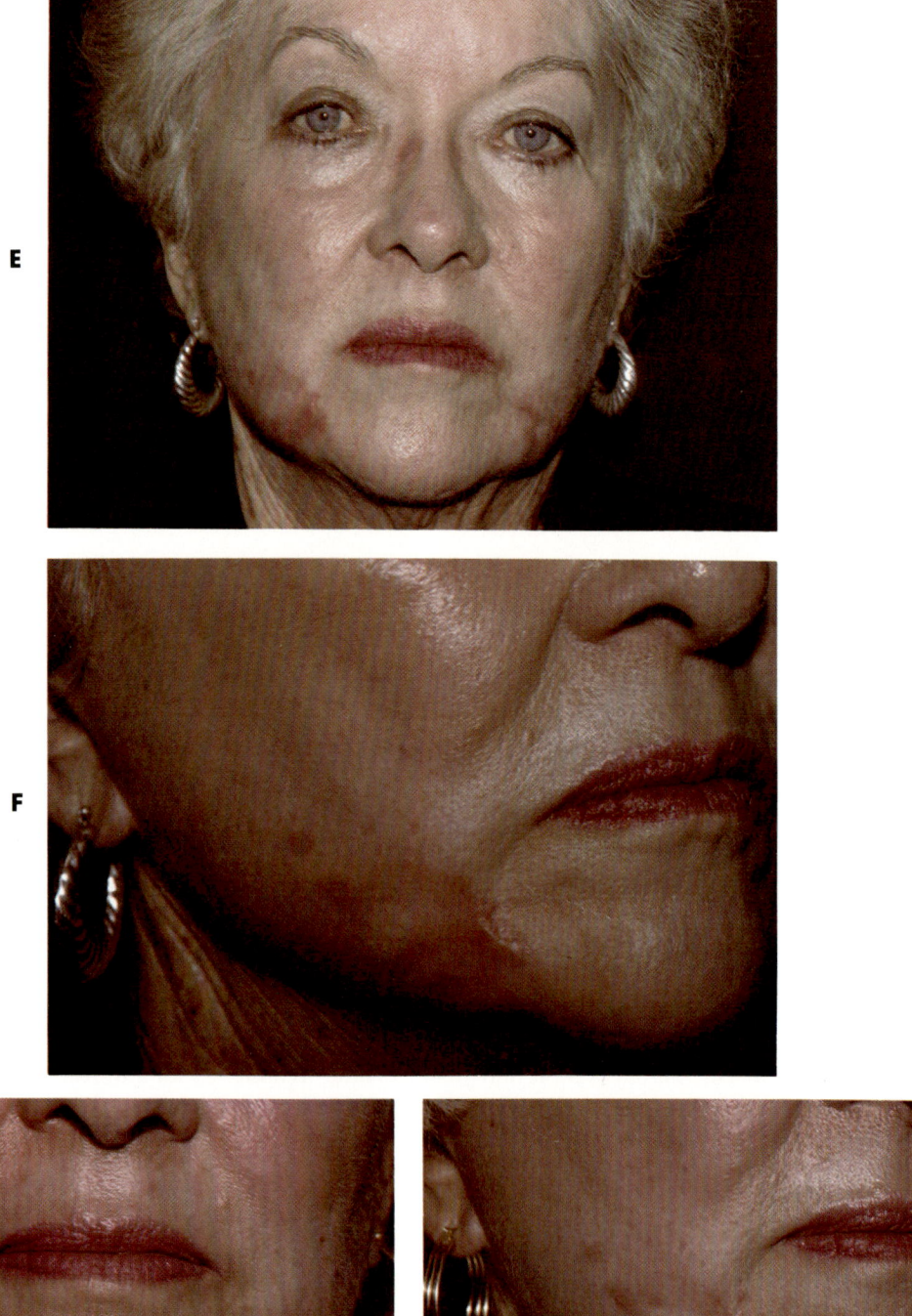

Case 5, cont'd. E and **F,** Eight months after peel the patient showed hypertrophic scarring of both anterior mandibular areas. She had failed to follow the routine postpeel visit schedule; had she sought attention earlier, this complication most likely could have been avoided. **G** and **H,** Appearance of the scars 60 days later after two treatments with steroid injections shows some improvement, but additional treatments to the anterior aspects of the right scar were indicated.

TEXTURE CHANGE

Not uncommonly, I have observed that within the first several weeks following rejuvenation, the skin appears to have a thickened, grainy, almost pigskinlike appearance, particularly in the areas where the skin is normally thicker, such as the midforehead and cheek area. Stegman, Tromovitch, and Glogau[109] considered this an uncommon complication, describing it as a "grainy, porous effect." Speculation as to the morphologic entity has included some temporary thickening of the stratum corneum.

In my experience, this has always been temporary, although when first encountered was quite disconcerting to the patient and physician. Patients become disturbed because they expect the new skin to be "smooth and fresh," as we promised them. Typically, this grainy texture occurs in the second or third week following the procedure and will abate within the same period of time, even if not treated. In those patients who demand that "something be done," we have prescribed Lacticare HC, which is a mild lactic acid and hydrocortisone preparation that acts as an exfoliant and antiinflammatory.* Since it appears that temporary thickening of the stratum corneum is responsible for the phenomenon, the lactic acid acts as a further mild peeling agent to promote reestablishment of a more normal-looking skin surface. This has proved to be reliable and effective in reversing this "coarseness" of the skin, as the patients refer to it.

The patients shown here both illustrate a salutary end result following no treatment.

*Upon the recommendation of dermatologist Jeffrey Marmelzat, M.D.

Case Presentations: Texture Change

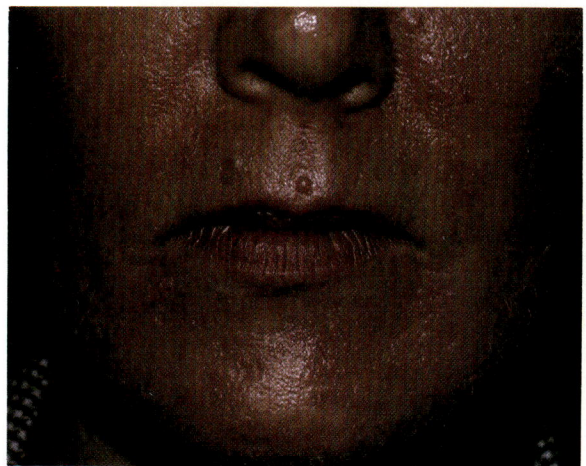
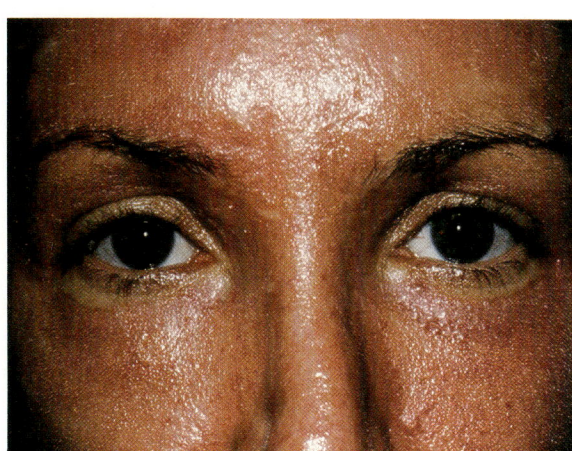

Case 1: Texture change—granular skin. A to C, This patient's skin had a grainy, pigskin-like appearance 21 days after an unoccluded Baker formula phenol peel performed elsewhere. (Note that the operator did not peel up to the lash margin, a technical error that is quite obvious to both the patient and the observer.) In my experience the grainy texture seen here almost always abates with conservative management; therefore no medical or surgical intervention was recommended and the patient was reassured that the condition would spontaneously improve.

Continued.

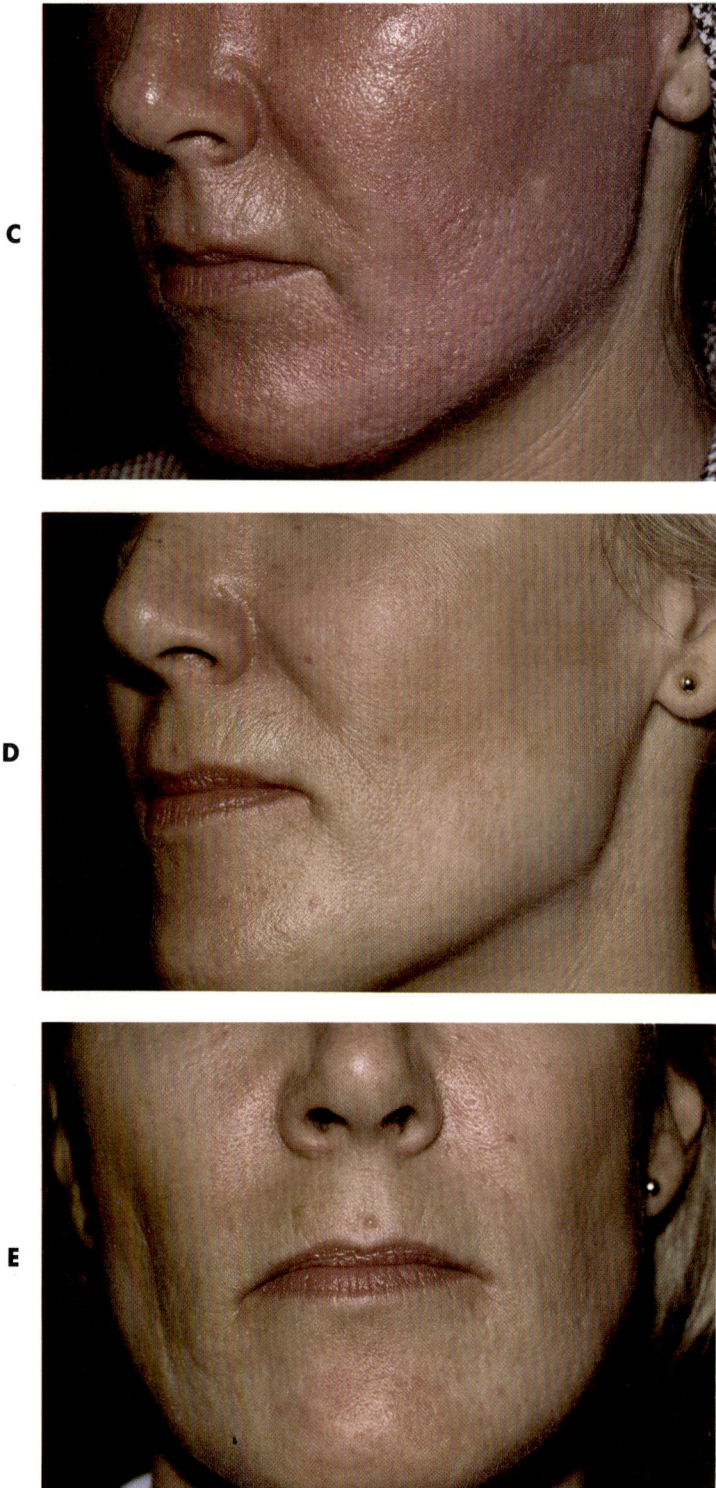

Case 1, cont'd. D and **E,** Views 420 days later show a reasonably satisfactory result with this conservative approach.

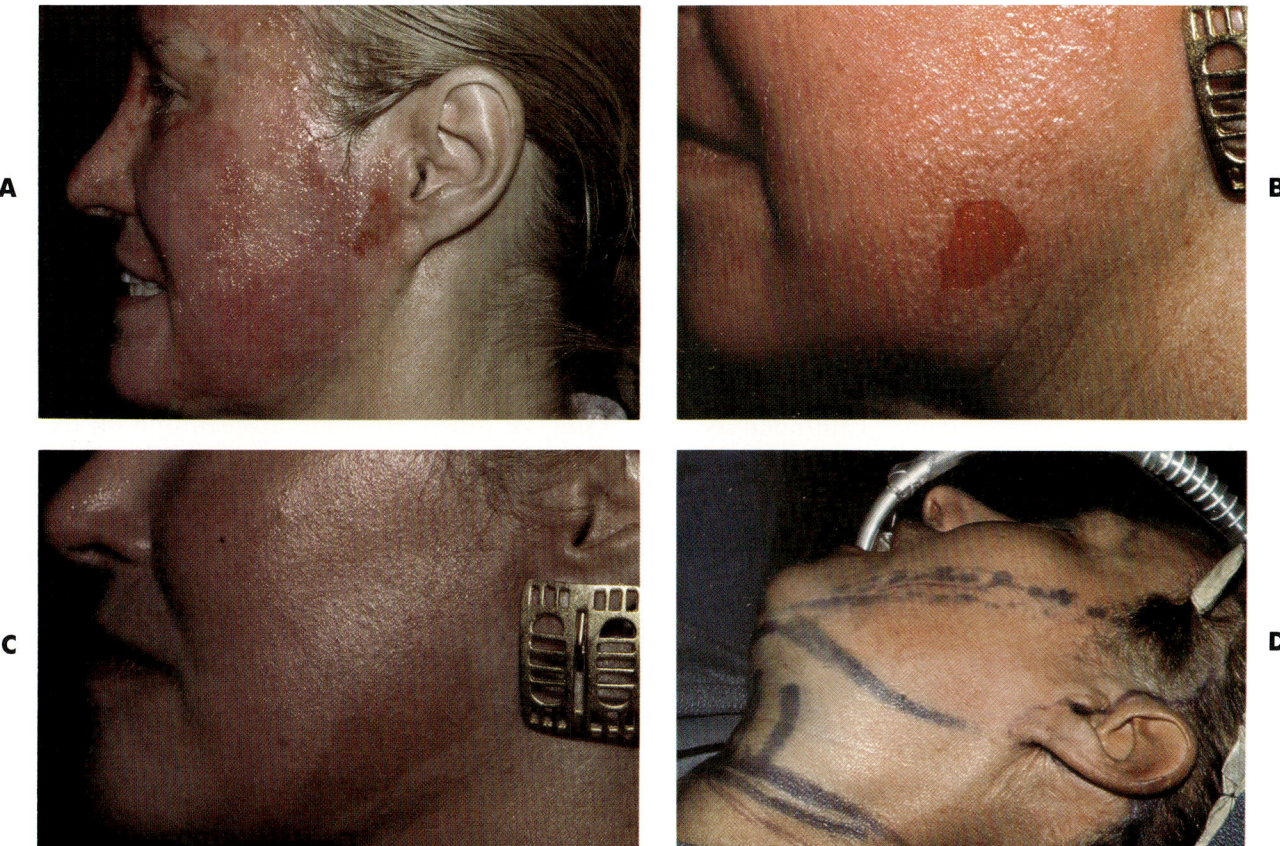

**Case 2: Delayed healing following factitious removal of hyperkeratotic skin.
A,** This ideal candidate's appearance was not unusual 1 week after skin peeling with Baker formula (no occlusion of cheeks). **B,** Ten days later, granular-appearing skin surrounded an area of the midmandible where she had manually removed a split-thickness portion of the temporarily hyperkeratotic skin. **C,** Thirty days later, with conservative management, the area had healed well but some postinflammatory hyperpigmentation was beginning. This abated with the use of the Kligman bleach cream. **D,** The view 2 months later shows the patient about to have face and neck lift performed; note that the postinflammatory hyperpigmentation has completely disappeared.

PIGMENTATION CHANGE/DEMARCATION LINE

It must be accepted that with more aggressive peel procedures there will be some change in the skin color, with hypopigmentation being most uncommon. Less commonly, some patients, deemed to be the ideal candidates with no evidence of predisposition to increased pigmentation, may develop focal or diffuse hyperpigmentation. Sam Stegman stated it well when he said, "The only thing which can be stated with certainty about color changes in chemical skin peeling is that there will be some." *
Lotter[72] studied pigmentation factors in skin peeling. She noted that certain drug classes such as the phenothiazines and psoralens, the latter particularly in conjunction with ultraviolet light, might induce increased pigment formation. Hormones known to affect pigmentation in humans are the pituitary melanocyte-stimulating hormones, adrenocorticotropic hormones, and, to a lesser degree, the male and female gonadal hormones and thyroid hormones. All these are capable of producing generalized hyperpigmentation through stimulation of melanogenesis. She further cautioned as to the effect of ultraviolet light and trauma on the skin.

Hyperpigmentation can manifest extremely early, even within the first 2 weeks of the procedure being performed. Usually, but not necessarily, the gradation in color change is related to the aggressiveness of the procedure.

At the first signs of increased pigment formation in the skin, the areas may be treated with topical steroids and/or topical bleaching agents such as hydroquinone. Our preference is to use a bleach cream compounded as follows:

> Retinoic acid 0.1% cream
> Hydroquinone 4%.
> Triamcinolone 0.1% cream or
>   hydrocortisone 2.5% cream

Each of the ingredients being combined is used in equal amounts (for example, 15 g, 15 g, and 15 g, to total 45 g). This formula for depigmenting skin was first devised by Kligman and Willis[60] in 1975. This triple-ingredient prescription is used for cases that defy the most conservative treatment. Obviously, sun exposure may precipitate development of hyperpigmentation, and therefore a nonsensitizing sun screen or sun block should be an essential ingredient in postpeel skin care. It is of the utmost importance that patients be aware of the hazards of sun exposure in the early posttreatment state, particularly during the summer months when sun intensity is strongest.

Patients whose skin has been particularly darkened and weathered by sun exposure will most often demonstrate a significant line of demarcation between the treated area of the face and untreated area of the neck. This disparity in color will be most noticeable when the patient's habitus is such that there does not exist a strong cervicomental angle whose shadow will conceal the line of demarcation. We are evaluating

---
*Personal communication.

the efficacy of TCA to "soften" the zone of transition; a band of 50% TCA is applied at the inframandibular line to create a transition between phenol-treated face skin and untreated neck skin.

Should one choose to peel the neck, the same dilemma of a line of demarcation at the cervical-thoracic junction exists. This line of demarcation may be even more difficult to conceal than that between the face and the neck. Therefore patients who usually cannot apply or will not consider applying cosmetics should be strongly advised against having the procedure performed.

Case Presentations: Pigmentation Changes

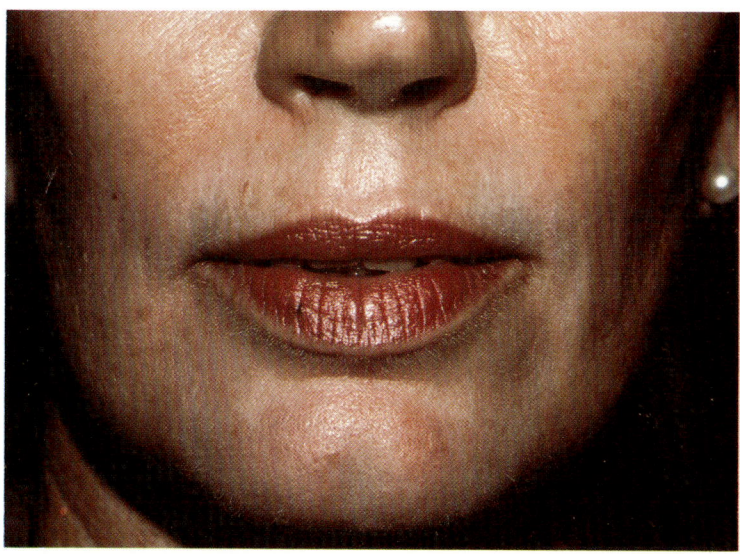

Case 1: Irregular pigmentation. This patient showed an irregular loss of pigmentation in the perioral area secondary to a phenol peel performed elsewhere. One would suspect uneven application of the peeling solution to be the cause.

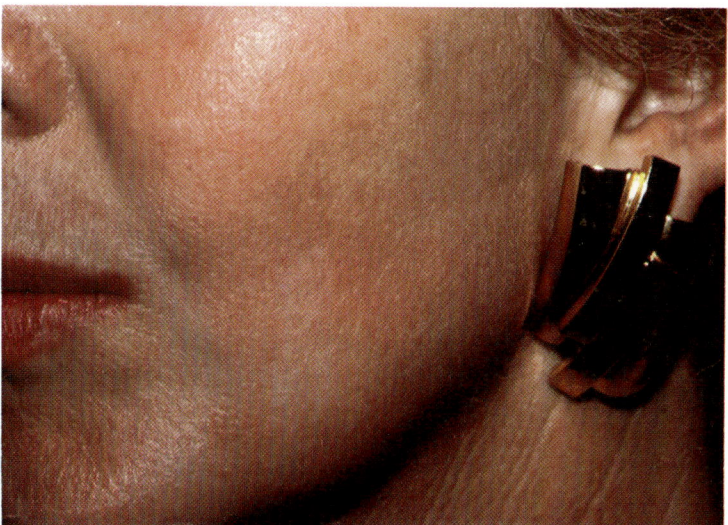

Case 2: Irregular pigmentation. This patient also showed an irregular loss of pigmentation, in this case in the midmandibular area.

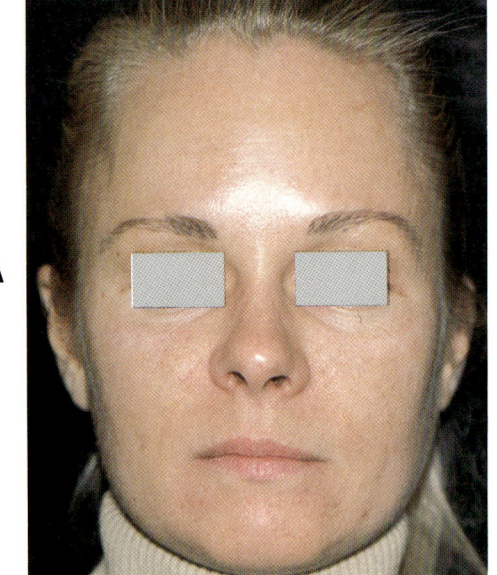
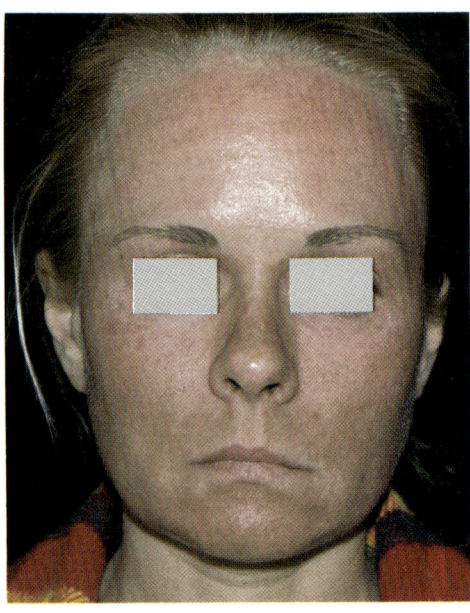

Case 3: Unanticipated postinflammatory hyperpigmentation. A, Because of the patient's fair complexion and pale blue eyes, one would expect her to be the least likely candidate for the development of postinflammatory hyperpigmentation, yet it occurred. **B,** The posttreatment view 35 weeks after the peeling procedure shows development of completely unforeseen postinflammatory hyperpigmentation. Unoccluded Baker formula.

Case 4: Postinflammatory hyperpigmentation—early intervention. This case demonstrates the merits of early intervention upon recognition of postinflammatory hyperpigmentation. **A,** Pretreatment view. **B,** Although this fair-skinned, blue-eyed patient was an unlikely candidate, hyperpigmentation occurred 8 weeks after her partially occluded Baker formula phenol peel. She was treated promptly with Kligman formula bleach cream with excellent results. This formula has been indispensable in the practice of chemical skin peeling. This case demonstrates the unpredictability of pigmentation. **C and D,** The patient's hyperpigmentation occurred diffusely in both areas that had been occluded (lower eyelids) and those that had not (cheeks). Note that the forehead, despite having been occluded, did not develop significant hyperpigmentation. Because unoccluded areas pigmented with the same degree of intensity as occluded areas after the peel, the presumably deeper penetration and stronger inflammatory response elicited by occlusion cannot be implicated exclusively. One wonders whether the patient may have sustained inadvertent sun exposure to the face after the procedure, inasmuch as her hair is styled in a manner that partially hides the forehead. Patients should be strongly cautioned against sun exposure for the first 2 to 3 months after a skin peel and should be encouraged to use hypoallergenic sunscreen products. The patient's use of her own brand of cosmetics, contrary to our advice to limit cosmetics to a recommended hypoallergenic brand with which we have had excellent results, also may have played a role. **E and F,** Three months later.

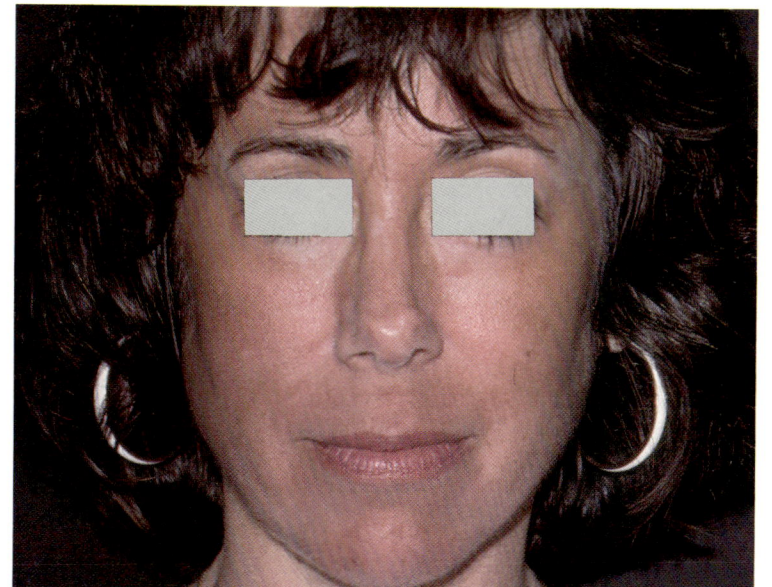

A

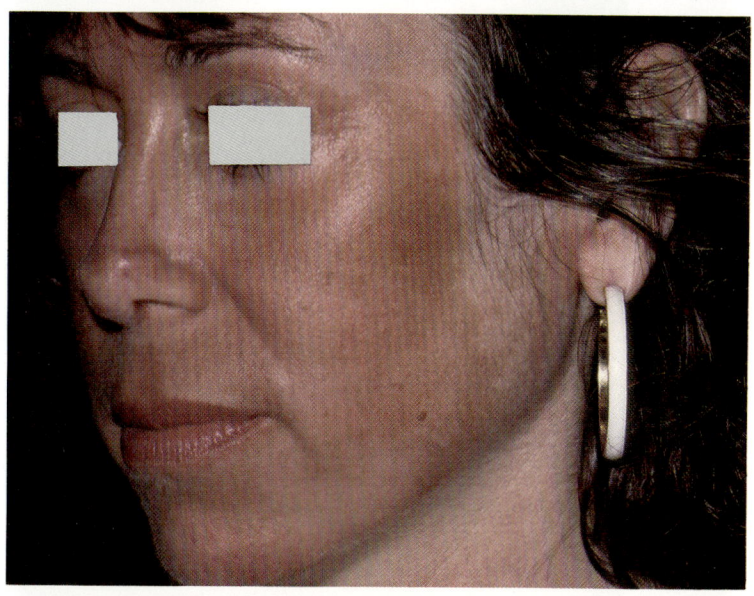

B

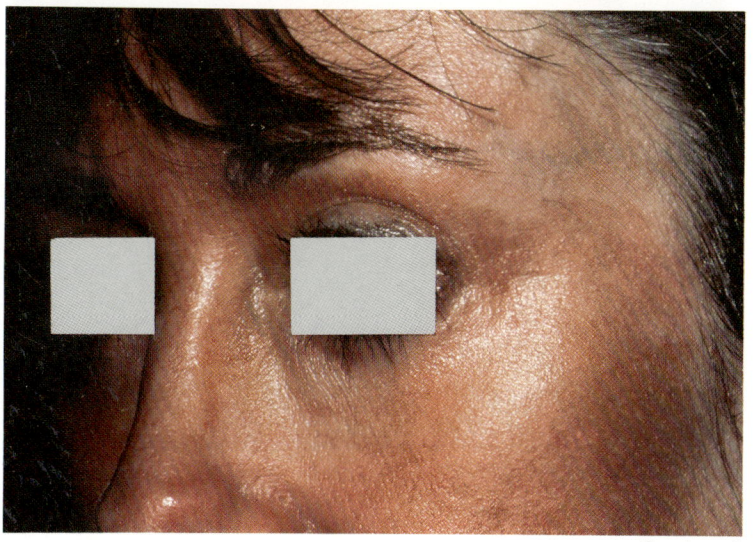

C

Continued.

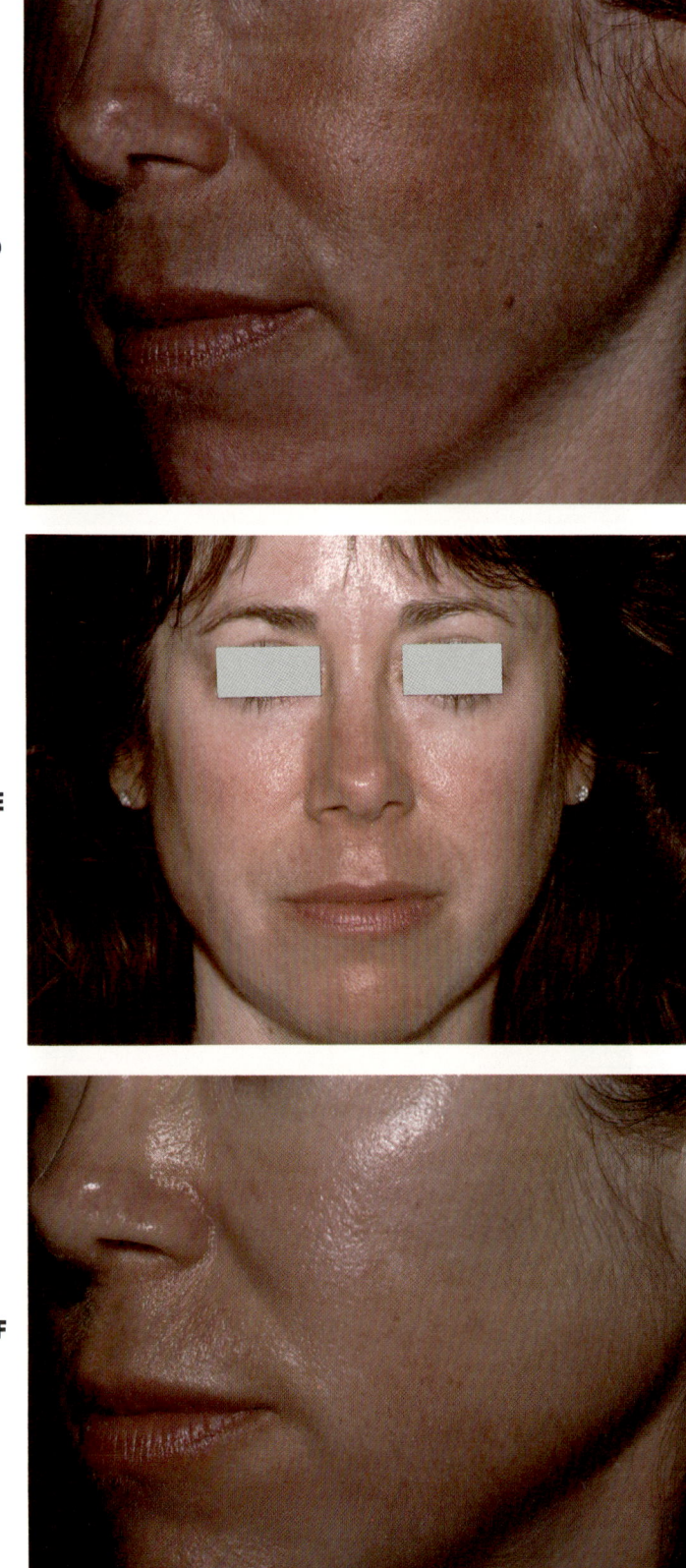

Case 4, cont'd. For legend see p. 160.

Treatment for Hyperpigmentation

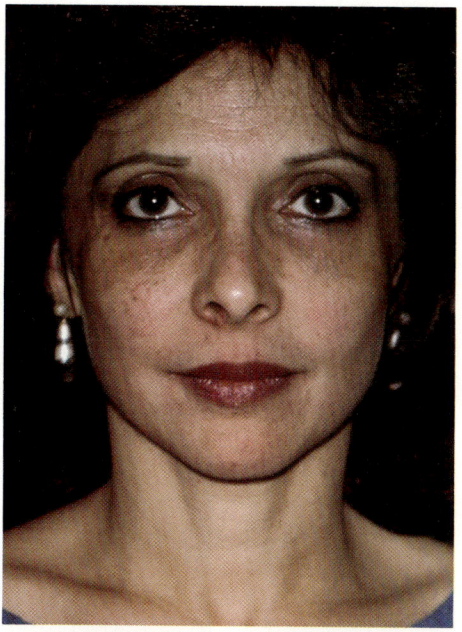

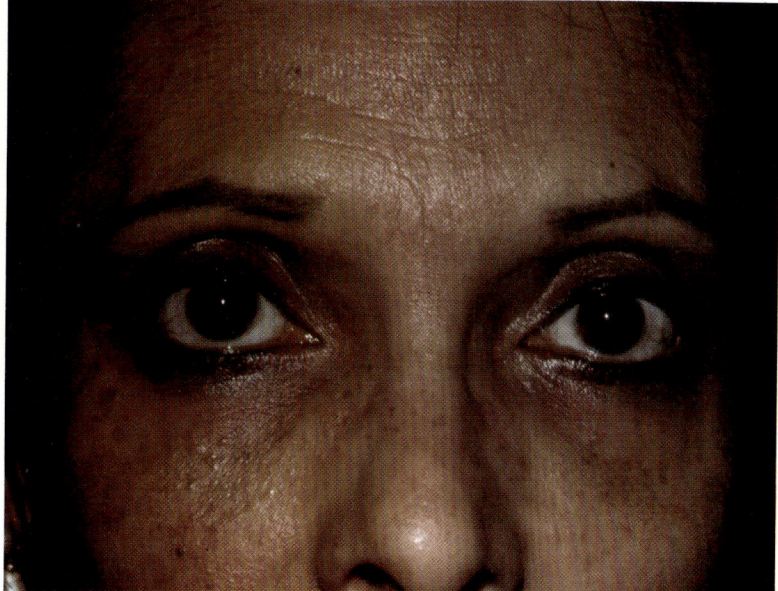

Case 5: Treatment for hyperpigmentation. Although chemical skin peeling can result in unanticipated postinflammatory hyperpigmentation, pigment changes after the procedure more often involve a loss of pigmentation. Occasionally, a peel is performed in the hope of deliberately inducing pigment loss. The cause of this patient's hyperpigmentation is uncertain. Her dark hair and eyes and Portuguese ancestry indicated a patch test before she underwent chemical skin peeling. The patch test results yielded an optimistic prediction for the outcome of the procedure and an unoccluded Baker formula phenol peel was performed. Patient is shown here before treatment.

Continued.

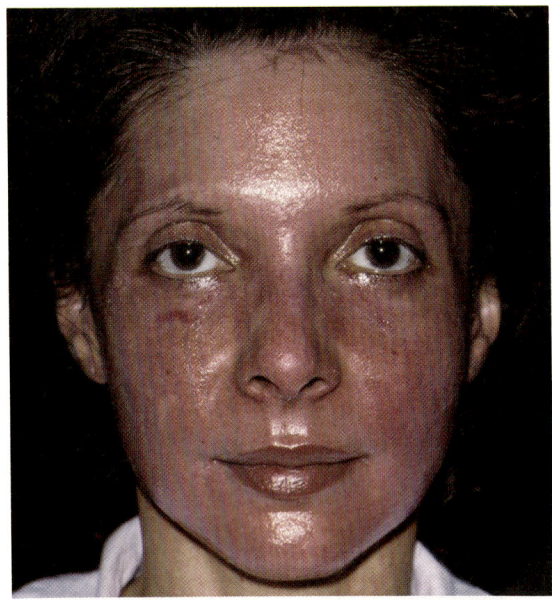
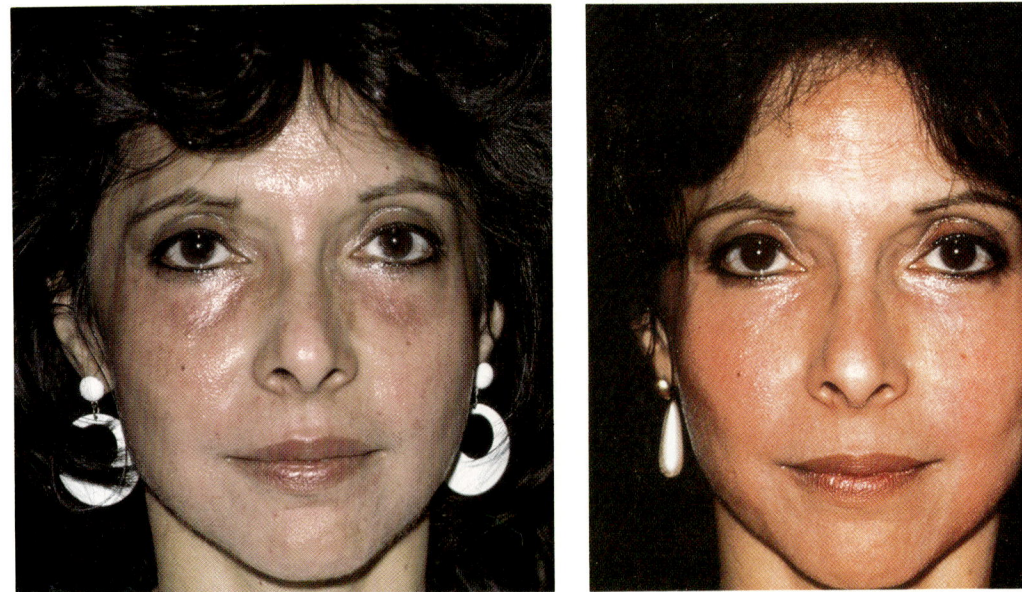

Case 5, cont'd. Results are shown at 7, 90, and 210 days after the procedure, respectively.

The Challenge of the Line of Demarcation

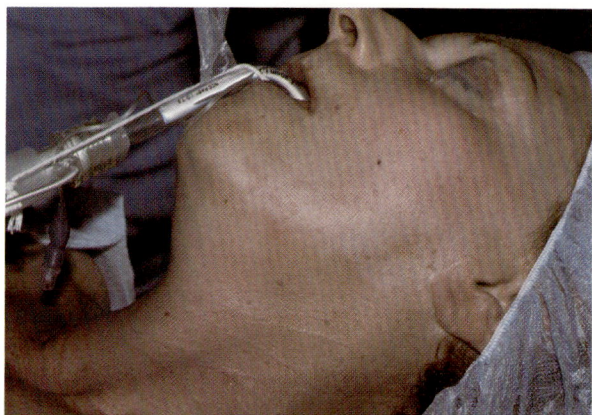
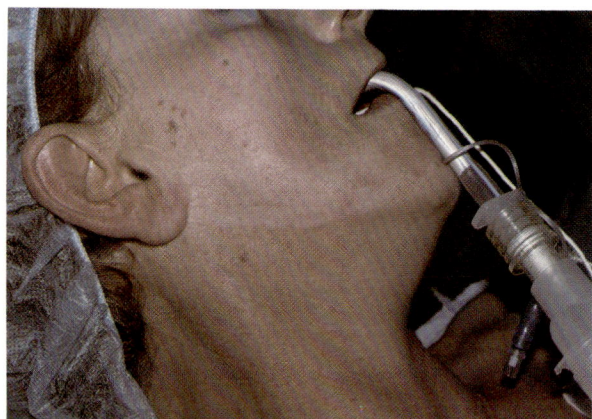

Case 1: Difference in line of demarcation. Despite the presumably identical technique employed (Baker formula, occlusion to jawline), this patient demonstrates a difference in the demarcation lines on either side of the face. The differentiation between the treated face and the untreated neck is much less noticeable on the left side.

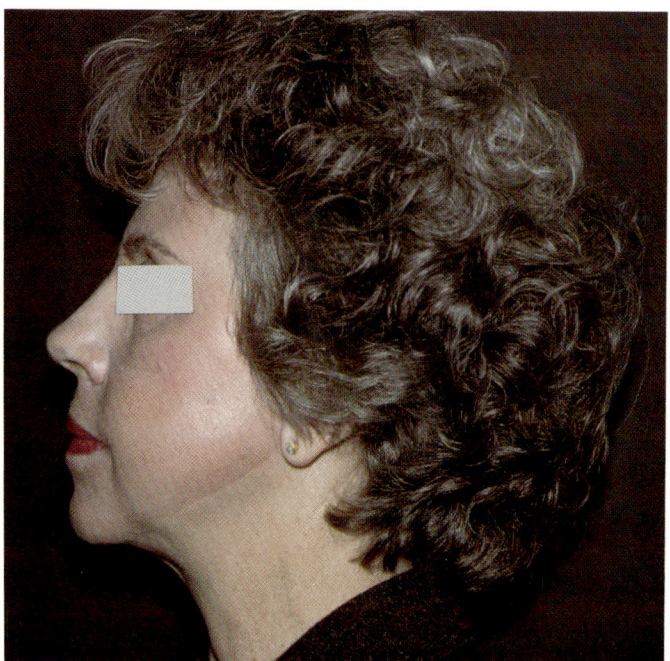

Case 2: Placement of line of demarcation. The line of demarcation is slightly higher than would have been ideal in this case. (Baker formula—occluded; 6 weeks after peel.)

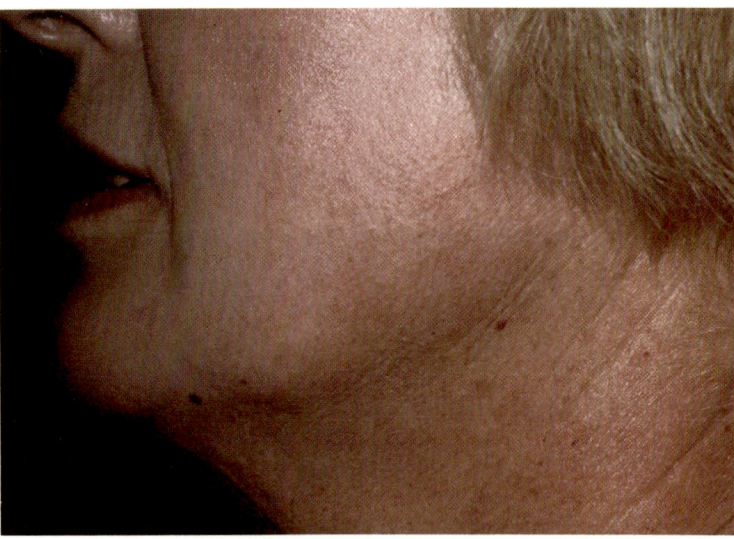

Case 3: Satisfactory "transition" between treated face and untreated neck. This case illustrates the unpredictability of the emergence or nonemergence of a distinct line of demarcation. Fortunately, a satisfactory transition has been achieved here. (One year after peel.)

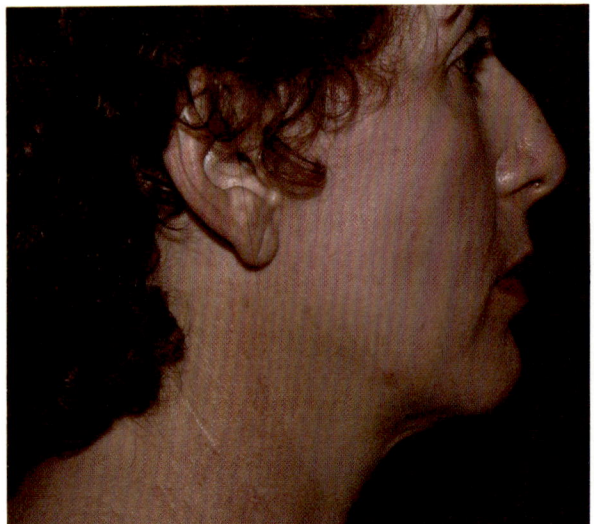

Case 4: Inconcealable line of demarcation. Despite satisfactory makeup technique employed on this patient's face, the eye can still discern the difference between the treated face and the untreated neck. (Three months after peel.)

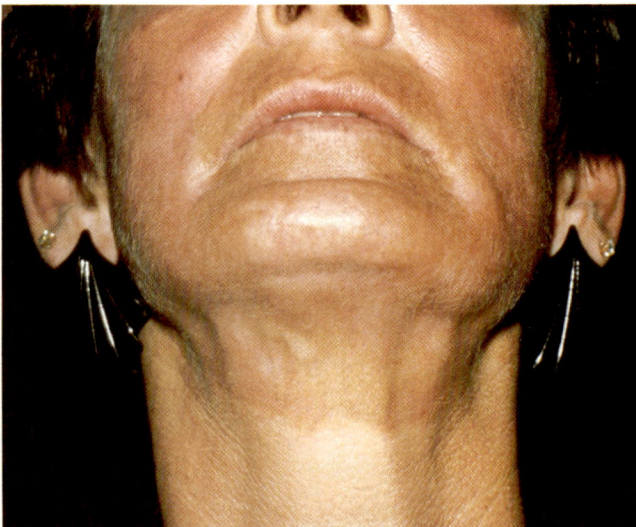

Case 5: Poor placement of endpoint. This patient had a peel performed elsewhere employing an unknown peeling agent. The poor placement of the endpoint for the peel has resulted in an obvious line of demarcation in the upper portion of the neck.

Minimizing the Line of Demarcation

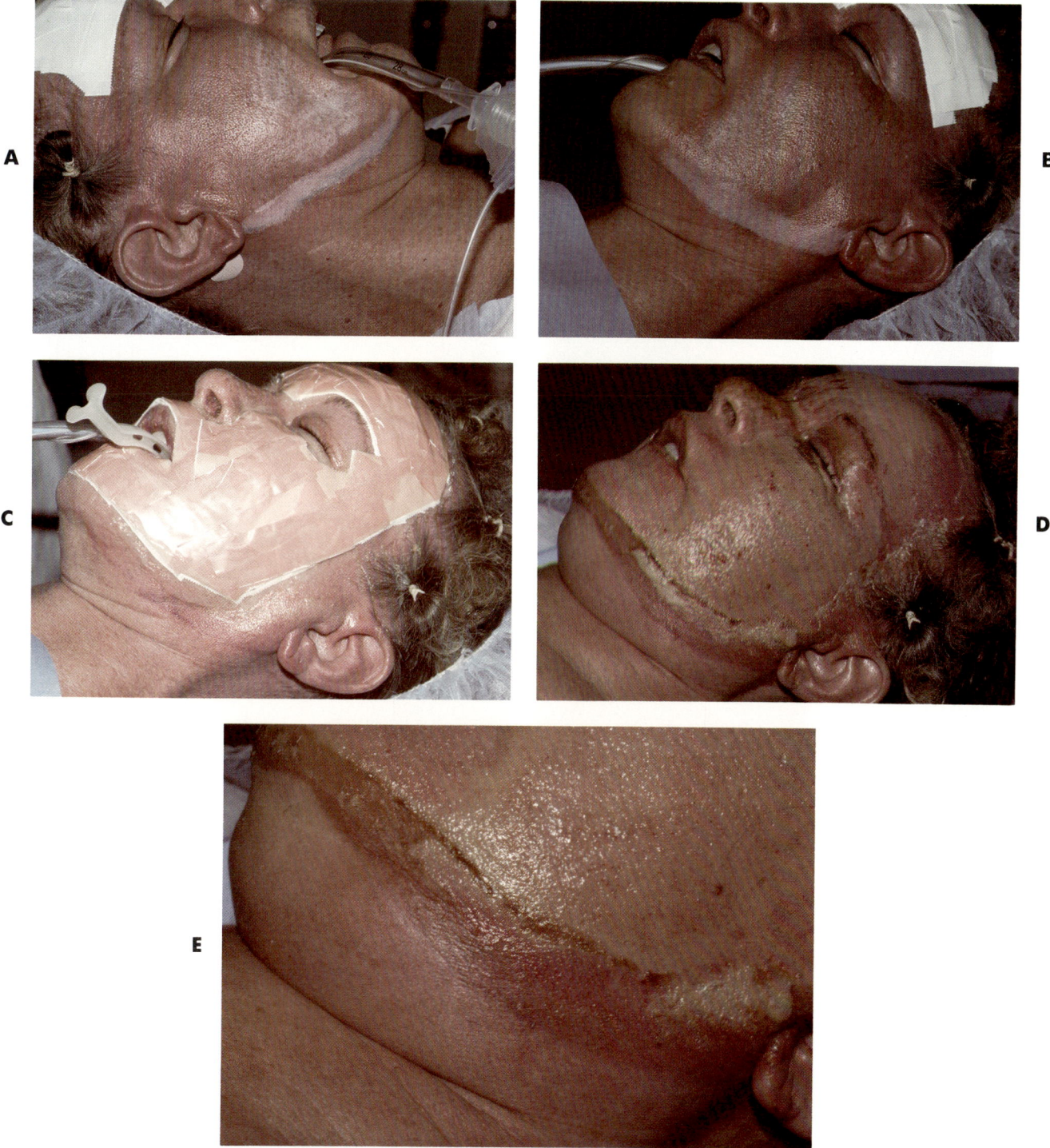

Case 6: Minimizing the Line of Demarcation. A and **B,** The face and cheeks have been treated with a Baker formula phenol solution, and 50% TCA has been applied just above the inframandibular line. **C,** After application of the peeling agents, tapes are applied to the phenol-treated areas, but the TCA-treated "strip" is not occluded. **D,** Note the difference in intensity of the peel between the area treated with occluded Baker formula and the unoccluded 50% TCA–treated area at the inferior margin, evident immediately after mask removal. **E,** Close-up view of **D.**

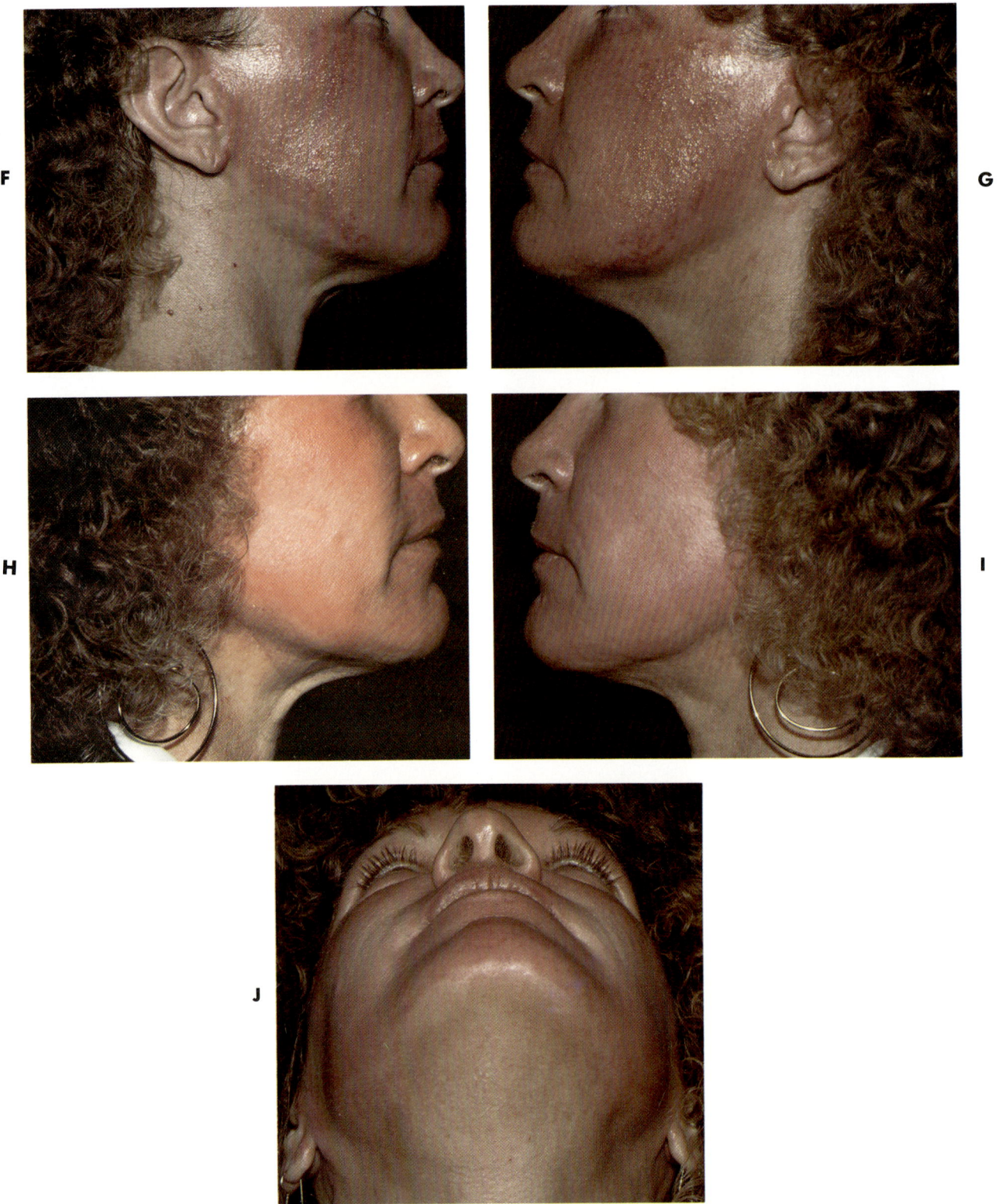

Case 6, cont'd. F and **G,** Patient is shown 6 days after the procedure. **H** and **I,** Lateral views at 17 days after peel show differential pink coloration of the skin at the mandibular margin, with the slightly lighter area at the inferior aspect of the peeled area corresponding to the TCA treatment zone. **J,** Basal view shows good transition between treated and untreated areas within the inframandibular shadow.

Continued.

PERSISTENT REDNESS/TELANGIECTASIA

Some patients will endure prolonged redness of the treated areas. This is generally related to the aggressiveness of the procedure. Nonetheless, even some patients on whom the procedure may have been more conservatively performed have persistent redness, which is a source of great consternation. Sun exposure and applications of photosensitizing agents, including cosmetics, may be responsible for the prolonged erythema.

Telangiectasia may develop after skin peeling, particularly when an aggressive technique has been employed. This is the appearance of a patient 1 month after a Baker formula peel with occlusion of the cheeks using white waterproof tape. Often, these may be precipitated by the patient using tissue paper to help cleanse the skin. Upon recognition of such a practice, patients are advised to refrain from the use of tissue which, because it is a wood pulp product, is inherently unkind to the extremely sensitive skin. Rather, they are advised to use a bare hand in washing the face. These resolve spontaneously within 4 to 6 weeks.

Whether topical steroids hasten resolution is uncertain. Patients who have the fairest skin are less likely to have prolonged redness and, conversely, those who are quite "ruddy" can anticipate prolonged redness. In our experience, 6 to 8 weeks is our minimum "fade time" prediction. A minority of patients will take up to 3 or 4 months. According to Brody,[27] however, "intermittency (of redness) may occur for as long as 2 years afterwards."

Case Presentations: Persistent Redness/Telangiectasia

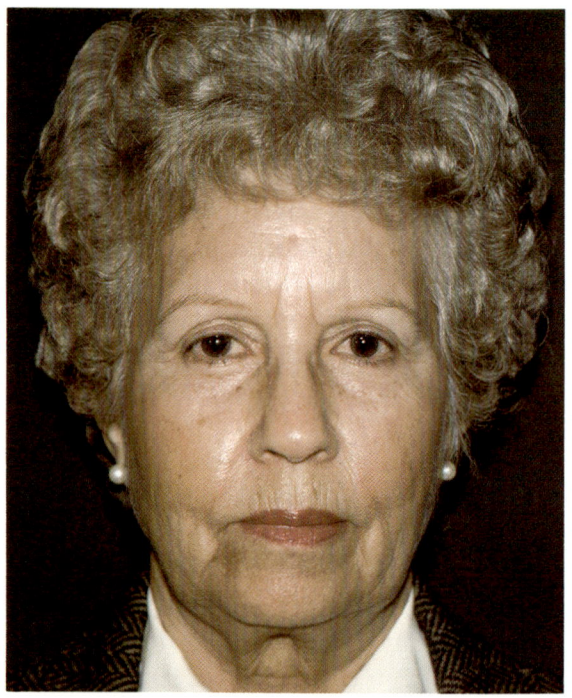
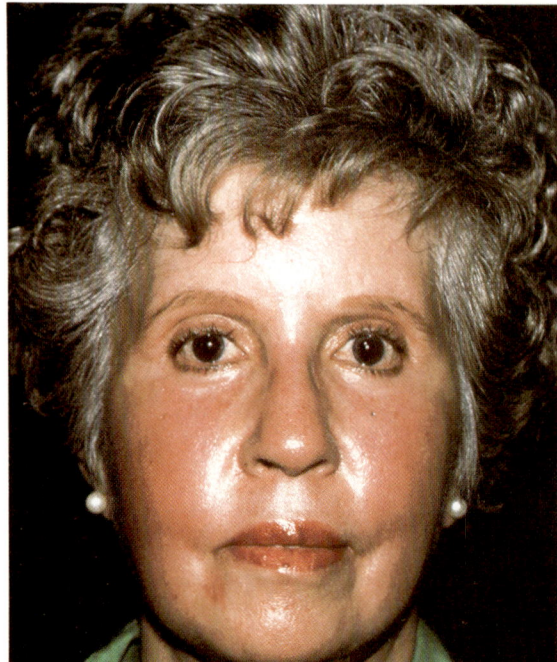
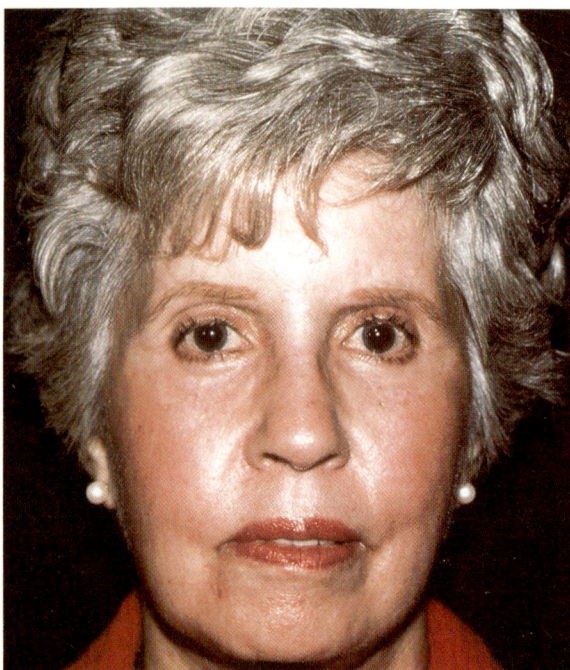

Case 1: Persistent redness. This Hispanic patient with dark hair and eyes "passed" a patch test before receiving an occluded Baker formula phenol peel. However, the hyperpigmented scar of the right portion of the chin seen in the pretreatment view resulted in an area of persistent redness that is present in these views 5 months and 8 months after peel.

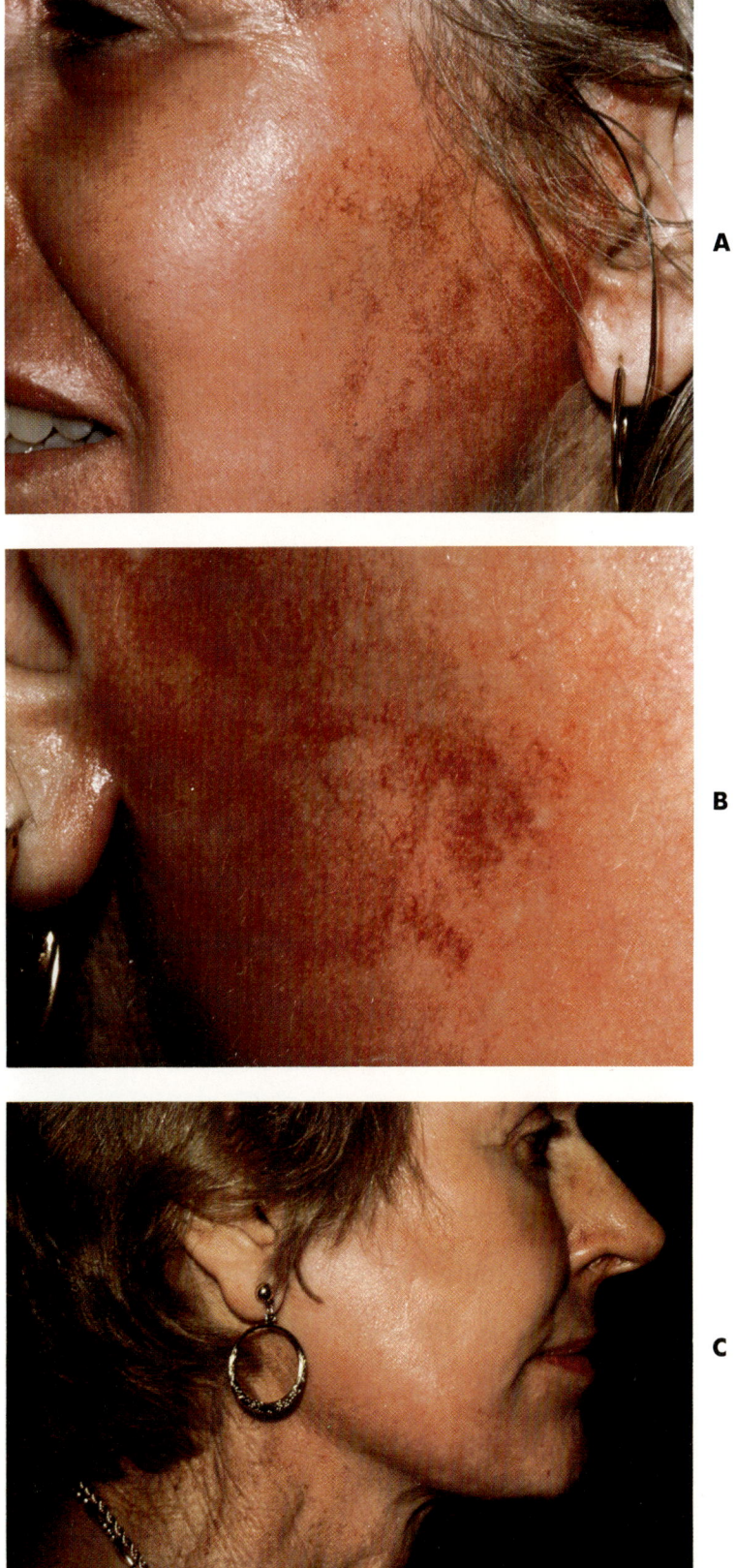

Case 2: Telangiectasia. Telangiectasia developed in the **A,** left preauricular and **B,** cheek area 30 days after a Baker formula phenol peel occluded with white waterproof tape. C, Within 2 months the telangiectasia had disappeared completely. In retrospect, I wish I had peeled this patient's neck as well, because the contrast between the treated face and the untreated neck is rather apparent.

Frontal view

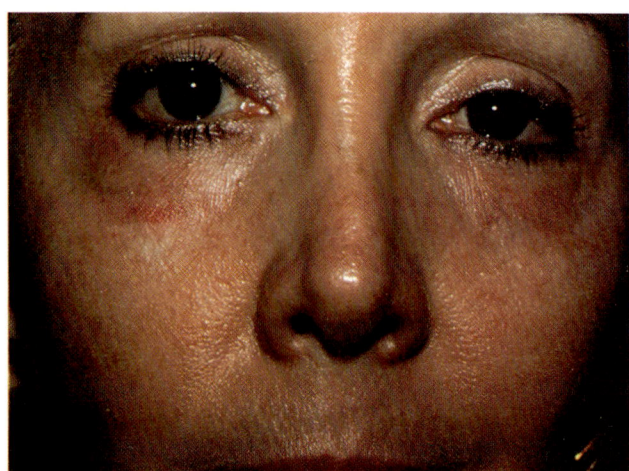

Oblique view

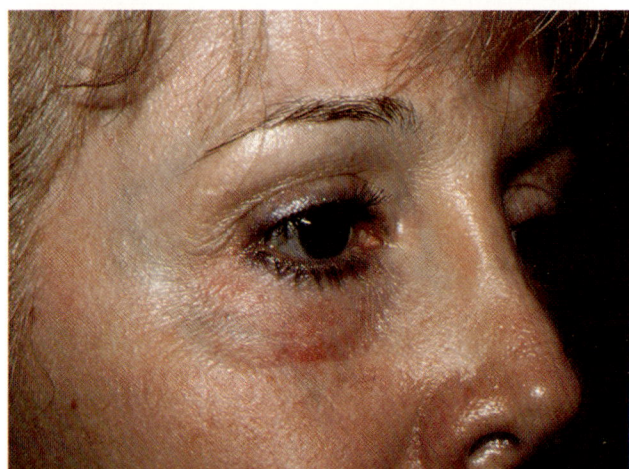

Case 3: Persistent redness. This patient reported having a 35% TCA peel performed elsewhere on the lower eyelids, which was deemed unsuccessful, and 2 weeks later had a "full-strength peel" performed on the same area. One month after the second peel, the patient was said to have had a "low-grade infection of the lower eyelids" and was treated with antibiotics. One month later she received "electrosurgery to the bilateral lower eyelid telangiectasias." Despite these treatments, redness of the area persisted. In retrospect, the patient may not have been well served by having two peel procedures within a short period of time, followed by a series of electrocautery treatments. Generally, the interval between peelings should not be less than 3 to 6 months, particularly in the case of the lower eyelids, which tend to be more sensitive to chemexfoliative procedures.

INFECTION
Herpetic Eruptions

Before the availability of oral acyclovir, the incidence of herpes simplex was not insignificant and a cause of great consternation to the patient and the physician.

Collins[35] endorsed a practical course of treatment to prevent herpetic eruption.

> "Patients with a positive history can be treated prophylactically with 200 ml of acyclovir (Zovirax)* three times daily, 24 hours prior to and for 4-5 days after peeling."

*Burroughs Wellcome Co., Research Triangle Park, NC.

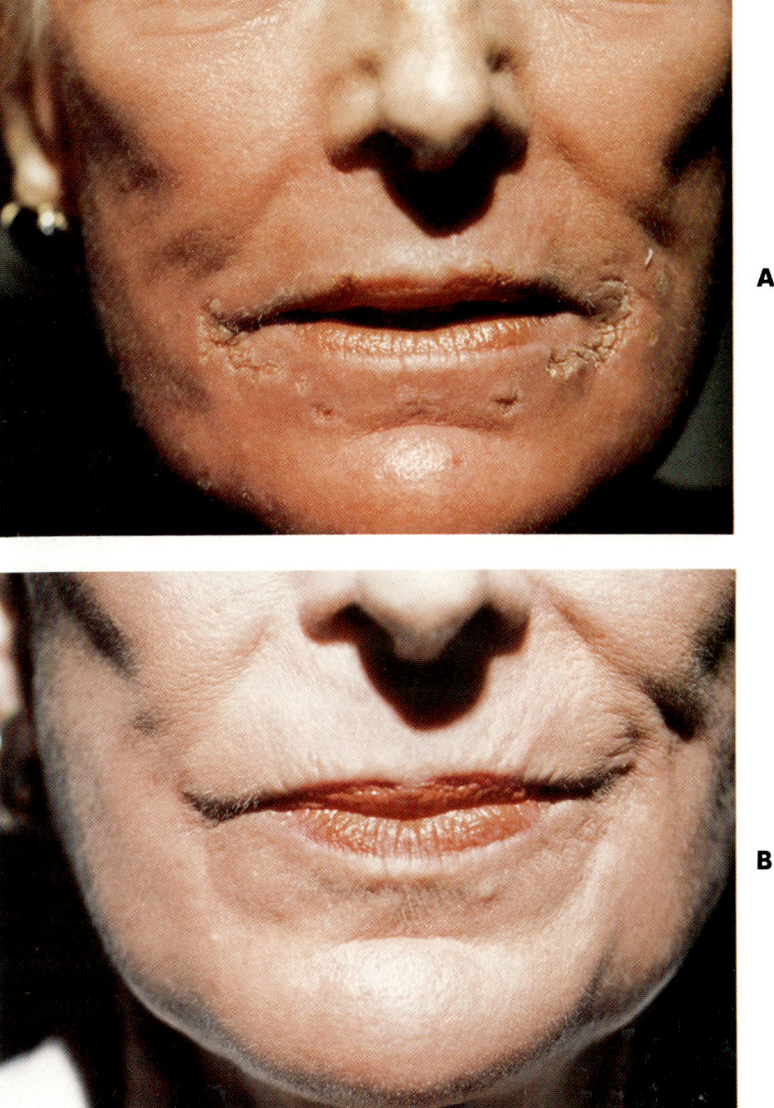

Case: Herpetic eruption. A, Classical herpes simplex lesions appeared approximately 10 days after chemical skin peel. This occurred in the pre-acyclovir (Zovirax) era. **B,** Appearance 60 days after routine wound care treatment is satisfactory.

In our practice, we continue administration of acyclovir through the tenth treatment day. This has almost totally eliminated the threat. Since adopting the technique, there was only one questionable eruption of the lip in over 200 consecutive cases.

Pain or severe pruritus commencing 5 to 7 days postoperatively may signal the onset of herpes simplex.[7] Should such manifest and if the patient is not taking acyclovir, I would recommend immediate prescription of the antiviral medication.

Pyogenic Infections

Pyogenic infections remain quite rare because of the inherent resistance of the facial skin to infection, particularly with the increased vascular supply attendant to the procedure. Should there be any signs of incipient infection, aggressive treatment with topical and/or systemic antibiotics is obviously indicated.

TOXIC SHOCK SYNDROME

Brody[27] reported three cases of toxic shock syndrome (TSS) since 1983 following one unoccluded and two occluded Baker's formula phenol face peels. He advised physicians to be alert for the patient developing fever, sinkable hypotension, vomiting, or diarrhea 2 to 3 days after the peel, accompanied in 2 to 6 days postpeel by scarlatiniform rash with subsequent desquamation. An antibiotic resistant to β-lactamase with large volumes of parenteral fluid to prevent vascular collapse is necessary. The syndrome may include myalgias, mucosal hyperemia, and hepatorenal, hematologic, or central nervous system involvement. The cause of the syndrome is always a strain of *Staphylococcus aureus*.

Dmytryshyn[42] reported on a case that was later reviewed in depth in *JAMA*.[45] This case was included in Brody's review. The patient was a 42-year-old transsexual male who underwent full-thickness chemical peel under general anesthesia. The peel ingredients included 3 ml of 89% phenol, 2 ml of tap water, 7 drops of Septisol, and 3 drops of croton oil.

Postoperative swelling was controlled for the first 4 days by continuous application of cool compresses and dexamethasone, 12 mg/day. On the fifth day, the patient experienced fever (temperature reaching 30° C), tachycardia, and hypotension. The facial swelling continued and was accompanied by a malodorous purulent discharge. The trunk and upper arms were marked with a diffuse nonpruritic macular erythroderma, and the patient was confused and somnolent.

Gram staining of the purulent material from the face showed +4 polymorphonuclear cells and +3 gram-positive cocci in clusters. Cultures yielded *S. aureus*. The organism was resistant to penicillin and methicillin by standard disk-diffusion susceptibility testing.

The patient was treated with cloxacillin (2 g every 4 hours), plus penicillin G, 2,000,000 units every 4 hours, intravenously, and was given

5% dextrose in saline, 200 ml/hr for the first 24 hours, then 125 ml/hr for the next 48 hours. In all, 10 liters of crystalloid was administered during the first 3 days.

The blood pressure returned to normal within 8 hours of initiation of fluids. Three days after appearance of the skin rash, skin desquamation—considered highly characteristic of TSS—occurred on the hands and feet.

The patient was discharged well, 15 days after admission to the hospital.

Dmytryshyn noted that possible risk factors in this case may have been colonization of nose, throat, axilla, and perineum with *S. aureus*. The large denuded area on the face could have allowed toxin absorption, and the risk for TSS could also have been heightened by use of continuous wet compresses on the infected area of the face and possibly by the use of diethylstilbestrol, which was being given to this patient to achieve feminization.

Dmytryshyn[42] noted that "approximately 2.5% of the 941 reported cases have been men." Dmytryshyn further noted that "most reported isolates of *S. aureus* from patients who have had toxic shock syndrome have been resistant only to penicillin and ampicillin sodium."

ACNEIFORM DERMATITIS

Not infrequently following peeling, we see an acnelike outbreak of the skin. It may be related to overzealous treatment of the skin with hydrocortisone ointments or other occluding preparations that we have prescribed to reverse dryness of the skin.

Several regimens have been used with success. The following recommendations made by dermatologist Jeffrey Marmelzat, M.D., have been quite effective.

1. Stop all moisturizers and cortisone-based ointments or creams.
2. Prescribe Purpose* soap or Cetaphil or Aquanil lotions to be used for washing the face several times a day.
3. Prescribe a topical antibiotic preparation (for example, Cleocin, Erymax solution or gel, or TS solution or gel).
4. Prescribe systemic antibiotics (for example, EES 400 qid or Minocin 150 mg/day tapering over 7 days).

Should the patient develop any problem with the topical antibiotic product, it should be discontinued.

We kiddingly remind the patients that "a small cost of looking young is the reemergence of teenage acne." But we seriously reassure the patient that this is a temporary condition that reverses with treatment and that will have no deleterious effect on the outcome.

---

*Johnson & Johnson, Inc.

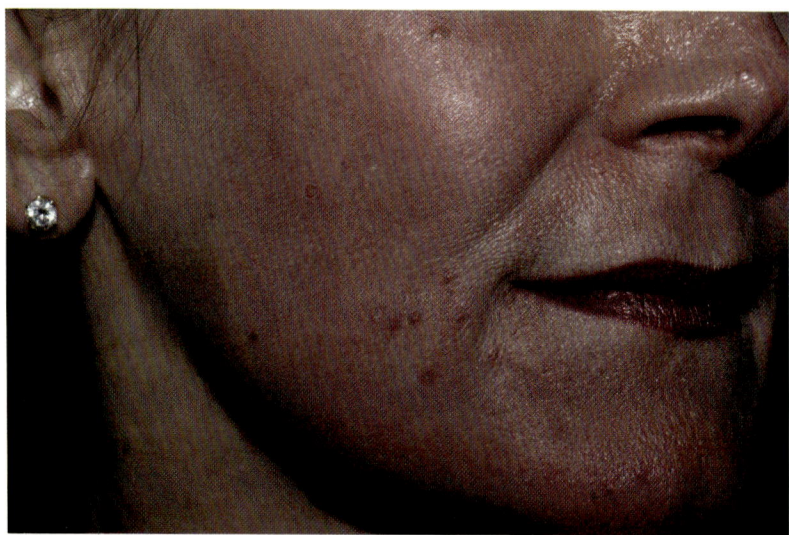

Case: Acneiform dermatitis. Close-up view of right mandibular area shows acneiform dermatitis that developed 6 weeks after chemical skin peeling. It responded successfully to the usual regimen.

EMERGENCE OF DARK NEVI

Infrequently following deep phenol peeling, there will be emergence of intensely pigmented yet superficial nevi. Often these will occur in locations where there had been none recognizable before.

Insofar as phenol is particularly toxic to melanocytes, it was somewhat paradoxic that these would emerge following peeling. Nonetheless, the emergence of these nevi may represent acceleration of the development of incipient nevi. The intense inflammatory process may engender a focal postinflammatory hyperpigmentation at a site where pigmented nevi may have emerged later in time. Using local anesthesia and a very light electrocautery, they are erased. I generally prefer to do this after the redness has subsided so as not to elicit further postinflammatory hyperpigmentation as a result of the treatment.

ITCHING AND BURNING

A significant number of patients develop annoying itching, usually in the first 2 weeks after treatment. Antihistamines may be effective. Topical steroids may reduce this postinflammatory reaction. Aspirin and nonsteroidal antiinflammatories may also help relieve the symptom. Most patients are reassured to know that it is a temporary phenomenon, generally peaking between 2 to 3 weeks after the procedure. Low-level pain medication is also advisable, and in some patients one must combine several or all of the above drug modalities to relieve this itching, which distracts from the pleasure of the result.

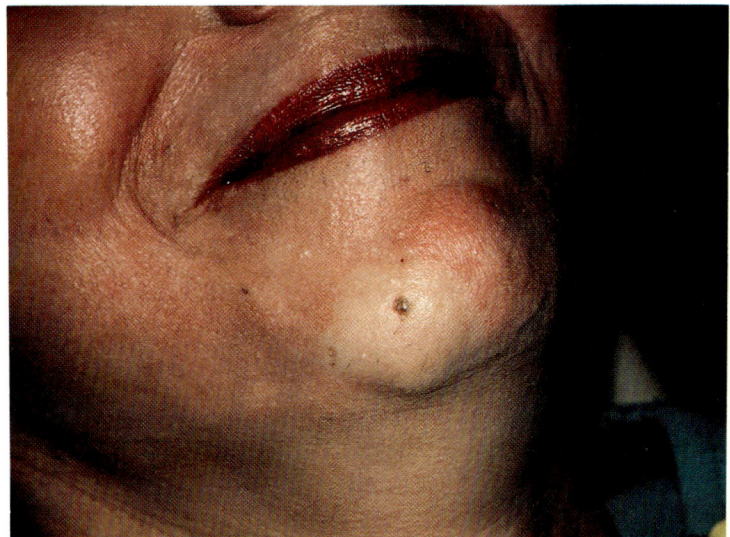

Case: Darkening nevi. Intensely pigmented nevi not infrequently appear after a chemical peel—particularly an aggressive phenol peel—often in areas where none had been noticed previously. Since phenol is somewhat toxic to melanocytes, it is paradoxical that nevi would emerge following a peel. It may be that incipient nevi, not yet apparent, are revealed by the planing effect of the peel. Furthermore, the intense inflammatory response following the procedure may cause a focal postinflammatory hyperpigmentation. If a patient is dissatisfied with the appearance of such nevi, they may be erased using light electrocautery under local anesthesia. I generally prefer to wait until after the postpeel redness has subsided to avoid eliciting further postinflammatory hyperpigmentation. The patient seen here had darkened nevi on the forehead, cheek, and chin 2 months following a tape-occluded phenol peel. A white "halo" that surrounds the chin nevus is due to the local effect of injected epinephrine.

MILIA

Milia, or small inclusion cysts, occur with unpredictable incidence. The peak incidence seems to be between 6 to 8 weeks after the process is performed. In some patients there may be 50 to 100 or more of these if the entire face has been treated. While most disappear spontaneously after several months, in those patients in whom they are unacceptable, each cyst must be "shucked" from its bed. The skin is then treated with topical antibiotics until reepithelialization has taken place.

Brody[27] noted that "the postpeel care of deeper peeling may produce milia by occluding the upper pilosebaceous units with ointments. Returning to gentle epidermabrasion . . . may retard their appearance."

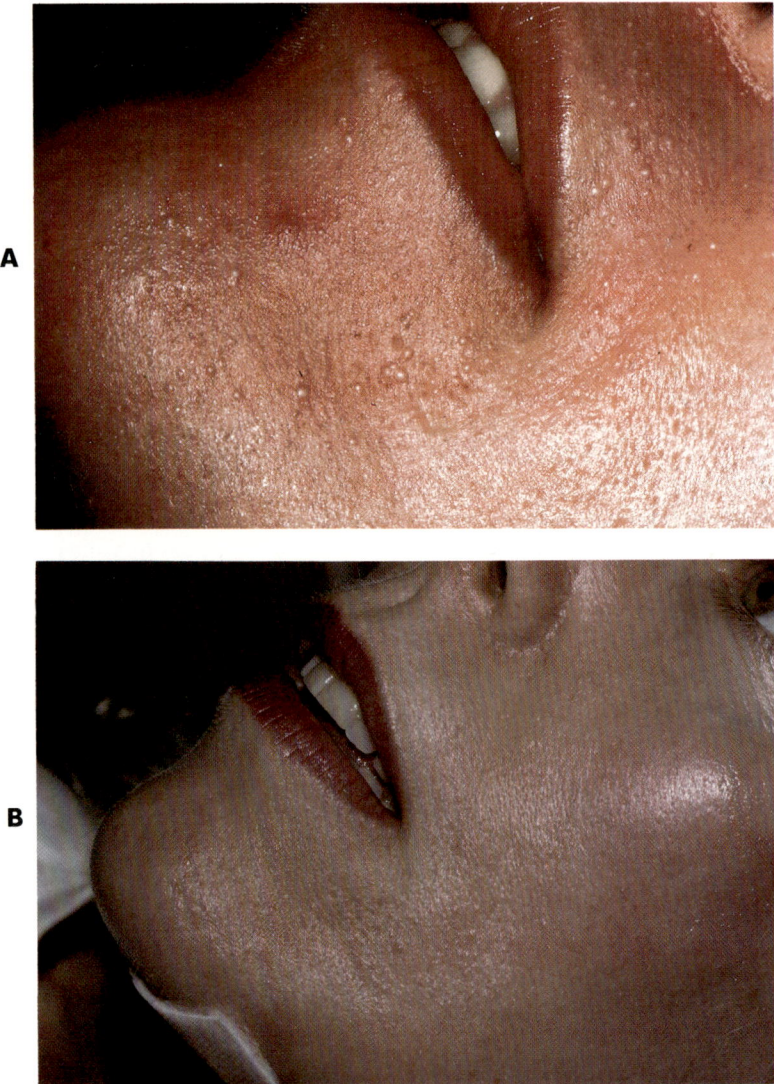

Case: Milia. This case demonstrates a classic development of multiple milia after an occluded Baker formula phenol peel. **A,** The patient is shown here 60 days after the peeling procedure and **B,** again 30 days after milia were individually uncapped. If untreated, milia generally will disappear within 60 to 90 days after first appearance. Frequently, however, impatient patients wish to have them removed.

HIRSUTISM

In my experience, I have observed an apparent increase in facial hair in three patients following facial peeling. In each case, the patient had the "maximum" technique, a Baker formula occluded phenol peel, performed. Each called attention to the complication themselves and evaluation of the pretreatment photographs confirmed their observations. Whether the increased facial hair growth eventually resolves without treatment is not known. It seems likely, however, that in the rare cases when it does occur it will be a permanent postpeel feature. A depilatory can aid in removing unwanted hair but is not indicated until all postpeel redness has resolved.

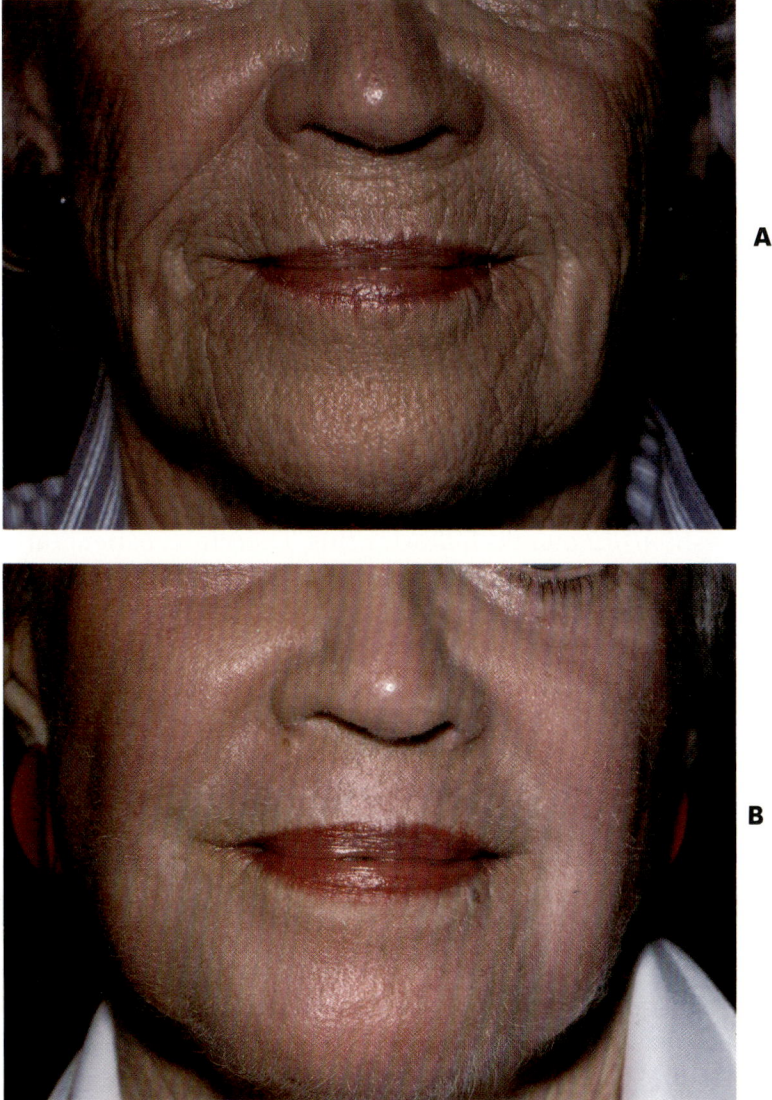

Case: Hirsutism. A, Pretreatment view. This patient had a maximum technique occluded Baker formula phenol peel with Salonpas applied as the first layer to areas of deepest wrinkling such as the perioral area shown here. **B,** The results were excellent; however, as seen here 5 months after the procedure, the patient showed increased facial hair growth in the chin area.

CHAPTER NINE

Repeeling

Repeeling is challenging for several reasons. If the previous peel was done relatively recently, the patient is somewhat dissatisfied with the result. There may also be less margin for error, although my experience shows that we have not seen a greater incidence of complication in repeels than in primary peels. It must be emphasized that significant time must elapse between the procedures to safely avoid complications. I never consider repeeling a patient if any residual redness remains from the primary peel. It usually takes 3 to 4 months for the redness to disappear completely following a peel. I prefer an additional cushion of 2 months following this. Therefore, patients are not considered for repeeling until at least 6 months following the previous peel.

The following case illustrates difficulties associated with repeeling. This patient had an aggressive peel performed with good results many years earlier by a competent and experienced practitioner. Although the patient sought additional treatment because of some persistent wrinkling of the medial lower eyelids, lower lip, forehead, and glabella, her skin still appeared to be quite satisfactory overall and I was therefore conservative in my approach. Rather than repeel the entire face with phenol, I performed the reverse of the standard procedure by treating the majority of the face with TCA and streaking only those areas that had etched lines with a Baker phenol solution. The result was inadequate, particularly on the forehead and medial lower lids. (The lower lids had not been taped.) At a third peeling session which followed my original repeel procedure by 6 months, the forehead, entire lower lids, upper lids, one transverse crow's foot, and the red/white lip junction of the lower lip were treated with the Baker phenol solution. The rest of the face was left untreated. Waterproof tapes were applied to the forehead, upper lids and infrabrow, crow's foot, medial lower lids, and the red/white lip junction.

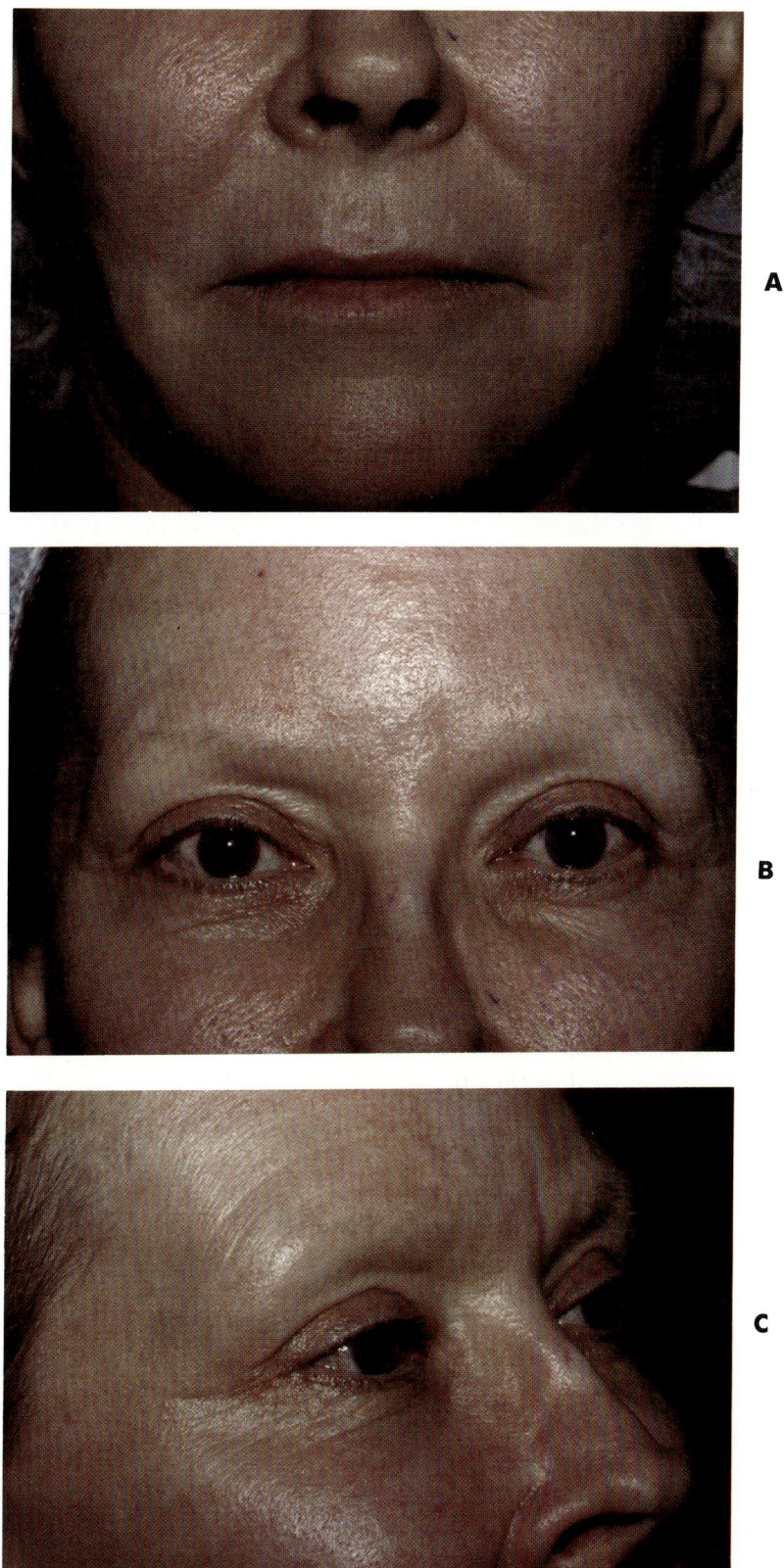

Case 1: Repeeling areas of persistent wrinkling. This patient had received two chemical skin peels previously but remained dissatisfied with some persistent wrinkling of the lower lip, medial lower eyelids, and forehead and glabellar lines. She was a very profound "eyebrow elevator," however, and was aware that skin peeling could not prevent recurrence of these lines of expression. **A** to **C,** Pretreatment views.

Continued.

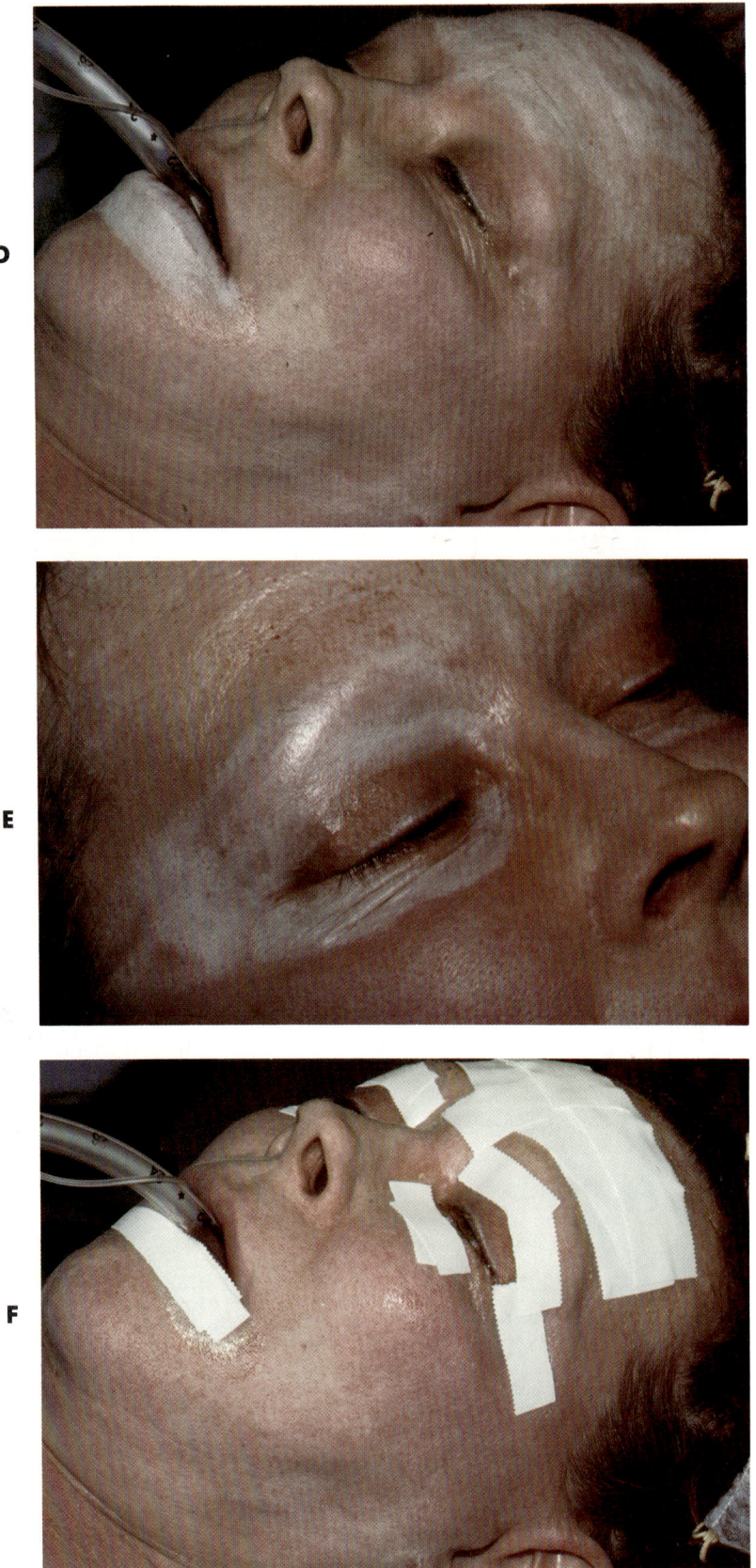

Case 1, cont'd. D and **E,** Baker formula phenol solution was applied to the forehead, glabella, infrabrow, lower eyelids, and lower lip areas. **F,** White waterproof tapes were then applied. In deference to the two previous peels and the skin's thinness, no Salonpas was used to occlude the treated areas—a rather conservative approach.

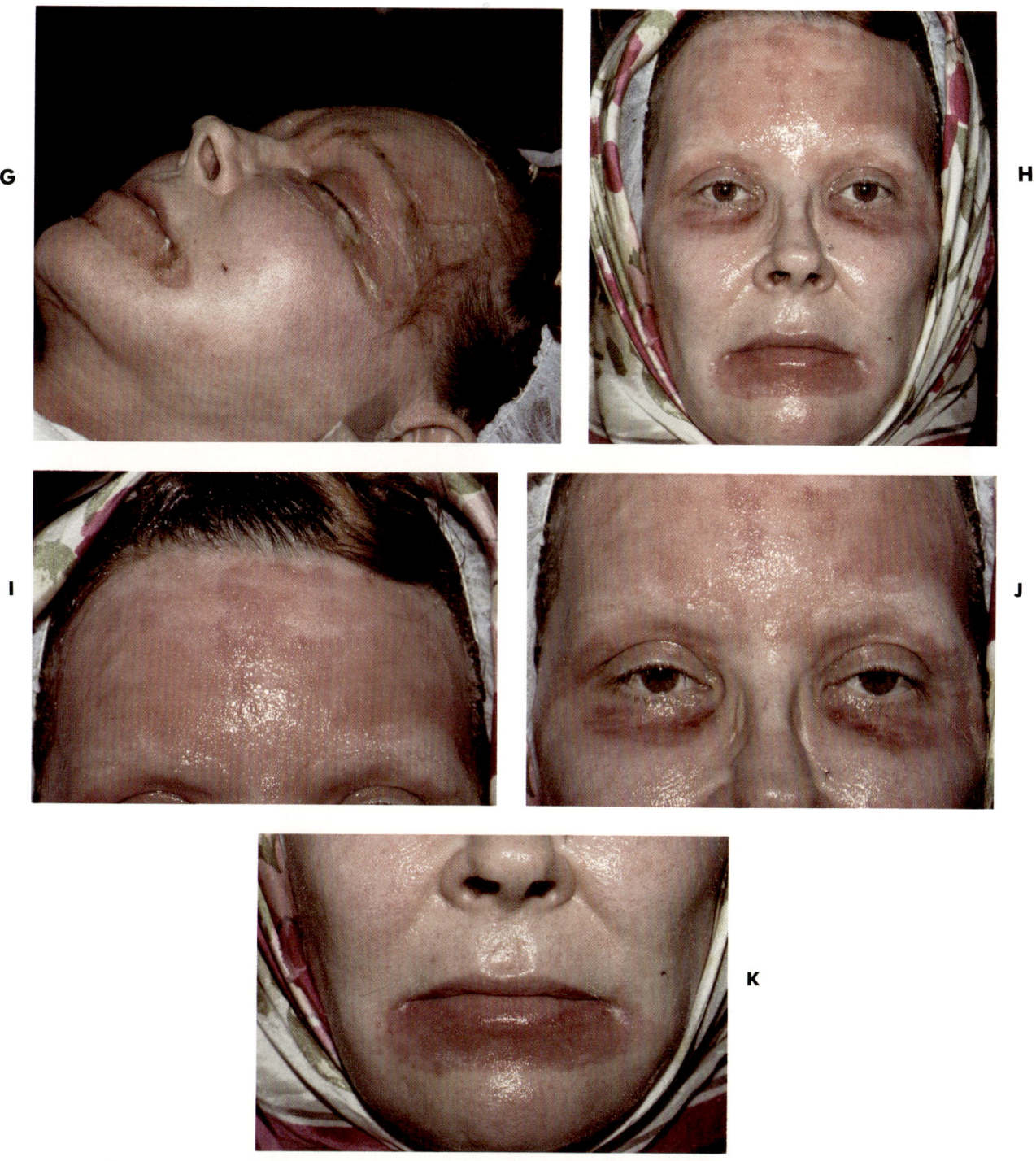

Case 1, cont'd. G, Two days after peel the tapes were removed. **H to K,** The appearance of the treated areas 6 days after the repeeling procedure looks promising.

184 CHEMICAL REJUVENATION OF THE FACE

Case 2 illustrates a situation where mild repeeling was indicated 8 years following a full-face Baker formula peel. At the time of the original peel the upper and lower lips, chin, and medial cheeks were occluded with Salonpas as the base layer, covered by white waterproof tape and then Hy-Tape.

Eight years later the patient complained of early wrinkling about the lower mouth and anterior cheek area, as well as some minimal rewrinkling about the eyes. I chose to treat her with unoccluded Baker solution over the lower eyelids and malar areas as well as the anterior cheeks, lower lip, and chin. Fifty percent TCA was used for the upper portion of the lower eyelids and the central portion of the upper lip. A rhinoplasty was performed at the same time with no concern since the areas of peeling and nasal surgery did not overlap.

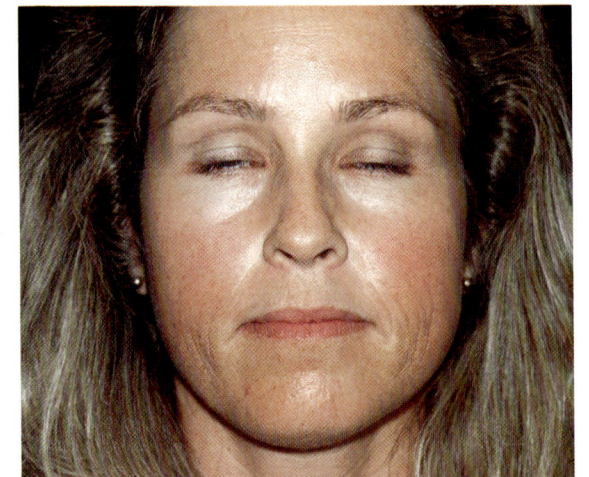
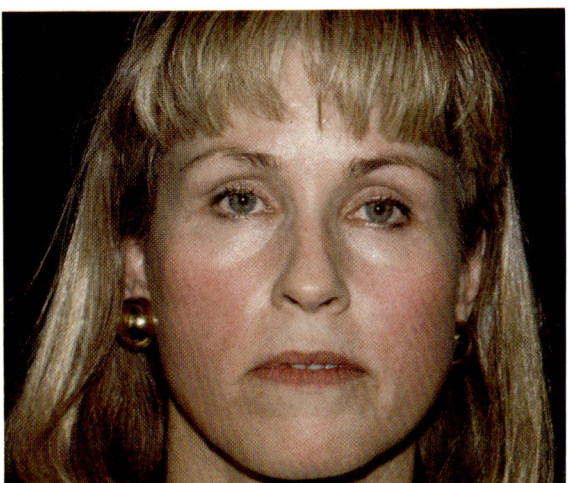
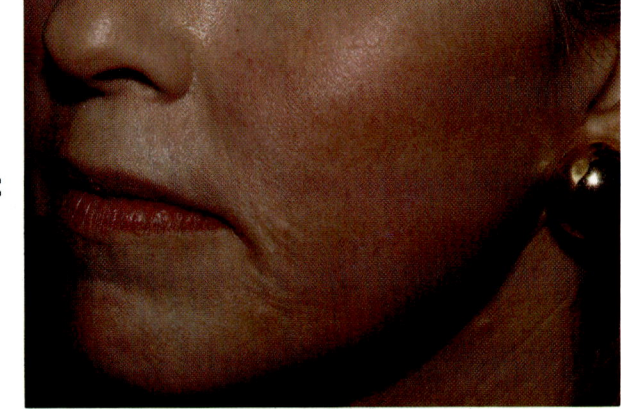

Case 2: Repeeling. The patient is shown here **A**, before and **B**, 8 years after her original chemical peel. **C**, Close-up view shows some persistent wrinkling about the mouth.

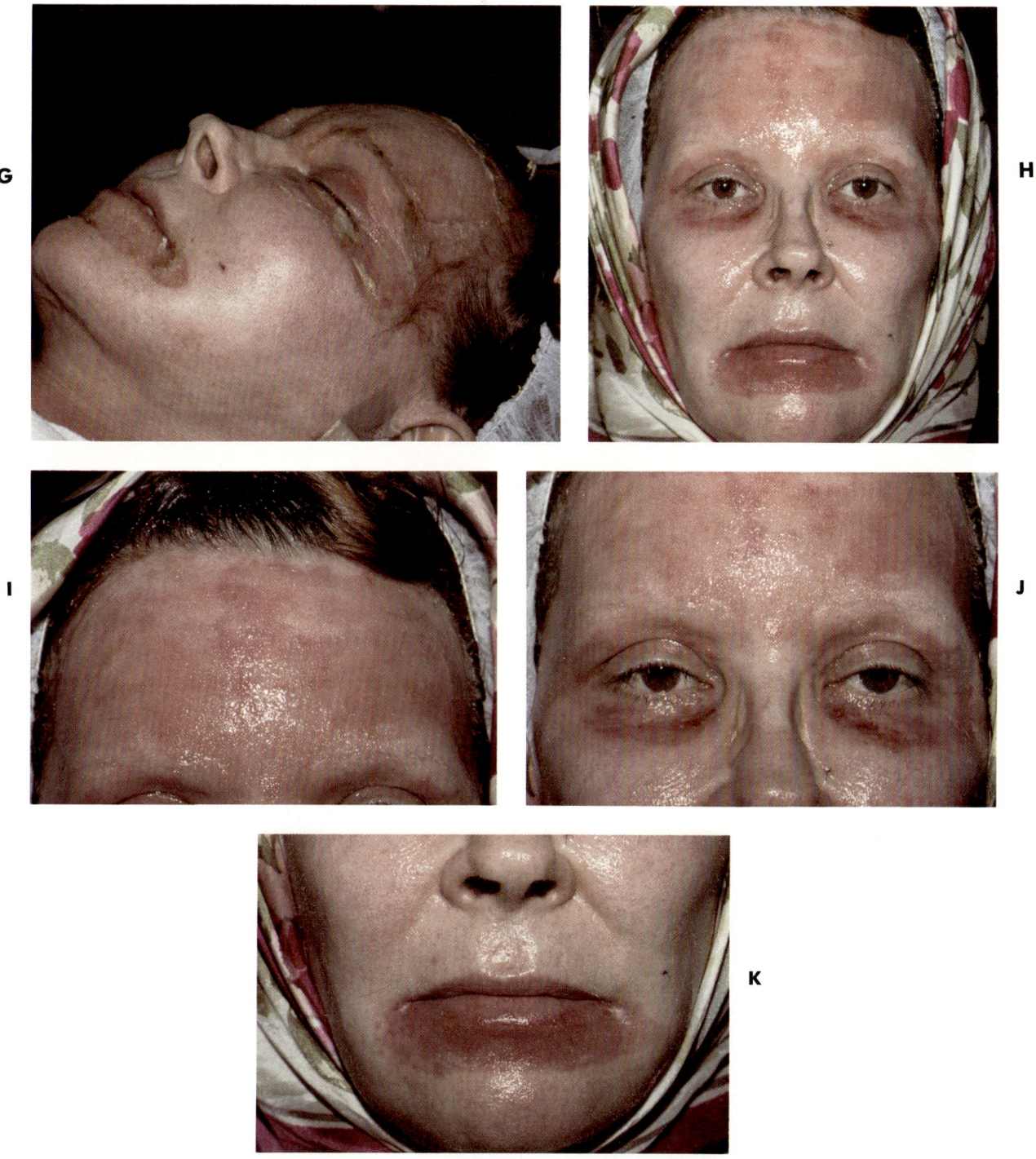

Case 1, cont'd. **G,** Two days after peel the tapes were removed. **H** to **K,** The appearance of the treated areas 6 days after the repeeling procedure looks promising.

Case 2 illustrates a situation where mild repeeling was indicated 8 years following a full-face Baker formula peel. At the time of the original peel the upper and lower lips, chin, and medial cheeks were occluded with Salonpas as the base layer, covered by white waterproof tape and then Hy-Tape.

Eight years later the patient complained of early wrinkling about the lower mouth and anterior cheek area, as well as some minimal rewrinkling about the eyes. I chose to treat her with unoccluded Baker solution over the lower eyelids and malar areas as well as the anterior cheeks, lower lip, and chin. Fifty percent TCA was used for the upper portion of the lower eyelids and the central portion of the upper lip. A rhinoplasty was performed at the same time with no concern since the areas of peeling and nasal surgery did not overlap.

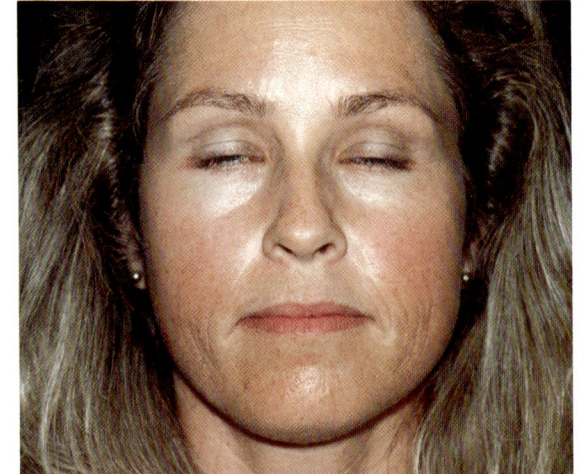
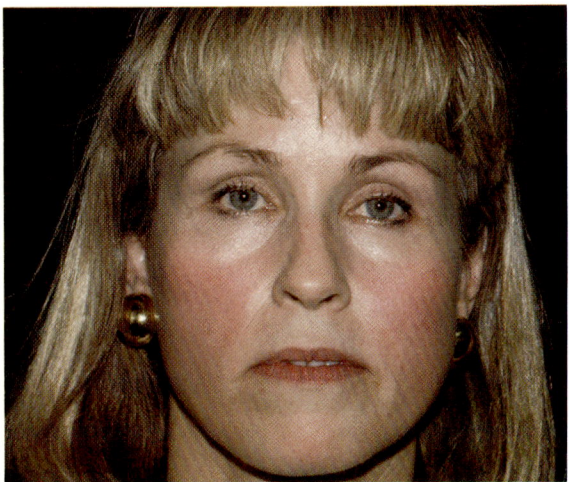
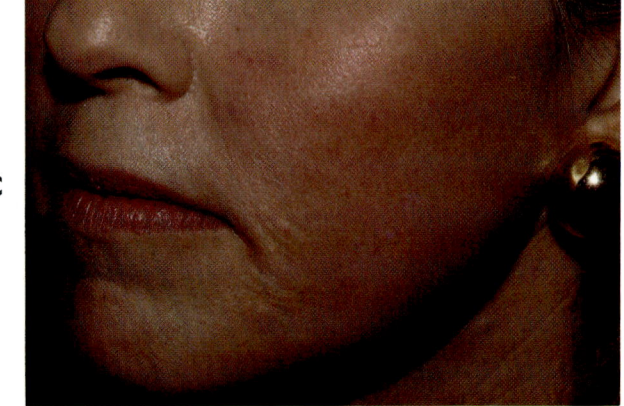

Case 2: Repeeling. The patient is shown here **A**, before and **B**, 8 years after her original chemical peel. **C**, Close-up view shows some persistent wrinkling about the mouth.

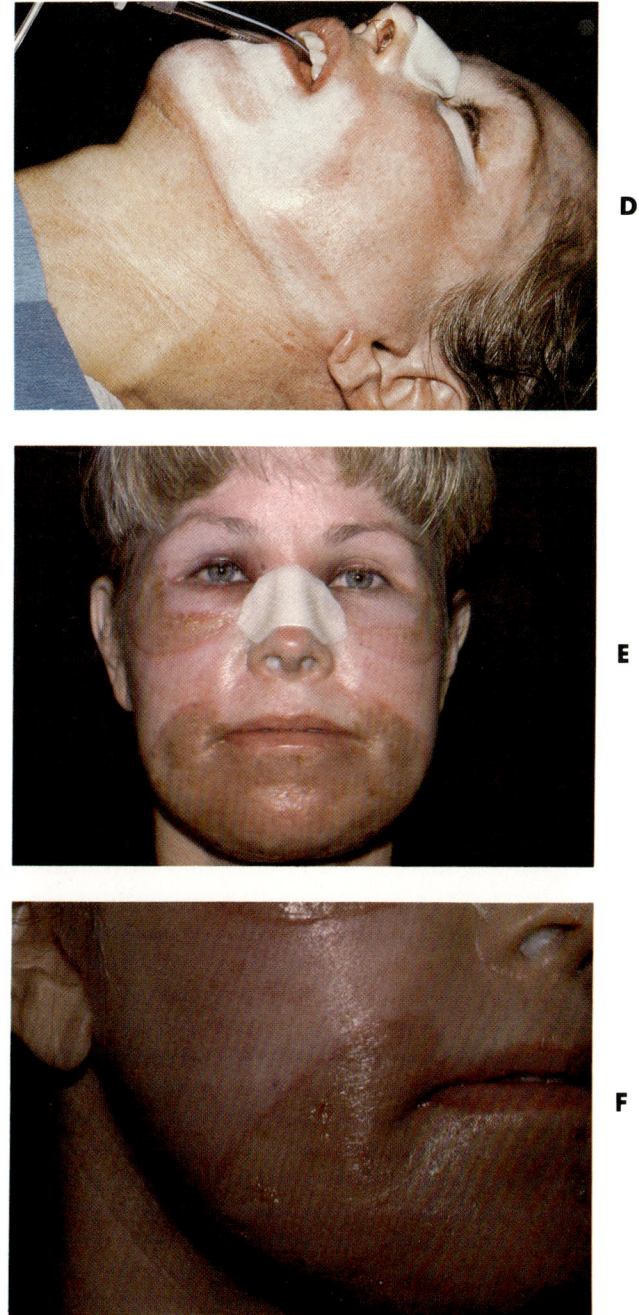

Case 2, cont'd. D, Retreatment of the area consisted of an unoccluded Baker formula phenol peel. **E** and **F,** The patient is shown 48 hours after the repeeling procedure. She had rhinoplasty performed at the same sitting.

CHAPTER TEN

Neck and Chest Peels

Neck and/or chest peels may be performed when it is necessary to match the color and homogeneity of the untreated neck with the treated face. The neck peel can be done at the same time as or separate from the face peel. We have not used phenol because of concerns for scarring but have used TCA in concentrations up to 50%. Ayres[8] noted that:

> "The neck is a 'difficult' area, as the skin is much thinner and less well supplied with cutaneous adnexa than that of the face, and the danger of excessive depth of destruction of the cauterant with resulting scarring is therefore much greater. However, at least some measure of improvement may be obtained and sometimes it is substantial."

Taping is never performed on the neck. Treatment with antibiotic ointment or a petrolatum may begin immediately after treatment or 1 or 2 days later when the epidermal slough becomes evident.

Some practitioners, using a variety of agents including Jessner's solution combined with 35% TCA, will treat the upper chest, particularly the "V zone," to avoid a stark contrast between the treated face and neck and untreated chest.*

---

*Personal communication, James Auerbach, M.D.

CASE PRESENTATIONS: NECK AND CHEST PEELS

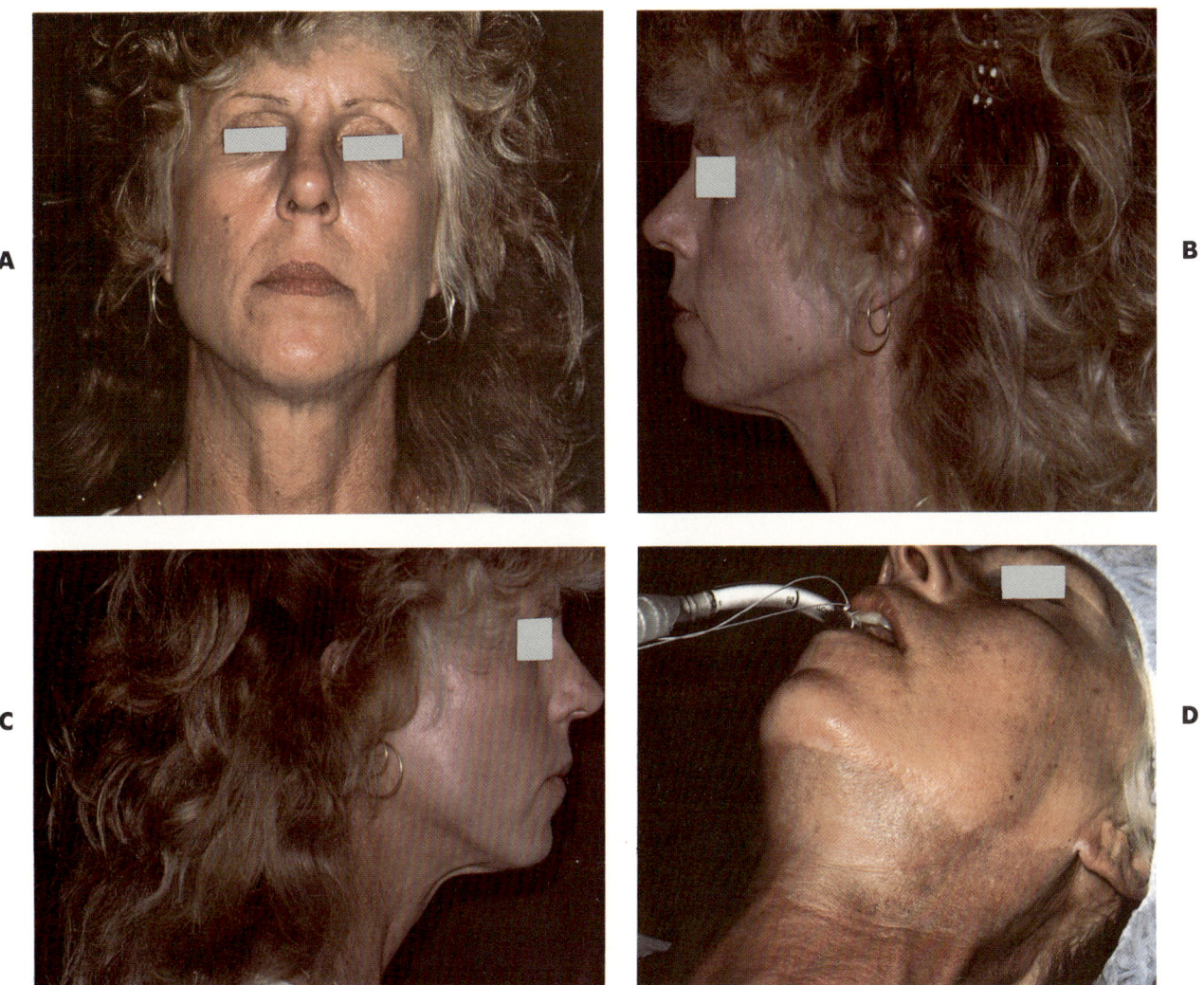

Case 1: Neck peeling. The patient is shown here before treatment. She had an occluded Baker formula phenol peel to the face 6 years previously. **A,** Frontal view with makeup. **B,** Left lateral view with makeup. **C,** Right lateral view with makeup. **D,** Patient immediately before treatment, wearing no makeup.

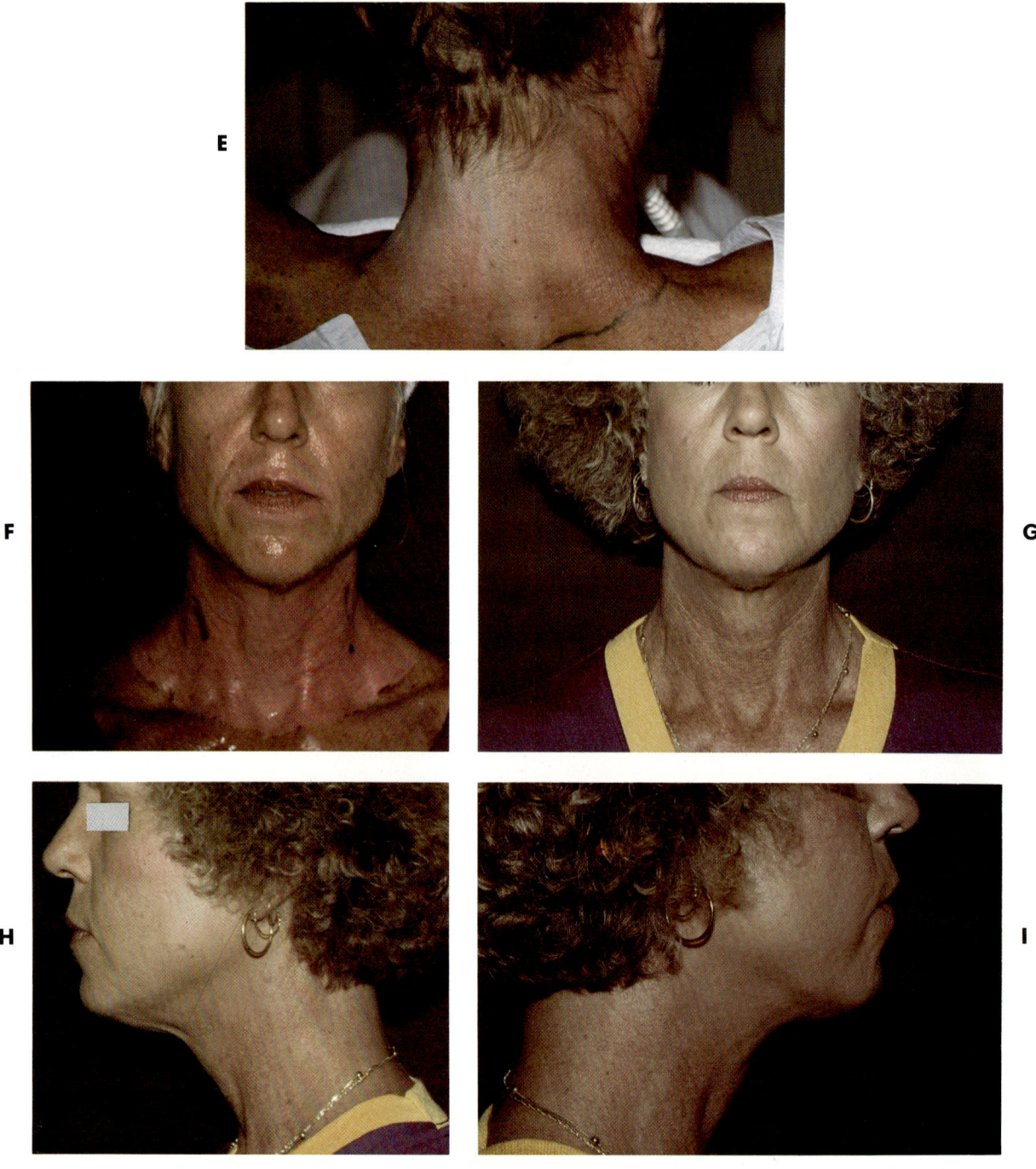

Case 1, cont'd. E, The patient is shown prepared for the neck peel. Note the designated limit of application. **F,** 50% TCA was applied to the anterior portion of the neck and was continued to encompass the entire posterior neck. **G to I,** The patient is shown 2 years after the neck peeling procedure. The contrast between face and neck has been improved. It should be noted, however, that some repigmentation of both the face and the neck has occurred. **G,** Frontal view; **H,** left lateral view; **I,** right lateral view.

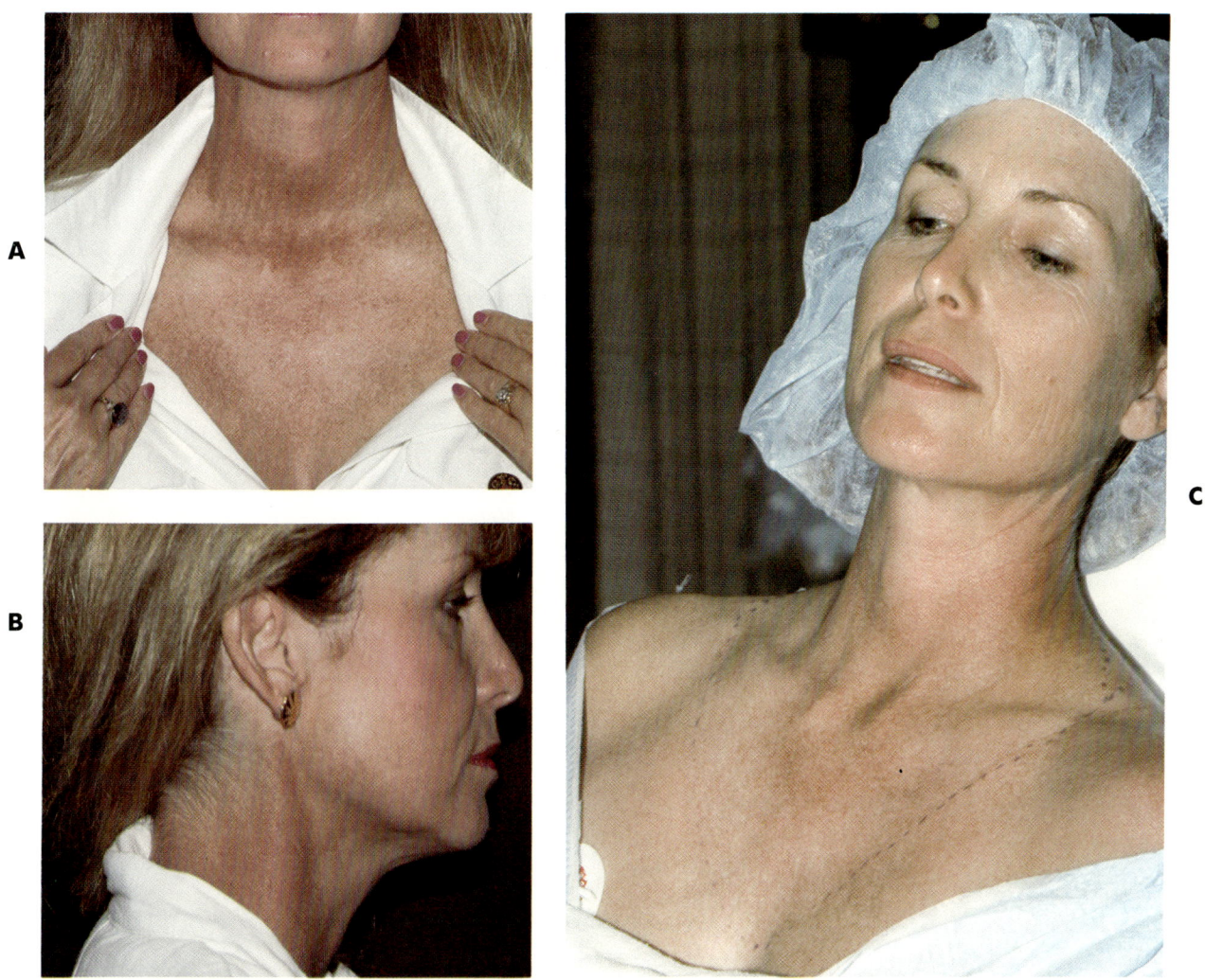

Case 2: Face, neck, and chest peeling. A to C, Pretreatment views. *Continued.*

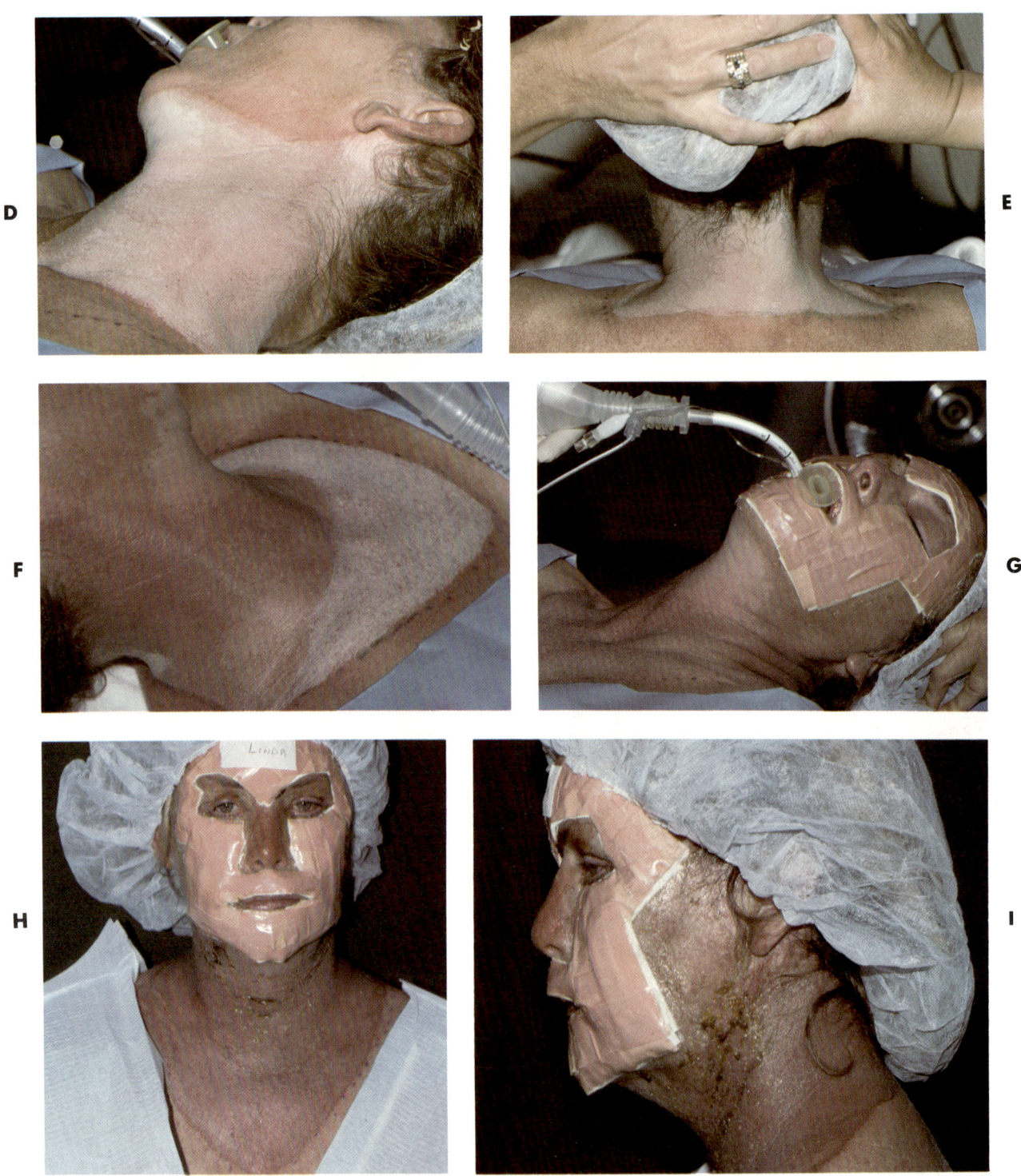

Case 2, cont'd. D and **E**, The neck was peeled with 50% TCA and the peel was extended completely around to the posterior neck. In combined procedures, the neck may be peeled during the intervals between applications of phenol peeling solution to the face. **F**, The upper chest was peeled with 35% TCA. **G**, At the conclusion of the face, neck, and chest peels only the face is occluded with tape. Our practice is not to tape the neck or chest. **H** and **I**, The patient is prepared for mask removal 48 hours postpeel. The name tag was placed on the patient's forehead since on the day of her procedure three occluded full face peels were performed and patient identification could conceivably be difficult.

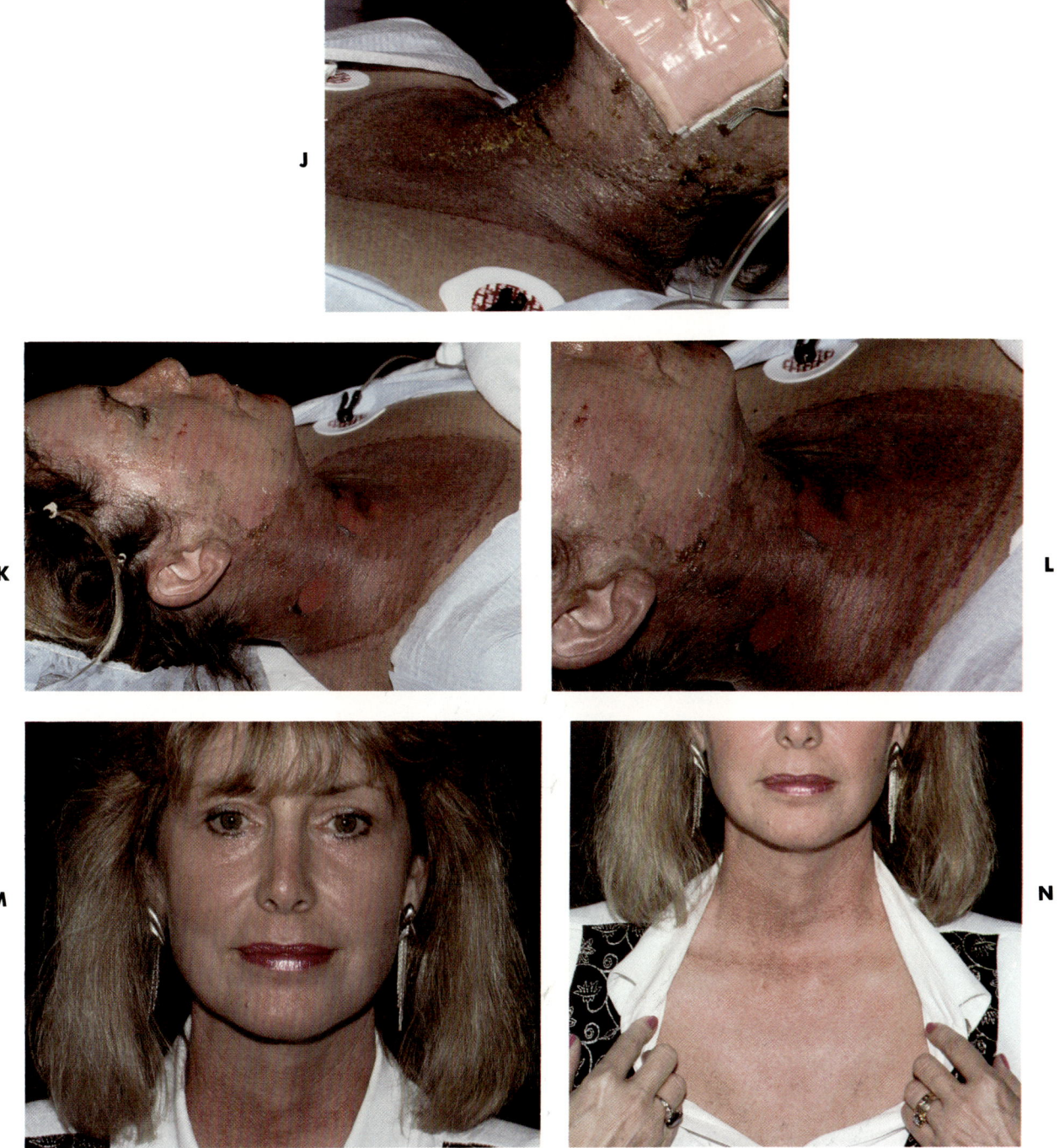

Case 2, cont'd. J, Note the gradation of skin necrosis between the more aggressively treated neck (50% TCA) and the chest (35% TCA). **K,** After mask removal from the face, the sloughed epidermis is removed from the neck. **L,** Close-up view of **K. M** and **N,** At 5 months postpeel, however, there is some unevenness in the color of the neck and chest, although there has been a significant improvement when compared with the pretreatment appearance.

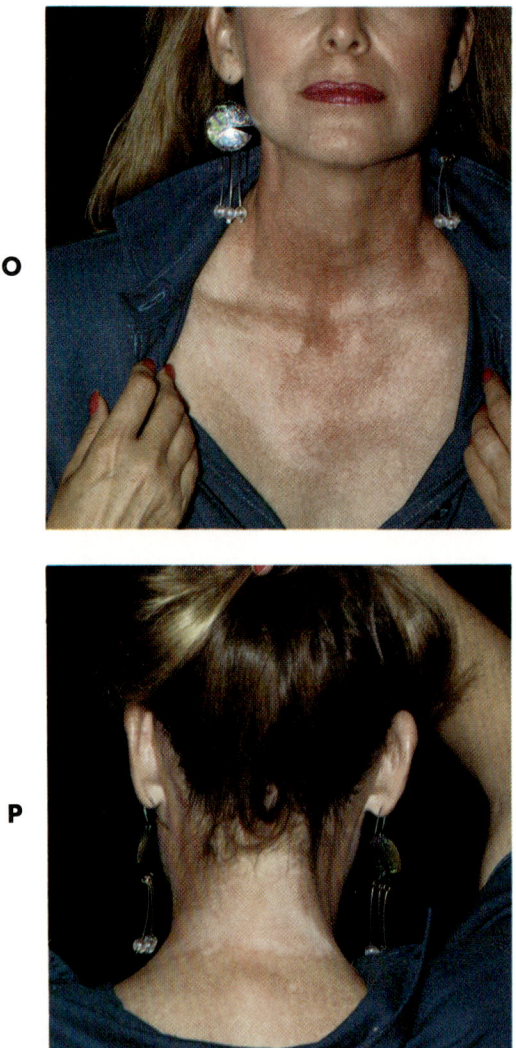

Case 2, cont'd. O, At 7 months after treatment there is still some inconsistency in the lightening effect of the peel both on the neck and on the chest. **P,** The posterior neck shows an area of marked hypopigmentation of unexplained origin, since a review of the intraoperative photographs shows homogenous application of the peel solution to the area.

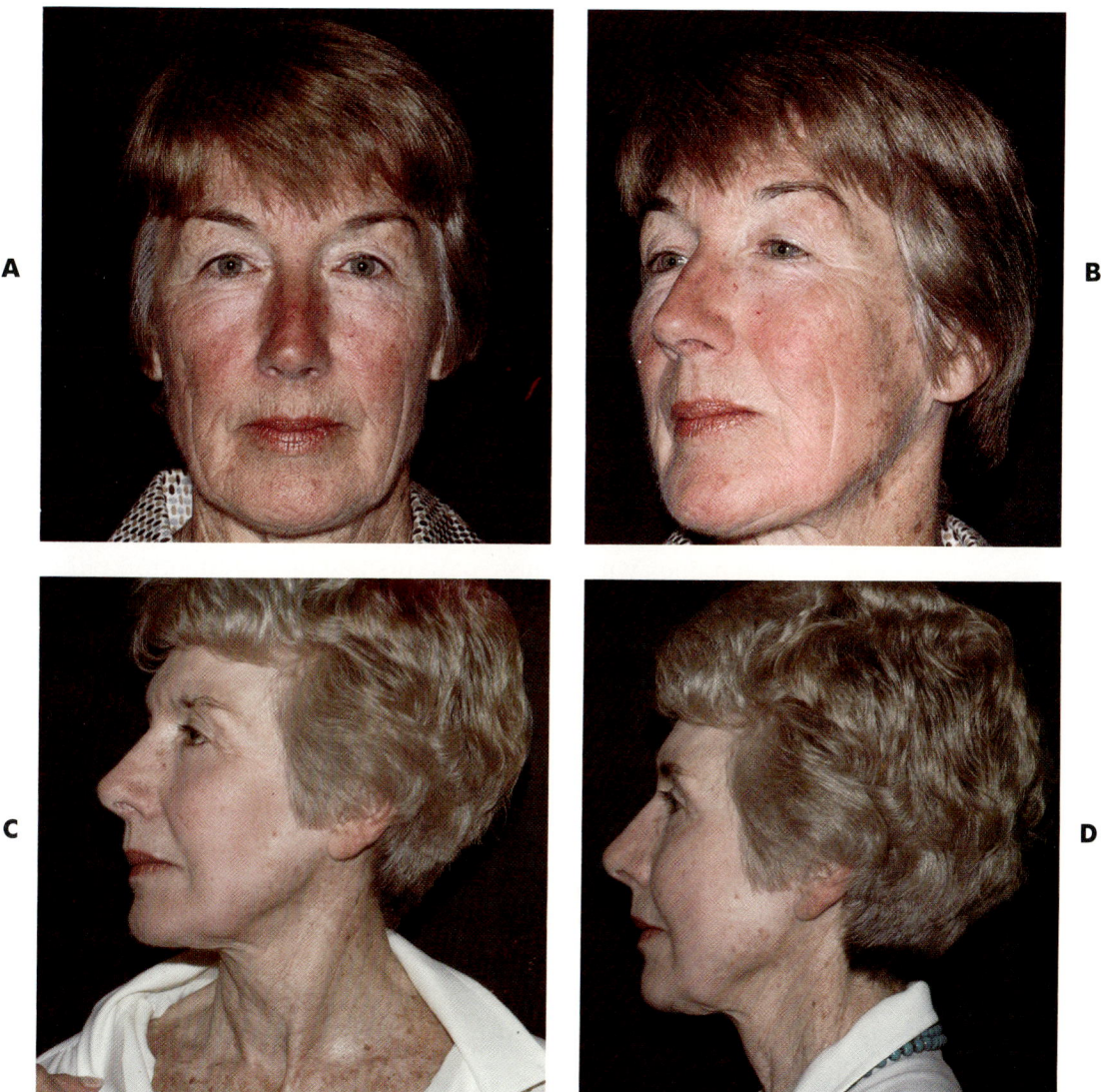

Case 3: Face and neck peeling. The patient is shown here before (**A** and **B**) and 7 years after (**C** and **D**) a combined face and neck peel. She was treated with an occluded Baker formula phenol solution on the face and 50% TCA on the neck. Good lightening was achieved with no short- or long-term complications. In C, note the contrast, however, between the treated face (occluded, Baker's solution) and neck (unoccluded, 50% TCA) and the untreated chest. A prospective patient in whom a distinct color difference between treated and untreated areas is likely to occur must be informed of this potentially unsatisfactory outcome. Such a patient should be given the option of a neck and/or chest peel to complement the primary peel. Photo examples of such color contrasts can be helpful as communication tools.

CHAPTER ELEVEN

Facial Peeling in Men

Facial peeling presents a much greater challenge in male patients than it does with female patients because of the unlikelihood that a man will wear camouflage makeup to conceal any resulting disparity in color between the treated and the untreated areas. In my experience, while male skin tends to wrinkle less prematurely than that of female patients, male wrinkling is often secondary to prolonged sun exposure with attendant sun-induced hyperpigmentation. While the peeling process can be expected to remove the wrinkles successfully, an undesired byproduct of the procedure will be some depigmentation of the skin in the treated area, which can range from mild to significant. One must then weigh the benefits of the procedure versus the generally unacceptable consequences.

Regional (i.e., not the entire face) peels are always fraught with concern over the potential color difference between treated and untreated areas, and this is particularly so when performed in men. With full-face peels, often the contrast between an aggressively treated face and an untreated neck is so profound that the resulting unnatural appearance is totally unsatisfactory to the male patient. Each case must be managed on its own merits; however, I would caution the neophyte practitioner to be extremely careful in selecting male patients for this procedure.

CASE PRESENTATIONS: FACIAL PEELING IN MEN

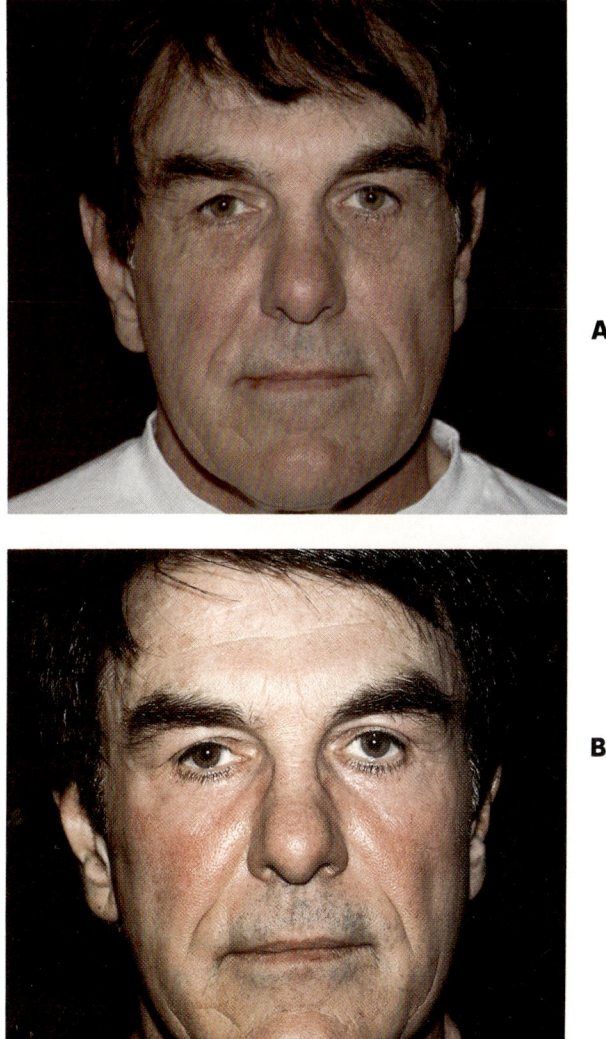

Case 1: The challenge of male peeling. A, This patient (shown before treatment) requested a lower-lid peel for the crepe-like appearance and spotted pigmentation found in this area. Note the asymmetric excessive skin of the upper eyelids. Regional peeling is always a challenge because of the potential for obvious color differences between the treated and the untreated areas, and this is a particular concern with peeling in men, who generally do not have the option of wearing camouflage makeup. In this case the view 5 months after peel **(B)** shows a very satisfactory color match between the treated area of the lower lids and the untreated face.

Continued.

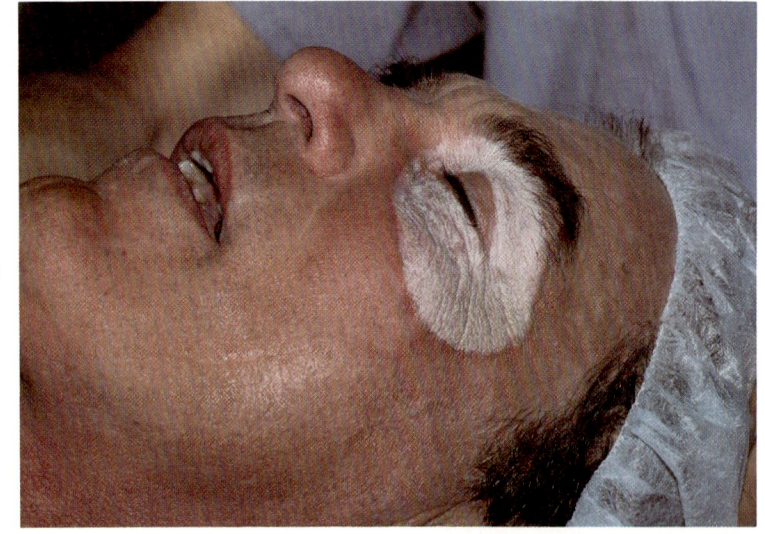

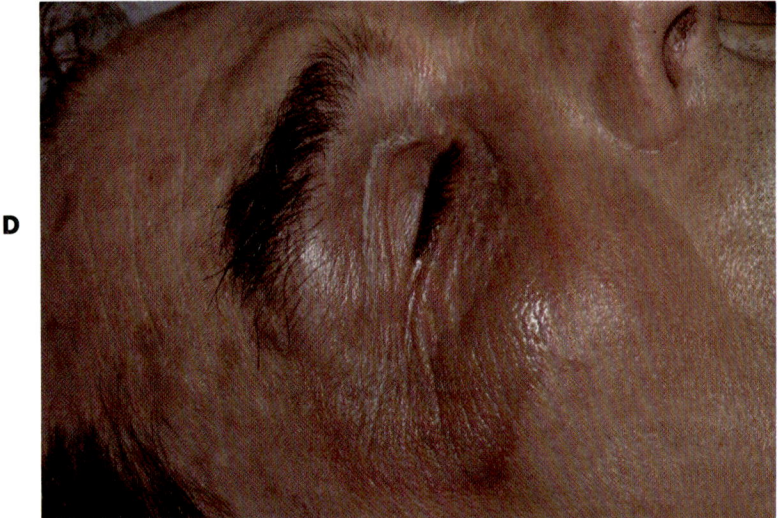

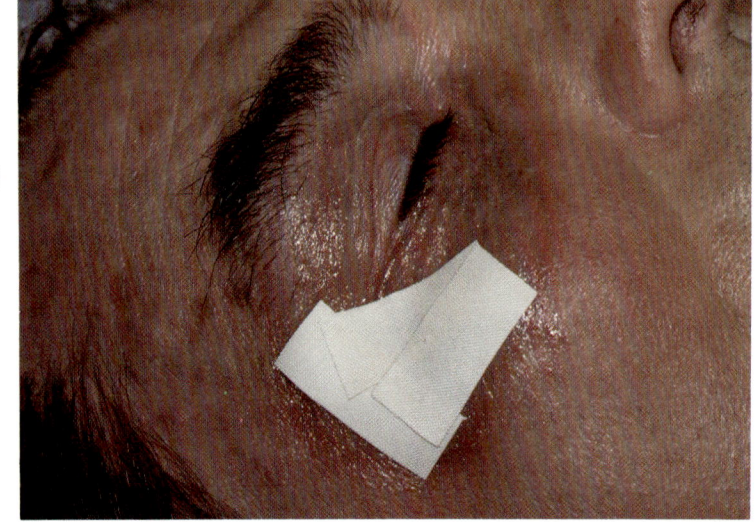

Case 1, cont'd. C and **D,** The technique used in this case included application of Baker formula phenol solution to the infrabrow and lower orbital areas. Note that the upper eyelid skin itself is not peeled but that application of solution to the infrabrow is carried inferiorly to the supratarsal crease. **E,** After application of the peeling agent, Salonpas is applied as the first occlusive layer and secured with rubber cement.

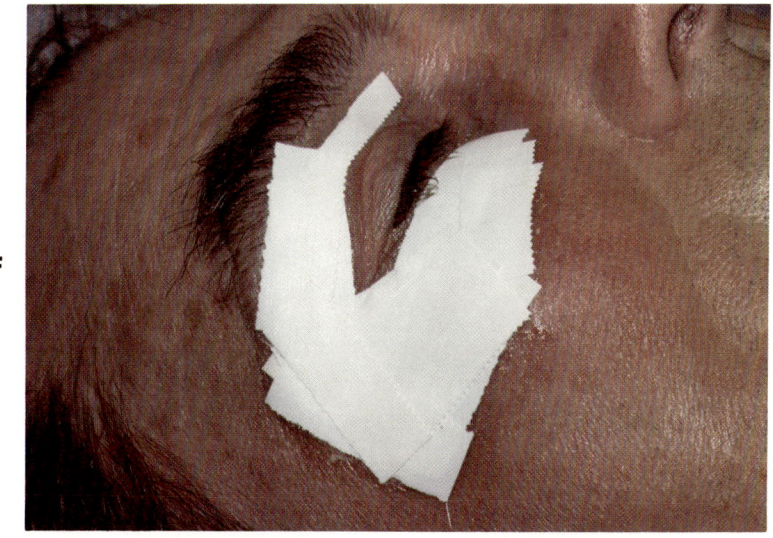

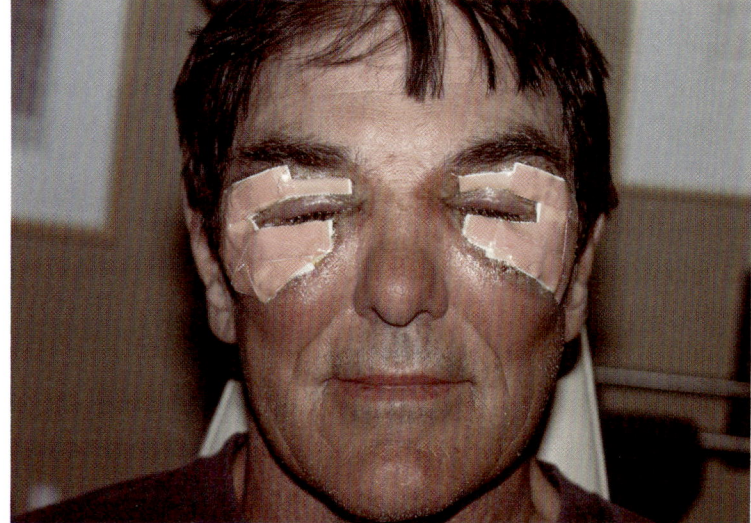

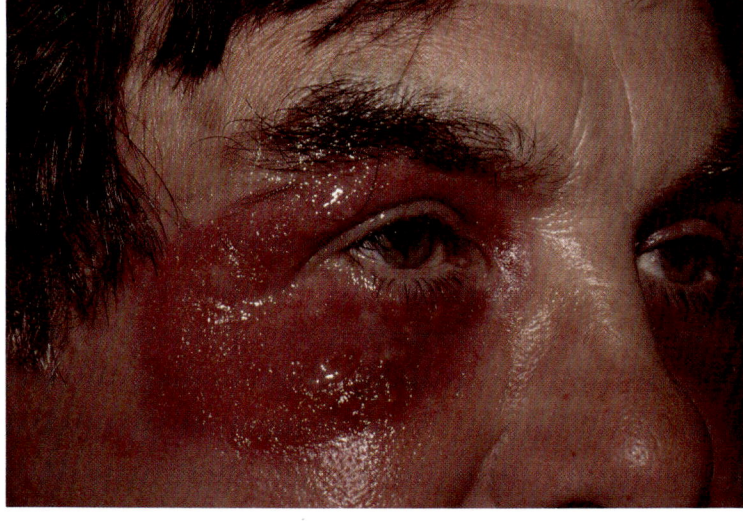

Case 1, cont'd. F, Waterproof tapes then are applied to the entire treated area. G, The patient's appearance 24 hours later shows some swelling of the eyelids, which is normal. H, The view 5 days after peel with the tapes removed shows that the swelling has abated.

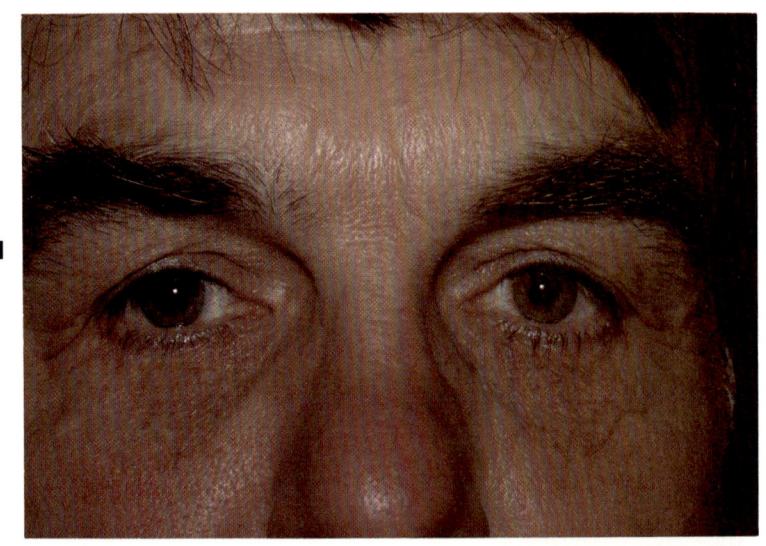

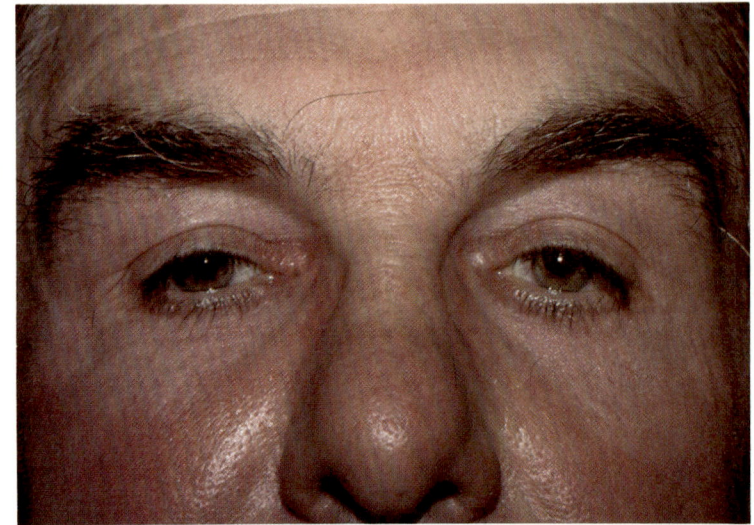

Case 1, cont'd. I and J, Comparison of before- and after-treatment views shows that the skin is slightly lighter in the peeled area, but this is not unacceptable to the viewing eye inasmuch as the skin of the lower lid tends to be lighter than the skin of the remaining face in many persons. The importance of observing anatomic boundaries during the application of peeling solution is, therefore, obvious. As a result of the peel there has been a significant improvement in the upper eyelid dermatochalasis, as well as the removal of the lower medial eyelid pigmentation. *Continued.*

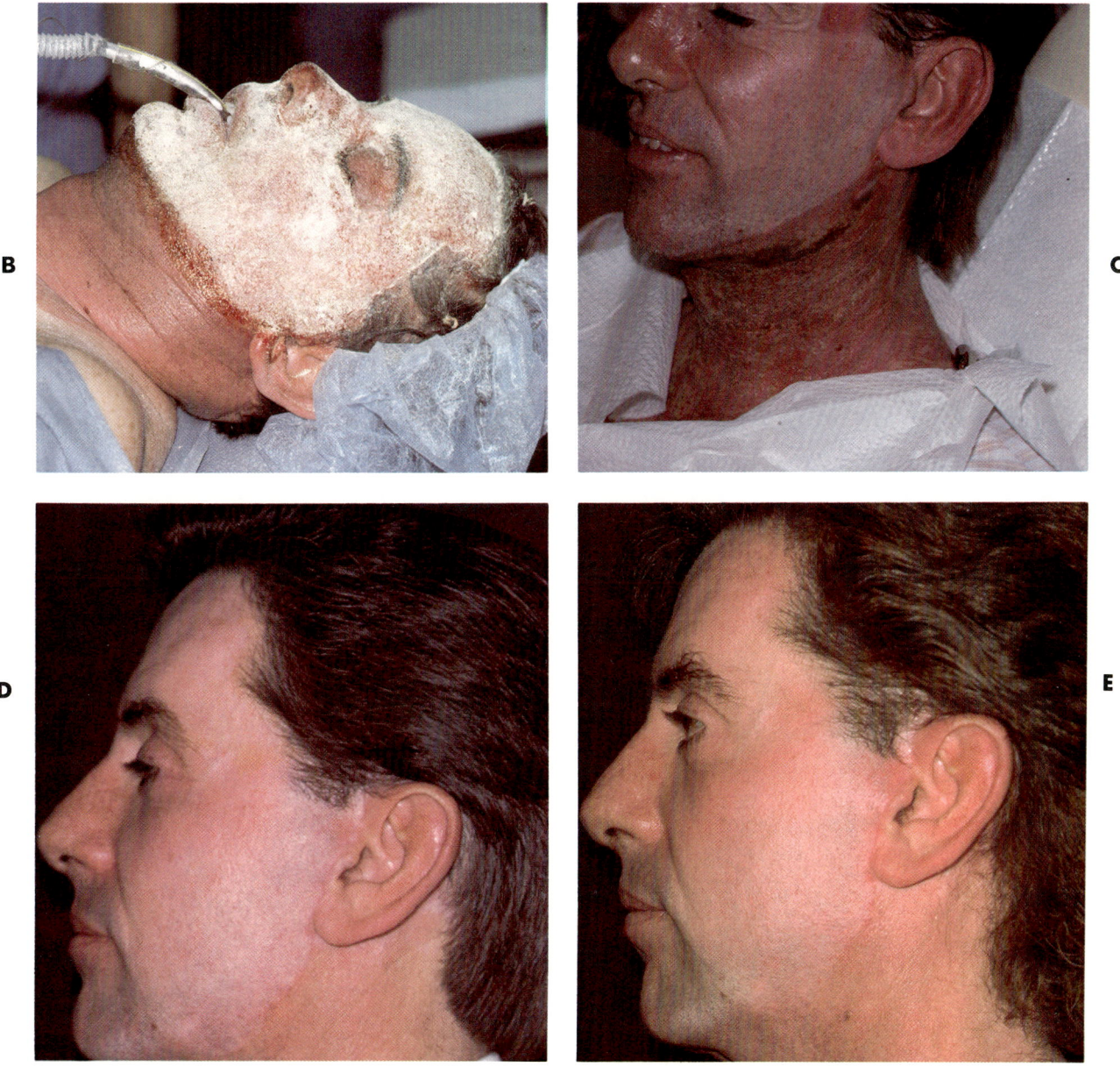

Case 2, cont'd. B, During the first procedure, in an effort to avoid an obvious color difference between the face and neck, the face was peeled with Baker formula phenol peeling solution and occluded while the neck was concomitantly peeled with 50% TCA. **C,** A noticeable color difference resulted nonetheless. **D,** A second neck peeling procedure was performed with 50% TCA again. Focal areas of the face were also retreated at that time with a phenol peeling solution to obtain a more even color. **E,** Despite these efforts, a marked color difference between face and neck persisted.

CHAPTER TWELVE
Technique: Step-by-Step

FACIAL PEELING IN MEN   199

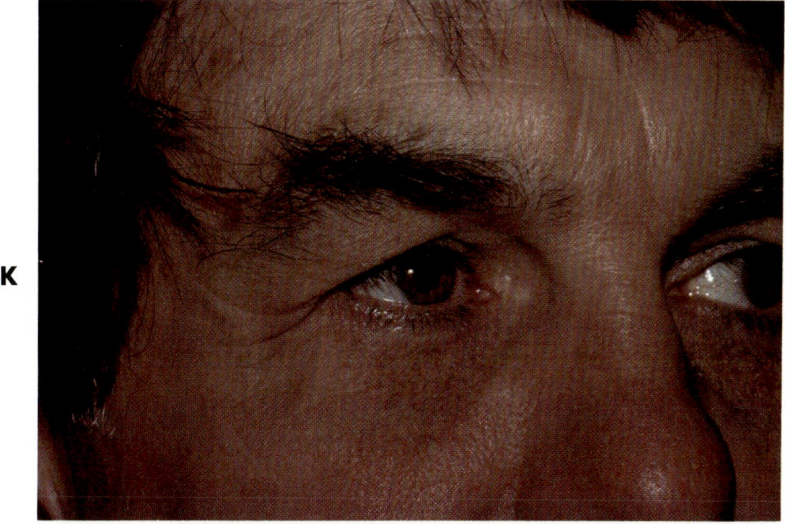

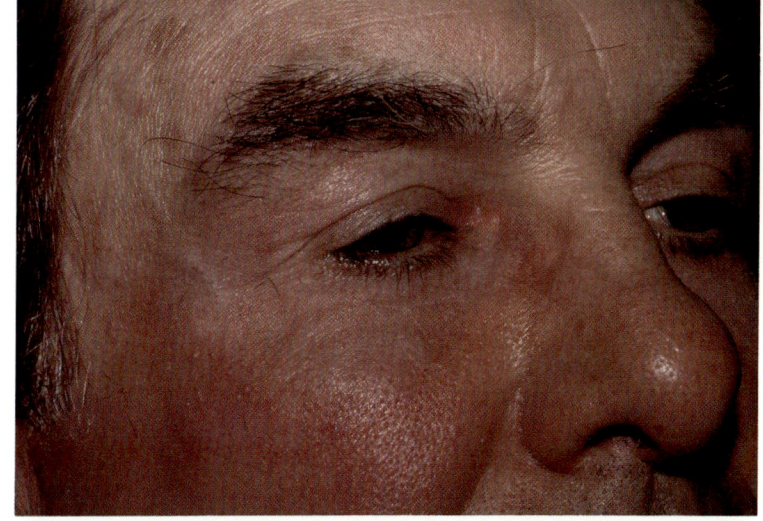

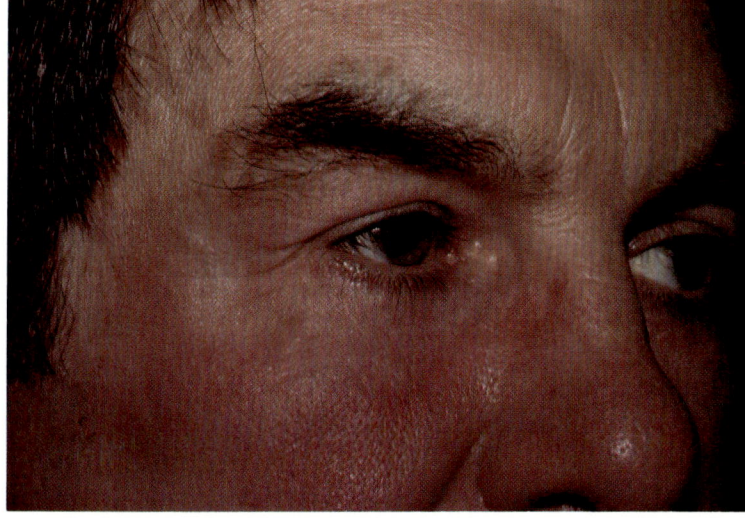

Case 1, cont'd. K, Pretreatment view. **L,** Note the development of several milia over the right malar eminence. A typical time interval for development of milia is 3 to 4 months after peel. **M,** A postpeel view at 5 months shows excellent healing after removal of the milia and a very satisfactory color match between the treated and untreated areas.

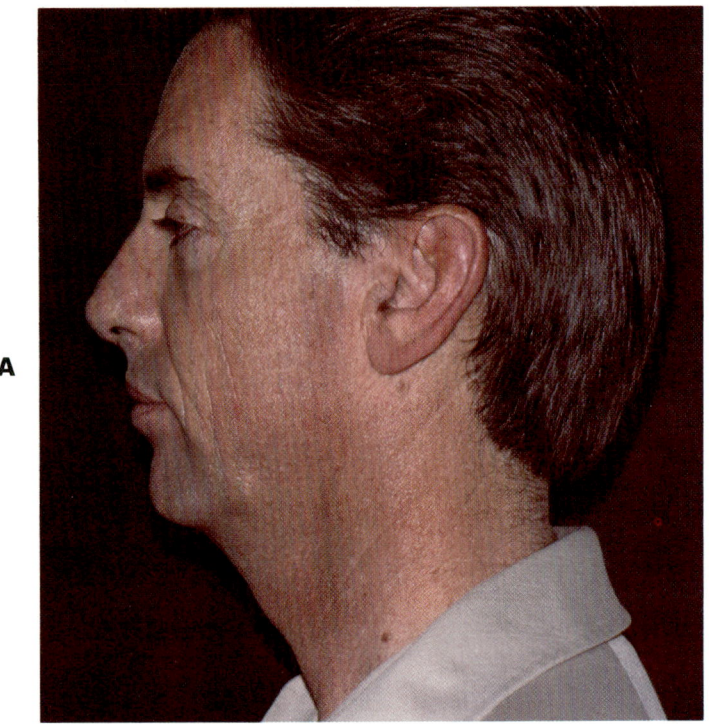

Case 2: Difficulties of male peeling—marked color difference. This case illustrates the great difficulty of using a phenol-based peeling agent for peeling the face of men. **A,** Pretreatment view. The patient certainly had the indications for a phenol peel, with prematurely wrinkled and sun-damaged skin. Anticipating a disparity in color between a treated face and an untreated neck, we chose to perform a 50% TCA peel to the neck at the same time as the face was treated with a phenol peel. Unfortunately, a significant color disparity did result, despite our best efforts to avoid it by peeling both face and neck. We therefore peeled the neck a second time with 50% TCA but achieved only a slight improvement in the color distinction between face and neck. Because of the difficulty in avoiding a noticeable color difference between an aggressively treated face and an untreated or lesser-treated neck, I would caution the neophyte practitioner to be extremely careful in selecting a man for a phenol face peel.

TECHNIQUE: STEP-BY-STEP

PREPARATION BEFORE PROCEDURE; APPLICATION OF PEELING AGENT AND OCCLUSIVE DRESSINGS

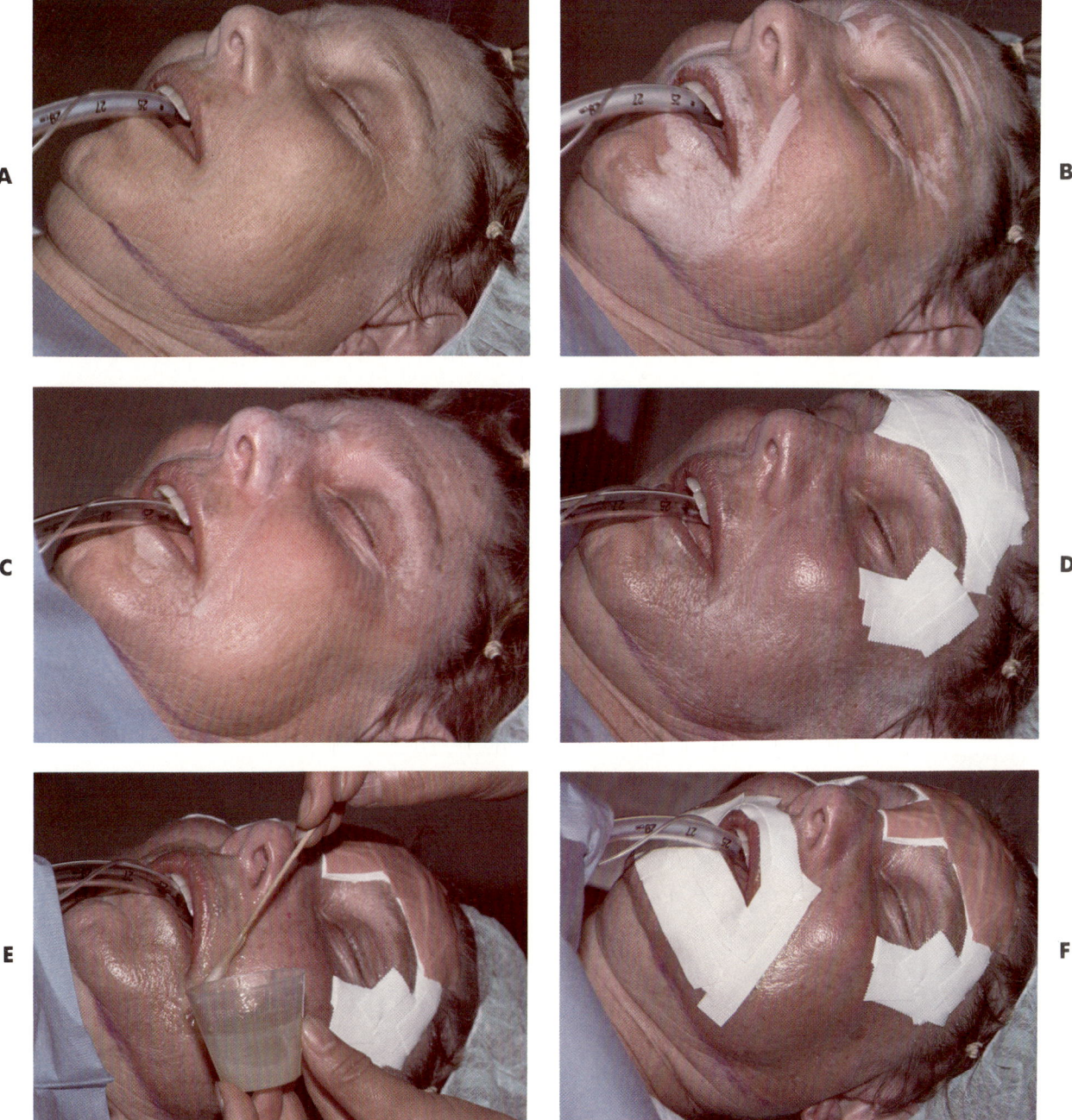

Preprocedure preparation. A, Patient under general endotracheal anesthesia is prepared for the procedure. **B,** Areas of deepest wrinkling are pretreated with 50% TCA.

Application of peeling agent and occlusive dressings. C, Phenol-based peeling solution is applied to the forehead, nose, and periorbital areas. Note the fading of frost where the 50% TCA has been applied. **D,** After application of the peeling solution, Salonpas tape is applied to the forehead and crow's-feet areas. **E,** Rubber cement is applied to the perioral area before placement of Salonpas dressings. **F,** Salonpas dressings are in place about the mouth.

MASK REMOVAL

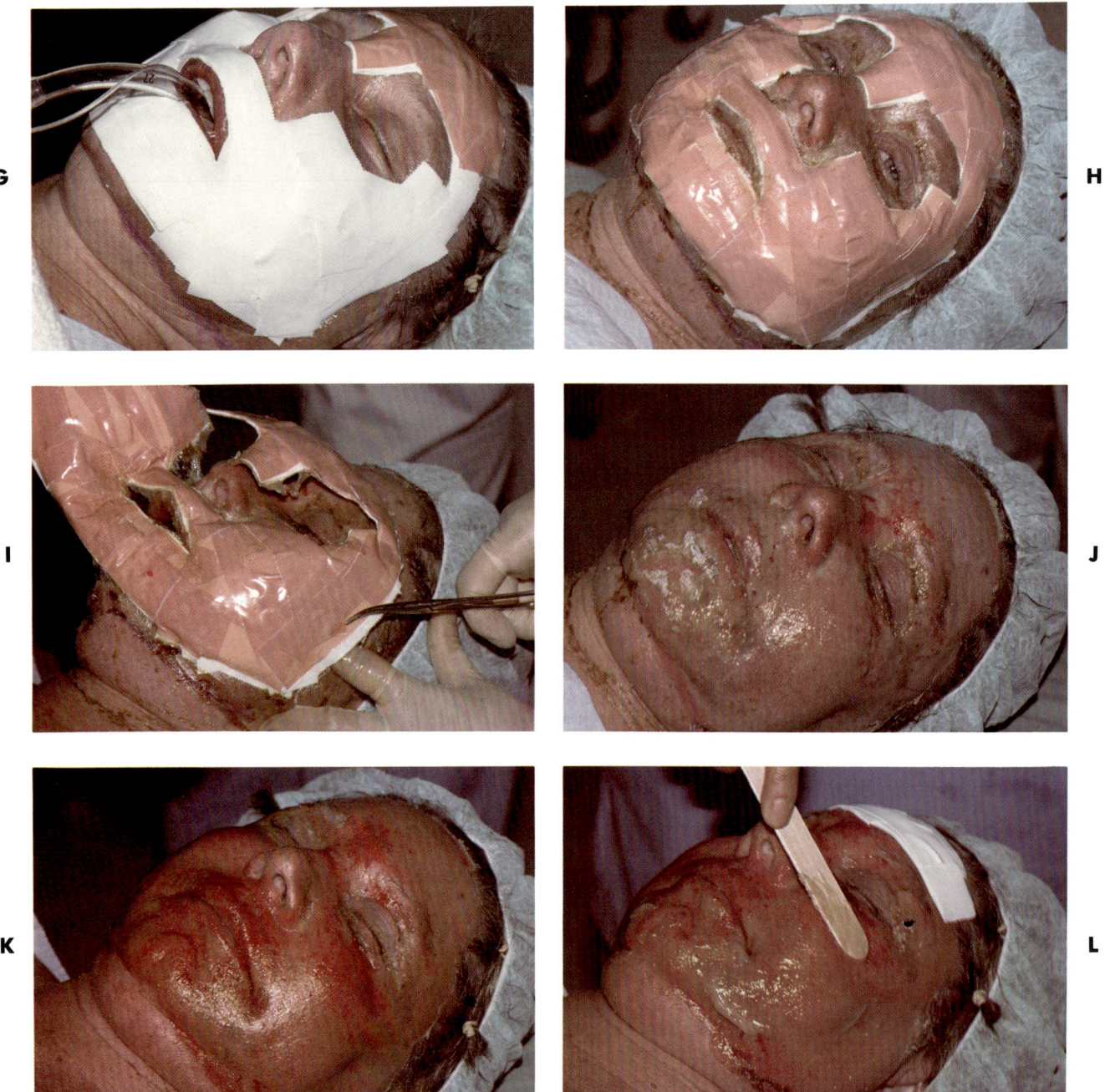

Mask removal. G, The occlusive mask is completed over the remainder of the face with white waterproof tape covered with Hytape. **H,** The patient returns for mask removal 48 hours after peel. **I,** The mask is gently lifted off the face, revealing **(J)** a raw and unreepithelialized skin surface, which requires tidying and drying **(K).**

Retaping deeply wrinkled areas. L, For maximum peeling effect, deeply wrinkled areas may require retaping after mask removal. In this case the forehead is retaped with waterproof tapes secured with rubber cement. Polysporin ointment is then applied to the remainder of the face.

POSTPEEL FOLLOW-UP

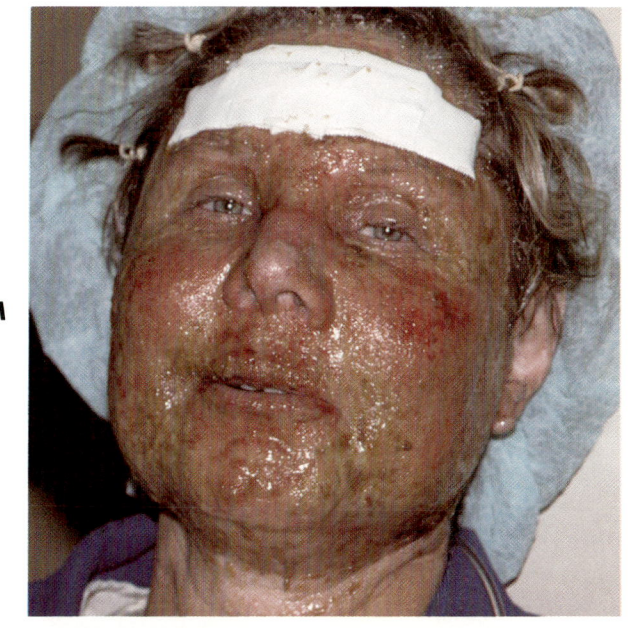

M

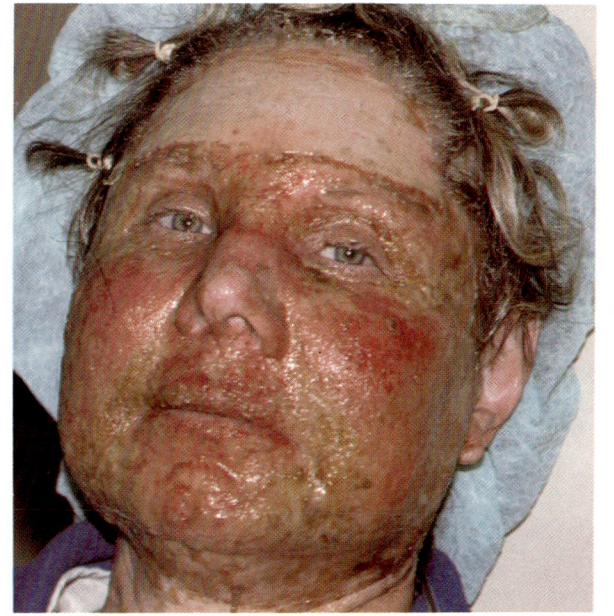

N

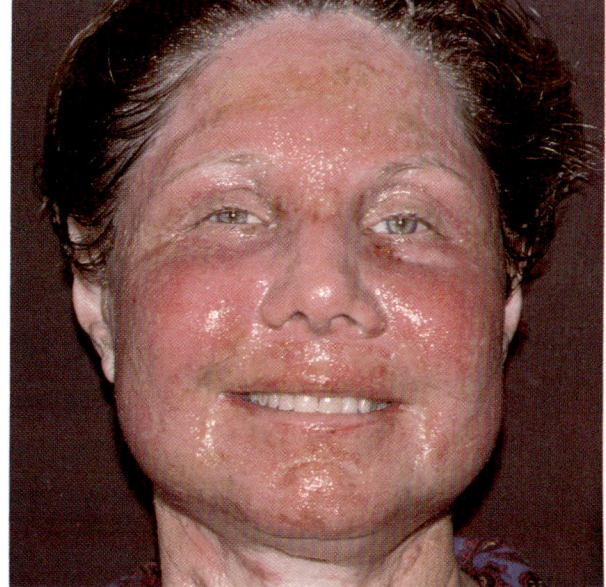

O

Postpeel follow-up. M and **N,** The forehead tape is removed 1 day later, 3 days after peel. **O,** The patient exhibits a happy face at the 1-week visit, in this case 6 days after peel and 3 days after removal of the forehead tape. Close-up views of the forehead **(P),** orbital area **(Q),** oblique right **(R)** and oblique left **(S)** orbitomalar areas, oblique left cheek **(T),** and perioral area and chin **(U)** show typical appearance of successfully peeled skin at this stage. Some reepithelialization is still to take place.

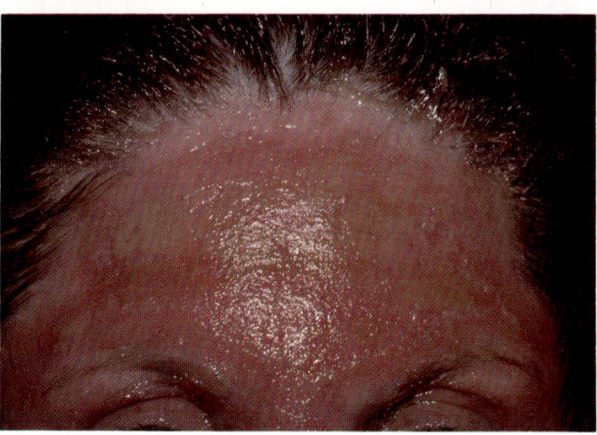

P

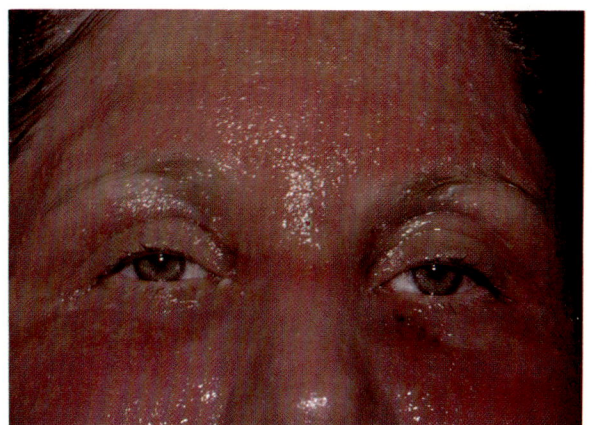

Q

POSTPEEL FOLLOW-UP

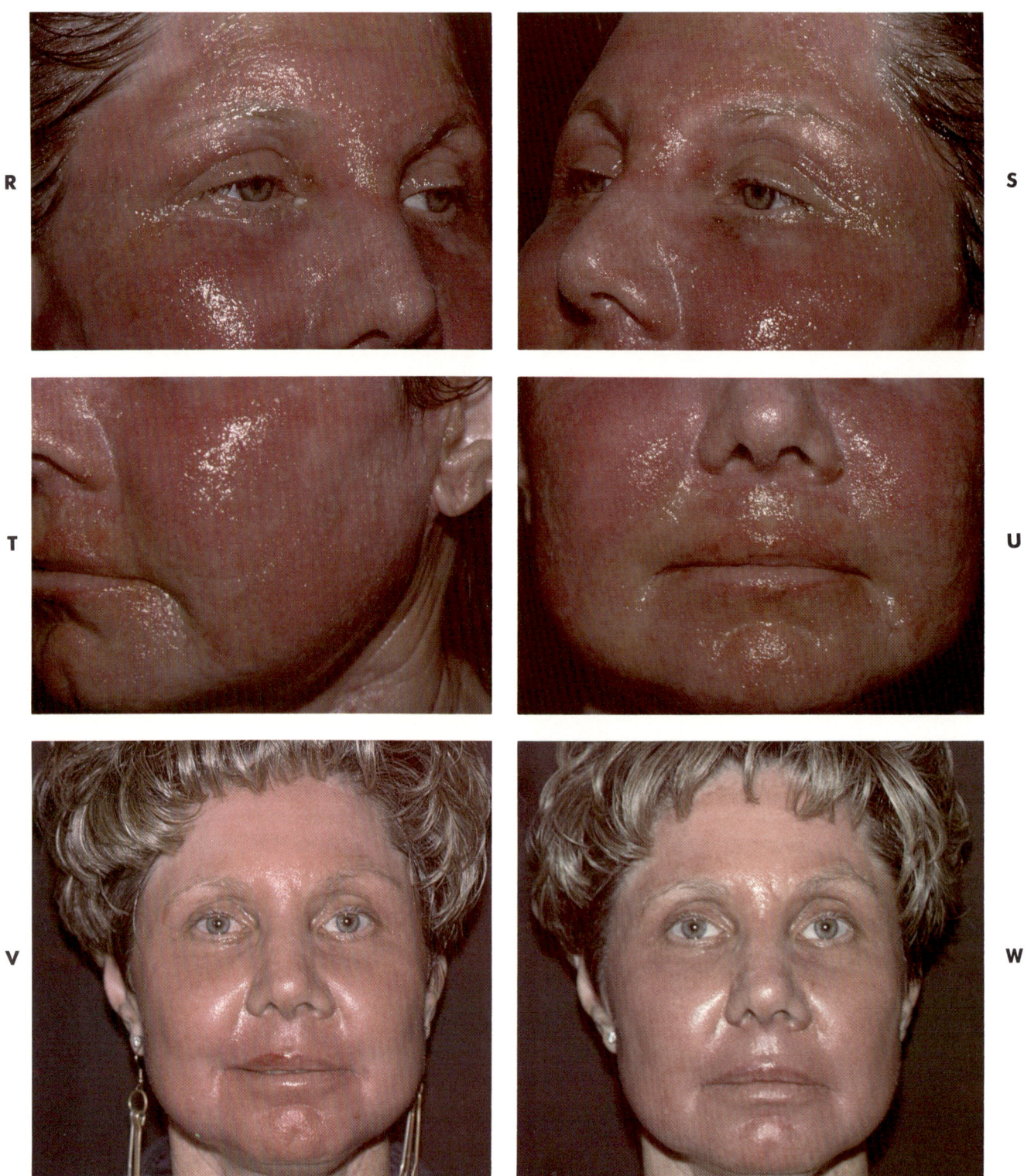

Postpeel follow-up, cont'd. The patient is seen here 13 days (**V**) and 24 days (**W**) after peel. The healing is proceeding smoothly and according to schedule, and the emerging results look very promising.

RESULTS AT 5 MONTHS

Before **After**

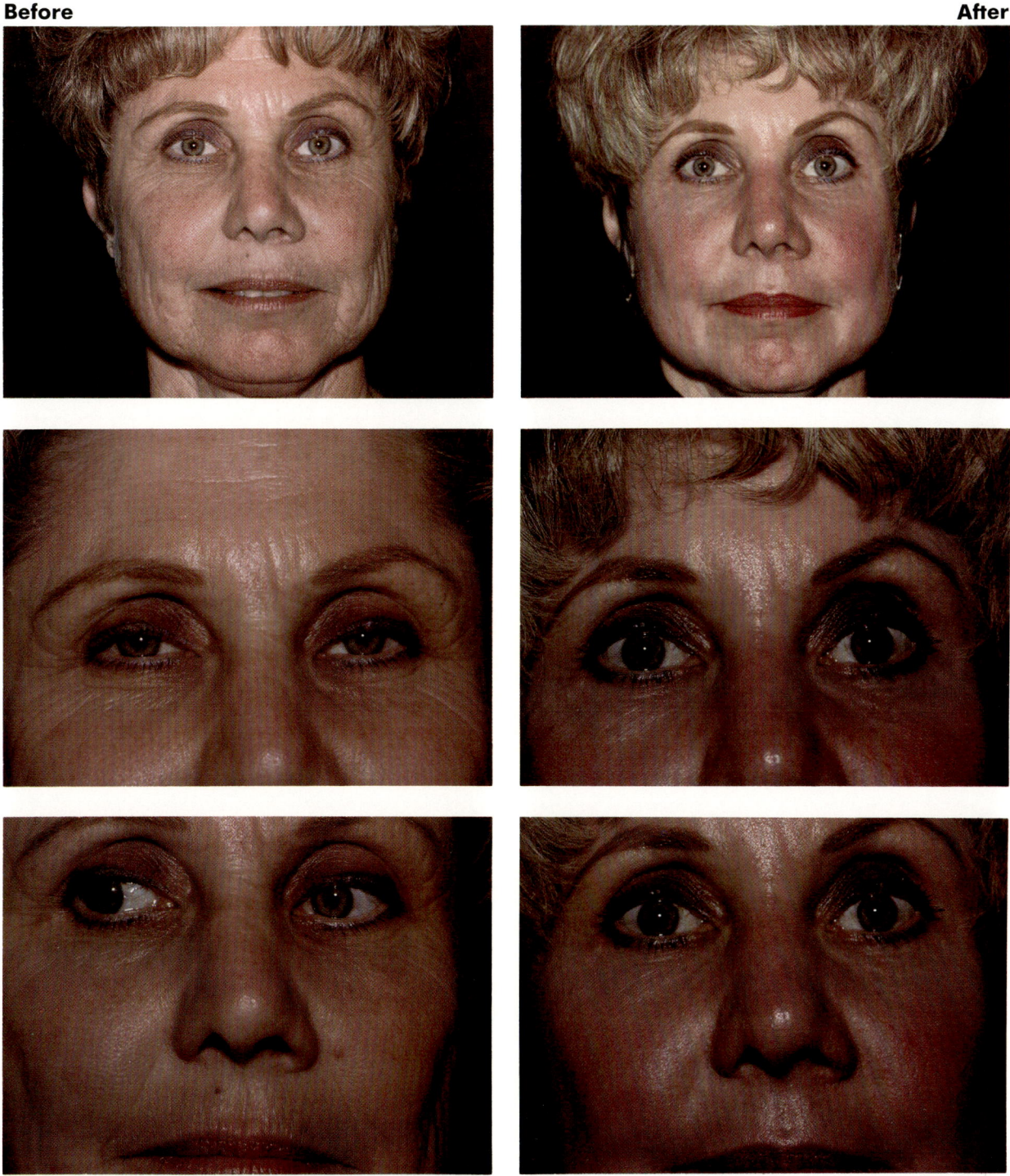

Results at 5 months. Views of the patient before treatment and 5 months after treatment show that good results have been obtained. The deep wrinkles of the forehead, crow's-feet, and periorbital area have been successfully removed with occlusion.

208 CHEMICAL REJUVENATION OF THE FACE

RESULTS AT 5 MONTHS

Before · After

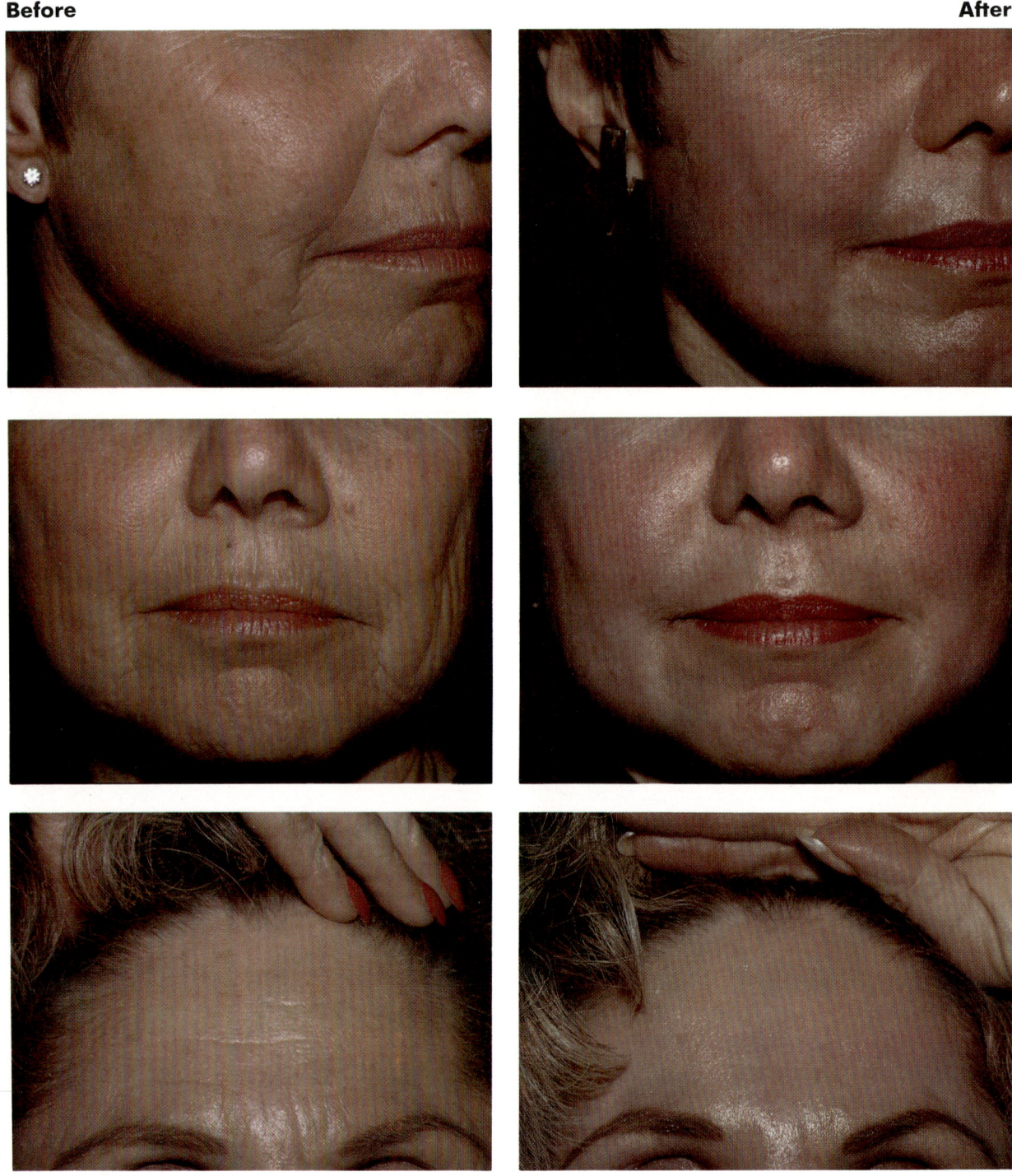

LONG-TERM RESULTS

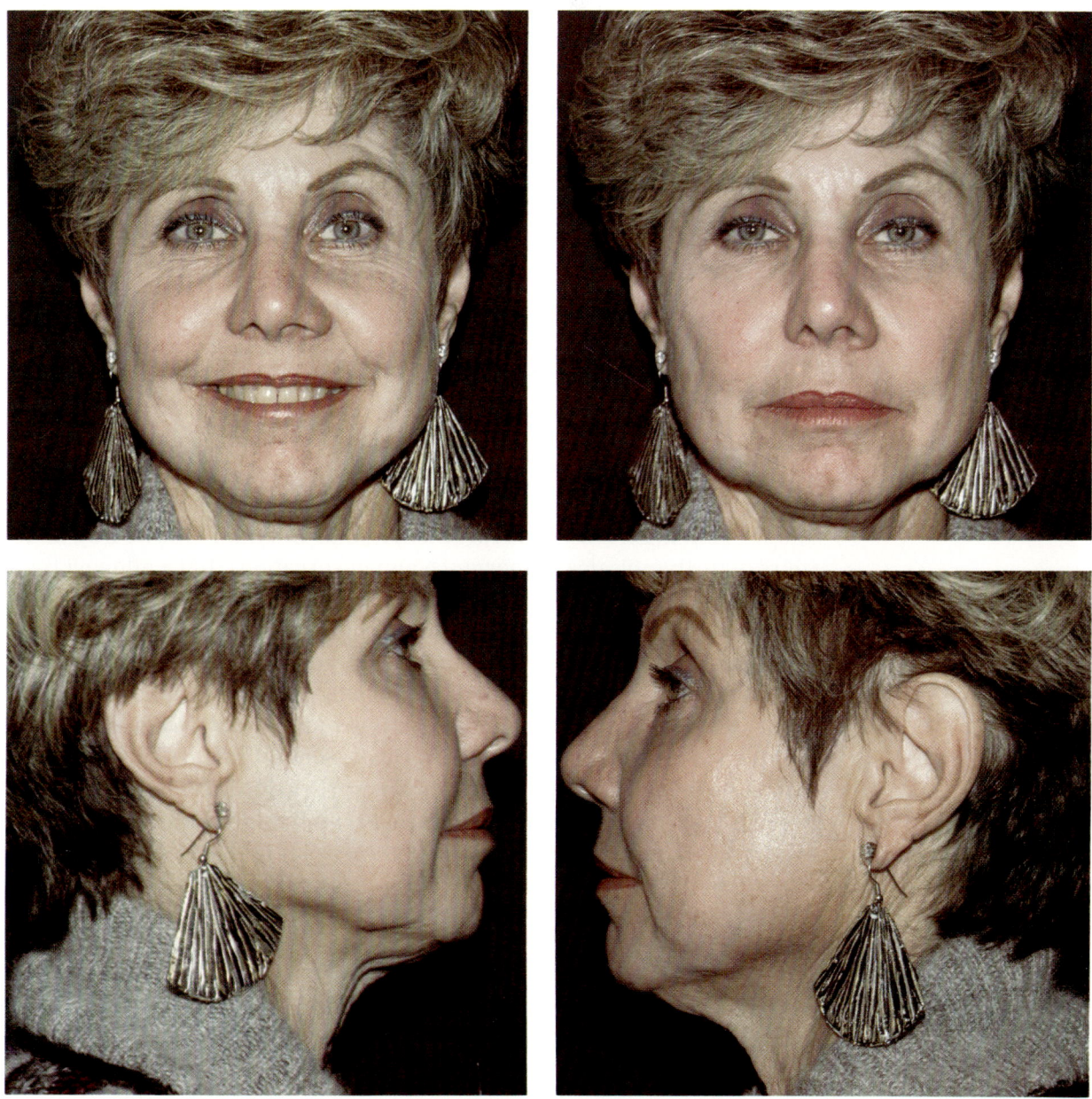

Long-term results. The final result is shown here 15 months after peel. Note the reasonable transition between treated face and untreated neck on the profile views. Cervical facial rhytidectomy is now indicated.

A Discussion with Thomas J. Baker, M.D.

No review of the subject of chemical skin peeling can be conducted without the recognition of and appreciation for the contribution of Thomas J. Baker, M.D., and his long-time associate, Howard Gordon, M.D. These men were visionaries in seeing the place for chemical skin peeling within the armamentarium of the cosmetic surgeon. Their initial clinical evaluations, followed by their laboratory and histologic evaluations of chemical skin peeling, and then followed by many years of further clinical experience and observations, have allowed their successors to bring this remarkable procedure to patients with safety and predictability. To them, as to many of the other pioneers of this art, should go the deep respect and appreciation of all current practitioners.

Recognizing the important contributions that Dr. Baker has made to the art and science of chemical skin peeling and wishing to draw on all his experience for the benefit of our readers, I asked Dr. Baker if he would participate in a question and answer session with me that would, hopefully, allow the reader of this book and student of the technique even greater insight into subtleties of this remarkable procedure.

This interview was conducted in September, 1990.

KOTLER: Dr. Baker, how did you become interested in chemical skin peeling?

BAKER: We got into it because there were lay operators here in Miami who were doing it when I came to town and we didn't know what they were doing. I went out and visited them and they showed me before and after pictures, but they were not informative.

We put two and two together. We saw the phenol, we dug out the literature, found out that people had used phenol peelings way back when, but not for rejuvenation—mostly for acne and other indications.

And then we checked out TCA and alpha-hydroxy acid and by talking to some of these lay operators, we finally came up with a solution that we experimented with and found the one that we are now using with the croton oil and the soap.

The first case we did was on a nurse that worked at our hospital—actually the first case I did was on my own forearm.

And then I did the forehead on a patient on whom I had done a facelift, a very elderly lady. I later did the rest of her face. That was my very first case of total peel.

Then one of the workers at the hospital said how great that lady looked and she wanted it done, so she was my second case. I have followed her for over 20 years.

KOTLER: Was the croton oil one of the ingredients the lay operators were using?

BAKER: Well, we do not know for sure. One of the employees told us that. We find that you can do peeling without the croton oil, but you get a little bit more penetration, a little more irritation with the croton oil.

KOTLER: What about the soap?

BAKER: We started using phenol and we knew it was buffered with something, so we assumed soap was a good thing, so we started using it with the soap.

KOTLER: What were your early major dissatisfactions?

BAKER: The major dissatisfaction? Early on, we did not know enough about the skin peel. We did not know what the long-term follow-up would be—we did not know what these people were going to look like. In the first article we said this might even be carcinogenic.

Perhaps it might make the skin too thin—this, that and the other, but it did not turn out to be that way.

We were very selective in patients and I did only a few and then the thing kind of caught fire, people started sending us patients from all over.

Unfortunately, we found out later on, we probably did a lot of people that now we would not do because of skin types. We now have a bit better knowledge.

KOTLER: Could you give us your "top" pearls?

BAKER: The top pearls? I think the number one, of course, is patient selection, like any plastic surgery procedure. We try to get the fair-skinned individual, although we do quite a few patients who are darker complexioned, we see patients who come to us with preexisting pigmentation problems.

The fair-skinned individuals are the best. It works on anybody, but the worst line of demarcation you get are the patients who have freckled, ruddy complexions. It takes the freckles away.

KOTLER: Would you peel a well-controlled diabetic?

BAKER: Yes.

KOTLER: Would you peel a patient with previous radiation?

BAKER: I have peeled patients with radiation and I would use the same criteria that I would use to decide if I were going to do a surgical procedure, or particularly a dermabrasion. I do not know how many patients we have done with radiation damage, but it is quite a few and we never had a problem.

KOTLER: There was a paper by Dr. Wolfe that reported much slower healing in a patient who had a large dose of radiation around the mouth and chin for carcinoma.

BAKER: I would expect slower healing. But they can still be peeled.

KOTLER: Would you peel a patient with eczema?

BAKER: I would be reluctant to do that. As far as major collagen disease, such as scleroderma, no. But if it is very mild, such as arthritis only, I would not hesitate to do that. If it were scleroderma, no.

KOTLER: Do you peel for dark circles under the eyes?

BAKER: Yes, we do it for that although now we are using TCA but if the circles are really dark, we will use the phenol peel and not tape them. That skin will bleach.

KOTLER: Do you find that there is some percentage of recurrence of the darkness?

BAKER: Yes. It is worth a try and sometimes you get very dramatic results. But I tell the patient this may not work.

KOTLER: One question apropos of that. Patients of Middle Eastern ancestry typically have this problem. Would you be as apt to do it in that patient as a very fair-skinned Northern European ancestored person, who just happens to have the dark circles?

BAKER: I prefer the patient of Northern European ancestry with darkness rather than the Mediterranean patient because pigmentation problems are more likely to occur with the latter.

KOTLER: Do you do face peeling for males?

BAKER: I do not do it at all. We have done it but males tend to have very oily skin. If you use a mask, the beard pushes the tape off after the first day anyway.

KOTLER: I have been very unhappy with a couple of cases because of the color difference.

BAKER: Yes. And I just do not have good luck with men, and I just finally said I am not going to do them anymore.

KOTLER: Management of the nonideal candidate?

BAKER: TCA peeling rather than phenol. We are using now 20%, 30%, and 35% TCA and in some cases 50% TCA. I still think that the phenol peel in our hands, around the mouth and in certain areas, is better and it's dependable.

KOTLER: What about peels in individuals of other ethnic origins, such as Asian, American Indian, or African-American?

BAKER: We do peel Asian patients. I have never peeled an American Indian because I never had an individual of this background request it. I would be very leery, for instance, of a South American person who has Indian blood. Peeling with phenol is simply contraindicated in black-skinned individuals, but TCA might be applicable.

KOTLER: Do you perform peels on Hispanic patients?

BAKER: I have done some. One of the best cases I have is in my book. She was a girl from Mexico who had hyperpigmentation from some bizarre peel. Our peel corrected this.

KOTLER: Is patch testing helpful?

BAKER: I do not do patch testing any more. I do not think it tells you anything.

KOTLER: Have you had cases where the results went contrary to the patch test?

BAKER: Well, if you are going to patch test, you going to patch test out on the face where it is going to be seen or up near the hairline. I do not think a patch test behind the ear where there is no exposure tells you anything. I do it if the patient requests it.

KOTLER: Could you describe your anesthesia technique?

BAKER: I start an IV on all patients. I usually use Versed and Demerol, or else Valium and Demerol.

I never use a general anesthetic. It is not necessary, but one thing we have found that helps us is if we do superorbital, infraorbital, and mandibular block along with the great auricular block. You can really make these people quite comfortable and we have been doing that routinely. We normally use Versed in the clinic because it is short acting, plus Demerol or another of the narcotics in place of Fentanyl because Fentanyl is short acting. You need a drug that is going to carry these people for 6 or 8 hours, such as Valium and Demerol.

KOTLER: Do you block with Marcaine for its longer duration?

BAKER: Yes.

KOTLER: Do you have the services of an anesthesiologist?

BAKER: Yes. We have an anesthesiologist working with us, but for years we did it ourselves.

KOTLER: What about anesthesia for the mask removal?

BAKER: I do not use any anesthesia for the dressing change.

KOTLER: Is cardiac arrhythmia a problem?

BAKER: We have never seen cardiac arrhythmias other than on an occasional PVC. I have those myself, so does my nurse, and so do a lot of patients. I do not think that if the peel is done slowly, over a couple of hours, that the phenol toxicity is important. I have never, in all the cases we have ever done, seen any evidence of systemic phenol toxicity whatsoever.

KOTLER: I think there is an unfounded fear of phenol in the medical community, particularly with respect to the arrhythmia issue.

BAKER: We calculated that we had used phenol in either total or partial procedures on over 5,000 patients. And we have never had a serious problem or had any systemic toxicity.

KOTLER: Could you discuss "to occlude or not to occlude"?

BAKER: As far as the Vaseline occlusion, we do use Vaseline most of the time now unless a person has really deep lines. If they are really deep ["corrugated cardboard"], we use the tape. Otherwise, we use just the Vaseline occlusive dressing but you could use an antibiotic ointment.
 Most of the peels we are doing now are without tape and the patients are more comfortable, plus you can see what is going on. I do think they reepithelialize quicker. There is a place for both.

KOTLER: Do you use Omniderm or other semipermeable dressings?

BAKER: I have had no experience with Omniderm or other semipermeable dressings, but I do not see any reason why you could not use them.

KOTLER: Do you have any caveats about repeeling?

BAKER: Patients who have been previously peeled—just like doing repeated dermabrasions—you have to use good judgment. We have repeeled patients or spot peeled them a number of times to try to get pigmentation homogeneous, but we have repeeled patients that have been peeled 5, 10, 15 years ago with no problems.

KOTLER: What is the maximum number of peels that you personally can attest to?

BAKER: I have never seen anybody have more than two. I think the results from the phenol peel are so permanent that they rarely need it for a long, long time.

KOTLER: What about intervals between peels?

BAKER: If I were to do spot peels, if I peel somebody and they get some blotching or some areas that did not take very well, I usually wait 3 or 4 months and then peel them again. As soon as all erythema is gone and the skin looks normal.

KOTLER: Can you give us an opinion on neck peels?

BAKER: I do not do them because the problems of hypertrophic scarring I have seen mostly have been in the neck. I have made a few exceptions. I have not had third degree losses but I have seen some from the lay operators and some that have been sent to me in which medical legal problems have been involved, so I just avoid the neck. They can, however, be peeled safely with TCA.

KOTLER: Could you describe postpeel management?

BAKER: Pain medication: Most of these people get along without a narcotic. If you get them through the first 6 or 8 hours, they will be all right.

KOTLER: Diet?

BAKER: I keep them on liquids until the mask is off, obviously. Then, as far as I am concerned, once the mask is off (if we use a mask) we let them have anything they want.

KOTLER: Do you routinely use a "recovery house"?

BAKER: As far as sending them to our recovery retreat, we send most of our patients there. I think that for the first day or two they need some encouragement and people to do things for them because often the eyes will swell shut. They need somebody to look after them.

KOTLER: Skin care after peel?

BAKER: Skin moisturizers? We use Crisco, we still use it—it is old fashioned, but it is pure vegetable oil and is excellent. As soon as the crust is all off we start them on that. If they have something else they want, fine. But with a perfumed product, they may have an allergic reaction. We prefer to keep it simple. I do not have any brand preferences. I do not use topical steroids initially. If they have prolonged erythema, I will put them on topical steroids.

KOTLER: How long is "prolonged erythema" in the ideal patient, for example?

BAKER: Eight or 9 weeks.

KOTLER: Do you use systemic antiinflammatories?

BAKER: I do not use antiinflammatories. Itching is a problem in probably 20% or 30% of the patients and I find there's three things that I tell them to do:
1. It happens almost always at night. I tell them to get out of bed and sit in a chair because the venous congestion in the face aggravates it.
2. I tell them to pack their face in ice, which gives temporary relief.
3. We use Temaril. It comes in a 2.5 mg size but they need to take more than that—5 or 7.5 mg. That with the ice and getting up usually will do it. The itching can last up to a week or 10 days, but usually if they will get on this routine it will clear up and it's never permanent.

KOTLER: Makeovers?

BAKER: I formerly used a personal makeup specialist in town. She was fantastic and I thought it was a good thing and I was recommending it.

KOTLER: What about the "rough skin" that appears in the second to third week?

BAKER: Some patients do exhibit this rough-to-the-touch skin that you describe. I do not know what it is but it disappears spontaneously.

KOTLER: Let's discuss complications.

BAKER: They are usually temporary—itching and burning or a pigmentation problem, primarily.

KOTLER: What about milia?

BAKER: Milia—aggravating but they go away.

KOTLER: Scarring?

BAKER: I have rarely seen hypertrophic scarring. And when you see it you have to treat it symptomatically. I had one case years ago and I still do not know why it happened. We have seen hypertrophic scarring, mostly along the mandibular line and on the upper lip, but I have not seen this in quite some time. I do not know why we do not see it much anymore, unless patient selection and management are better. It certainly is a possibility. We even have it on our consent form, we discuss it with the patient.

KOTLER: Is scarring more likely to occur with a more aggressive technique?

BAKER: I think so.

KOTLER: There is less tape occlusion now than years ago. Perhaps that is a factor?

BAKER: I think it is. I have not seen hypertrophic scarring in all areas of the face. I have never seen it on the forehead. And I have not seen it on the eyelids, on the lower or upper eyelids. I have seen it mostly along the mandibular border, just under the mandible and some in the perioral area.

KOTLER: Do you think it is related to movement? The most movable parts of the face are in the lower third.

BAKER: Seems logical. I have not seen a single hypertrophic scar or even a suggestion since we have gone to the Vaseline.

KOTLER: Depigmentation?

BAKER: As far as depigmentation, when you peel you do get some loss of pigment. I do not think there's much difference in occlusion or nonocclusion techniques, they still show some depigmentation. I tell every patient, "If you are going to get rid of your lines—whatever I do, dermabrasion or peels—you are going to lose some of your pigment. We hope it will not be very much, but it could be." I discuss this very thoroughly.

KOTLER: Any secrets about concealing the line of demarcation?

BAKER: I do not know how to decrease the line of demarcation. We talk about extending the peel beyond the tape, but now that we are not using the tape, I do not know how to do that.

KOTLER: Do you have suggestions for reversing hyperpigmentation?

BAKER: Hyperpigmentation is still a problem just like it is with dermabrasion. I just go back and peel again. The worst cases of hyperpigmentation I have seen have been people from Central and South America. I do not see it much in pure Caucasians.

I do not know how to prevent it except to tell them to stay out of the sun.

KOTLER: Do you prescribe a sun screen routinely? Without PABA?

BAKER: I do not avoid PABA. I go into a thorough discussion about sun screens. I think anything 15 SPF or better is enough, but many of my patients are tennis players and golfers and I try to get them to use water soluble or invisible sun screens. If they want a makeup base, Clinique's Continuous Coverage is very good. It is very heavy and it stays in place. Johnson & Johnson makes Sundowner 15 which is very good; you can just put it on like after shave lotion and you cannot tell it is there.

KOTLER: Do you advise patients to stop female hormones?

BAKER: I do not advise patients to get off their female hormones.

KOTLER: Infection?

BAKER: I have never seen an infection. Undoubtedly there is surface contamination, but I have never seen an infection. I do give patients antibiotics, I guess as much for my own peace of mind as much as anything. We put them on Keflex.

KOTLER: For how long?

BAKER: One day before and 4 days after. I cannot prove it is bad or good.

KOTLER: I have cultured the exudate at mask removal. It had multiple contaminants.

BAKER: Yes. I have done that too. But they do not get systemic shock.

There was a case locally at a lay clinic. A peel patient developed a fever a day or two after her peel and she started feeling poorly. She got worse but was sent home. They did not do anything about it. She developed subacute bacterial endocarditis and died.

KOTLER: How do you prevent herpetic outbreaks?

BAKER: We put patients on Zovirax—if they develop the eruption—both topically and internally. About 5% or 10% of the patients who have peels will get herpes, so I think if you put everybody on it, prophylactically, I do not think you can be faulted for that.

KOTLER: Actually, that's what we have been doing for about the last 3 years. The patient starts the day before and we keep them on it for 10 days.

BAKER: Have you ever seen anybody develop herpes after they have been on it?

KOTLER: Since routinely using Zovirax, I've seen only one very minor outbreak—a small area on the lip. However, I certainly had seen several, which were very extensive, prior to Zovirax.

KOTLER: What do you do for milia?

BAKER: Most of the time they will go away. And then an occasional patient I bring in and put under magnification and pop some of them. Usually, it is just a matter of patients riding it out.

KOTLER: Persistent erythema?

BAKER: I have seen perhaps a half dozen cases and it lasted up to a year. And I have no miracle cures. We try antiinflammatory agents, topical steroids, and systematic treatment. I have never seen it persist ad infinitum. I have seen it last a long time.

KOTLER: Has anybody demonstrated increased hair growth?

BAKER: When you do a perioral peel, often it appears that there is more hair on the upper lip. I think that is probably just because the patient is not washing regularly to take care of it. It is hard for me to believe that it would promote hair growth. I have not had anyone come back and complain about it, but I have noticed that myself. Some patients, 8 or 10 weeks afterward, see a little hair growth on the upper lip and want to know when they can use a depilatory. It can be used after the erythema disappears.

KOTLER: Postpeel acne?

BAKER: As far as an acnelike condition, I have seen a rare case that develops some breaking out of the skin later on and we just treat it like acne. We prescribe tetracycline and regular skin care.

KOTLER: Do you use Retin-A as a pretreatment?

BAKER: I do not always use it, but it is probably a good routine if TCA is to be used. I think it is critical to prepare the skin with Retin-A for 4 to 6 weeks.

KOTLER: Do you use Retin-A after a phenol peel?

BAKER: A patient could start using it again when the erythema is gone.

KOTLER: Do you have an opinion on alpha-hydroxy acids as peeling agents?

BAKER: I have not had any experience with alpha-hydroxy acids. I think that people like you and me and others who are doing a fair amount of peeling are now looking at more than just a single-peel technique. I think there is going to be a lot more TCA used. I think we have put it on the back shelf for a long time. I am happy with it, but it is not in the same league as phenol. I believe if we all put our heads together, with histologic and some well-controlled studies, researching a variety of techniques, strengths, and methods, we can come up with something that really will be valuable to our colleagues.

KOTLER: Now that there is acceptance of the peel as a process and there is more public awareness, I think we probably have to offer a greater menu.

BAKER: Yes, I think we have a menu. We now can use Retin-A and TCA and we can use some of the other peeling agents. We can use phenol without a mask and we can use phenol with the mask.

We can now look at our patients and have four or five modalities we can use for different kinds of skin.

KOTLER: Thank you for sharing your enormous experience with our colleagues.

BAKER: My pleasure.

References

1. Alt TH: Complications of chemical peeling easily avoided by careful administration, *Dermatol Times* 16:990-991, Nov 1981.
2. Alt TH: Occluded Baker-Gordon chemical peel: review and update, *J Dermatol Surg Oncol* 15:9, Sept 1989.
3. Ariagno RP, Briggs DR: Chemexfoliation as an adjunct to facial rejuvenation, *Trans Am Acad Ophthalmol Otol* 80:536-539, 1975.
4. Aronsohn RB: Facial chemosurgery, *Eye Ear Nose Throat Monthly* 50:20-27, 1971.
5. Aronsohn RB: Complications of chemosurgery, *Eye Ear Nose Throat Monthly* 51:48-56, 1972.
6. Aronsohn RB: Hand chemosurgery, *Am J Cosmetic Surg* 1(3):24-28, 1984.
7. Asken S: Unoccluded Baker-Gordon phenol peels—review and update, *J Dermatol Surg Oncol* 15(9):999, Sept 1989.
8. Ayres S: Dermal changes following application of chemical cauterants to aging skin, *Arch Dermatol* 82:578-585, 1960.
9. Ayres S: Superficial chemosurgery in treating aging skin, *Arch Dermatol* 85:385-393, 1962.
10. Ayres S: Superficial chemosurgery, *Arch Dermatol* 89:395-403, 1964.
11. Baker TJ: Video tape discussion on chemical skin peeling. In Goulian DM, Courtiss E, editors: *Symposium on surgery of the aging face*, St Louis, 1978, Mosby–Year Book.
12. Baker TJ: Chemical peel. In Courtiss EH, editor: *Male aesthetic surgery*, St Louis, 1982, Mosby–Year Book.
13. Baker TJ, Gordon HL: Chemical face peeling and rhytidectomy, *Plast Reconstr Surg* 29(2):199-206, 1962.
14. Baker TJ, Gordon HL: Chemical face peeling and dermabrasion, *Surg Clin North Am* 51(2):387-401, 1971.
15. Baker TJ, Gordon HL: Chemical peeling as a practical method of removing rhytides of upper lip, *Ann Plast Surg* 2:209-212, 1979.
16. Baker TJ, Gordon HL, Mosienko P: Chemical peel. In Courtiss EH, editor: *Aesthetic surgery trouble: how to avoid it and how to treat it*, St Louis, 1978, Mosby–Year Book.
17. Baker TJ, Gordon HL, Seckinger DL: A second look at chemical face peeling, *Plast Reconstr Surg* 37(6):487-493, 1966.
18. Baker TJ, Gordon HL, Mosienko P, Seckinger DL: Long-term histological study of skin after chemical face peeling, *Plast Reconstr Surg* 53(5):522-525, 1974.
19. Balin A, Pratt L: Physiological consequences of human skin aging, *Cutis* 43:431-436, 1989.
20. Batstone JH, Millard DR: An endorsement of facial chemosurgery, *Br J Plast Surg* 21:193-199, 1968.
21. Beeson WH, McCollough EG: Chemical face peeling without taping, *J Dermatol Surg Oncol* 11(10):985-990, 1985.
22. Behin F, Fuerstein SS, Marovitz S, Arch WF: Comparative histological study of mini pig skin after chemical peel and dermabrasion, *Arch Otolaryngol* 103:271-277, 1977.
23. Botta S, Straith R, Goodwin H: Cardiac arrhythmias in phenol face peeling, a suggested protocol for prevention, *Aesth Plast Surg* 12:115-117, 1988.
24. Brodland DG, Cullimore KC, Roenigk RK, Gibson LE: Depths of chemexfoliation induced by various concentrations and application techniques of trichloroacetic acid in a porcine model, *J Dermatol Surg Oncol* 15(9):967-71, 1989.

25. Brodland DG, Roenick RK: Chemexfoliation for actinic keratoses, *Mayo Clin Proc* 63:887-896, 1988.
26. Brody HJ: Medium depth peel achieved with CO_2/TCA, *Dermatol News*, May 1986.
27. Brody HJ: Complications of chemical peeling, *J Dermatol Surg Oncol* 15(9):1010-1019, Sept 1989.
28. Brody HJ: The art of chemical peeling, *J Dermatol Surg Oncol* 15(9):918, Sept 1989.
29. Brody HJ: Variations and comparisons in medium-depth chemical peeling, *J Dermatol Surg Oncol* 15(9):953, 1989.
30. Brody HJ, Hailey CW: Medium-depth chemical peeling of the skin, *J Dermatol Surg Oncol* 12(12):1268-1275, 1986.
31. Brown A, Kaplan L, Brown M: Cutaneous alterations induced by phenols: a histological bio-assay, *J Int Coll Surg* 34:602, 1960.
32. Brown AM, Kaplan LM, Brown ME: Phenol-induced histological skin changes: hazards, technique and uses, *Br J Plast Surg* 13:158-169, 1960.
33. Burks JW: Dermabrasion and chemical skin peeling, Springfield, IL, 1979, Charles C Thomas.
34. Collins PS: Trichloroacetic acid peels revisited, *J Dermatol Surg Oncol* 15(9):933-937, Sept 1989.
35. Collins PS: The chemical peel, *Clin Dermatol* 5(4):57-73, 1987.
36. Collins PS, Farber GA, et al: Superficial repetitive chemosurgery of the hands, *J Dermatol Surg Oncol* 11:22-24, Oct 1985.
37. Combes FC, Sperber PA, Reisch M: Dermal defects; treatment by a chemical agent, *NY Physician Am Med* 56:36, Aug 1960.
38. Deichmann WB, Keplinger ML: Phenols and phenolic compounds. In Clayton GD, Clayton FE, editors: *Patty's industrial hygiene and toxicology*, ed 3, New York, 1981, John Wiley.
39. Deichmann WB, Schafer L: *Phenol studies*, Kettering Laboratory of Applied Physiology, pp 129-143.
40. Deichmann WB, Witherup S: Phenol studies: acute and comparative toxicity of phenol and O-, M-, and P-cresols for experimental animals, *J Pharmacol Exp Ther* 80:233, Mar 1944.
41. Del Pizzo A, Tanski E: Chemical face peeling—malignant therapy for benign disease? *Plast Reconstr Surg* 66(1):122-123, 1980.
42. Dmytryshyn JR, Gribble MJ, Kassen BO: Chemical face peel complicated by toxic shock syndrome, *Arch Otolaryngol* 109:170-173, 1983.
43. Duffy D: Informed consent for chemical peels and dermabrasion, Dermatologic Therapy II, *Dermatol Clin* 7(1):183-185, 1989.
44. Duffy DM: Tattoo not removal method determines final outcome, *Dermatol News*, May 1986, p 19.
45. Eller JJ, Wolf S: Skin peeling and scarification, *JAMA* 116(10):934-938, 1941.
46. Farber G: Chemical peeling. In Burks J, editor: *Dermabrasion and chemical peel*, Springfield, IL, 1979, Charles C Thomas.
47. Farber G, Collins PS, Wilhelmus SM: Update on chemical peel, *J Dermatol Surg Oncol* 10(7):559-560, 1984.
48. Fredericks S: Chemical peel. In Kaye BL, Gradinger GB, editors: *Symposium on problems and complications in plastic surgery of the face*, St Louis, 1984, Mosby–Year Book.
49. Goldman PM, Freed MI: Aesthetic problems in chemical peeling, *J Dermatol Surg Oncol* 15(9):1020-1024, Sept 1989.
50. Goulian DM, Courtiss E, editors: *Symposium on surgery of the aging face, videotape discussion: chemical peel procedure*, St Louis, 1978, Mosby–Year Book.
51. Gross BG: Cardiac arrhythmias during phenol face peeling, *Plast Reconstr Surg* 73(4):590-594, 1984.
52. Gross BG, Maschek F: Phenol chemosurgery for removal of deep facial wrinkles, *Int J Dermatol* 19:159-164, 1980.
53. Hanke CW, Balin PL: Current trends in the practice of dermatologic surgery, *J Dermatol Surg Oncol* 16:2, Feb 1990.
54. Hayes DK, Berkland ME, Stambaugh KI: Dermal healing after local skin flaps and chemical peel, *Arch Otolaryngol Head Neck Surg* 116:794, 1990.
55. Holzberg M, et al: The Ehlers-Danlos syndrome, recognition, characterization and importance of a milder variant of the classic form, *J Am Acad Dermatol* 19:656-666, 1988.
56. Horvath PN: The light peel, *Bull Assoc Milit Dermatol* 18:5, 1970.
57. Klein DR, Little JH: Laryngeal edema as a complication of chemical peel, *Plast Reconstr Surg* 71:419-420, 1983.
58. Kligman AM, Baker TJ, Gordon HL: Long-term histologic follow-up of phenol face peels, *Plast Reconstr Surg* 75(5):652-659, 1985.
59. Kligman AM, Leyden JJ, Kligman LH, et al: Retinoic acid is said to reverse aging effects, *Dermatol News* 18(10):1-10, 1985.
60. Kligman AW, Willis I: A new formula for depigmenting human skin, depigmenting human skin, *Arch Dermatol* 3:40-48, 1975.

61. Koopman CF: Phenol toxicity during face peels, *Otolaryngol Head Neck Surg* 90:383-384, 1982.
62. Korcok M: Untoward effect of a face peel: toxic shock syndrome, *Med News* 248(1):23, 1982.
63. Kotler R: Phenol peeling. In Parish L, Lask G: *Aesthetic dermatology,* New York, 1990, McGraw-Hill.
64. Letessier S: Chemical peel with resorcin. In Roenig RK, Roenig HH, editors: *Dermatologic surgery: principles and practice,* New York, 1988, Marcel Dekker.
65. Litton C: Chemical face lifting, *Plast Reconstr Surg* 29(4):371-380, 1962.
66. Litton C: Observations after chemosurgery of the face, *Plast Reconstr Surg* 32(5):554-556, 1963.
67. Litton C, Fournier P, Capinpin A: A survey of chemical peeling of the face, *Plast Reconstr Surg* 51(6):645-647, 1973.
68. Litton C, Szachowicz EH, Trinidad GP: Present day status of the chemical face peel, *Aesthetic Plast Surg* 10(1):1-6, 1986.
69. Litton C, Trinidad G: Complications of chemical face peeling as evaluated by a questionnaire, *Plast Reconstr Surg* 67(6):738-743, 1981.
70. Lober CW: Chemexfoliation—indications and cautions, *J Am Acad Dermatol* 17(1):109-112, 1987.
71. Lorincz A: Chemexfoliation. In Putterman AM, editor: Cosmetic oculoplastic surgery, New York, 1982, Grune & Stratton.
72. Lotter AM: Human pigment factors relative to chemical face peeling, *Ann Plast Surg* 3(3):231-240, 1979.
73. LoVerme WE, Drapkin MS, Courtiss EH, et al: Toxic shock syndrome after chemical face peel, *Plast Reconstr Surg* 80(1):115-118, 1987.
74. MacKee GM, Karp FL: The treatment of post-acne scars with phenol, *J Dermatol* 64:456-459, 1952.
75. Mandy SH: Tretinoin preoperative and postoperative management of dermabrasion, *J Am Acad Dermatol* 15:878-879, 1986.
76. Matarasso SL, Glogau RC: Chemical face peels, *Dermatol Clin* 9:1, Jan 1991.
77. McCollough EG, Beeson WH: Chemical peel—aesthetic surgery of the aging face (some material taken from McCollough EG, Hillman RA: Chemical face peel), *Otolaryngol Clin North Am* 13(353):182-212, 1980.
78. McCollough E, Gaylon E, Hillman R: Chemical face peel, symposium on the aging face, *Otolaryngol Clin North Am* 13(2):353-365, 1980.
79. McCollough EG, Langsdon PR: *Dermabrasion and chemical peel—a guide for plastic surgeons,* New York, 1988, Thieme Medical Publishers.
80. Monheit GD: The Jessner's + TCA peel: a medium-depth chemical peel, *J Dermatol Surg Oncol* 15(9):949-950, Sept 1989.
81. Montagna W, Carlisle K, Kirchner S: Epidermal and dermal histological markers of photodamaged human facial skin, Shelton, CT, 1988, Richardson-Vicks.
82. Mosienko P, Baker TJ: Chemical peel, *Clin Plast Surg* 5(1):79-96, 1978.
83. Mullins JF, Lettieri MF: Chemosurgery of facial wrinkles, *Tex Med* 59:488-495, 1963.
84. Murad H: Use of AHAs add new dimensions to chemical peeling, *Cosmetic Dermatol* 3(5):32-34, May 1990.
85. Murad H: Something old, something new: the story of alpha-hydroxy acids, personal communication.
86. Pascher F: Systemic reactions to topically applied drugs, *Bull NY Acad Med* 59:613-619, 1973.
87. Price NM: EKG changes in relationship to the chemical peel, *J Dermatol Surg Oncol* 16:1, Jan 1990.
88. Rae V, Falanga V: Wrinkling due to middermal elastolysis, *Arch Dermatol* 125:950-951, 1989.
89. Resnik SS: Chemical peeling with trichloroacetic acid, *J Dermatol Surg Oncol* 10(7):549-550, 1984.
90. Resnik SS, Lewis LA: The cosmetic uses of trichloroacetic acid peeling in dermatology, *South Med J* 66(2):225-227, 1973.
91. Resnik SS, Lewis LA, Cohen BH: Trichloroacetic acid peeling, *Cutis* 17:127-129, 1976.
92. Sperber PA: Chemexfoliation: a new term in cosmetic surgery, *J Am Geriatr Soc* 11:58-62, 1963.
93. Sperber PA: Chemexfoliation in the aging skin, J Med Assoc Ala 33(5):121-130, 1963.
94. Sperber PA: Chemexfoliation in treatment of acne scarring, *Tex State J Med* 59:496-501, 1963.
95. Sperber PA: Chemexfoliation and silicone infiltration in treatment of aging skin and dermal defects, *J Am Geriatr Soc* 12:594-601, 1964.
96. Sperber PA: Chemexfoliation for aging skin and acne scarring, *Arch Otolaryngol* 81:278-283, 1965.
97. Sperber PA: *Treatment of the aging skin and dermal defects,* Springfield, IL, 1965, Charles C Thomas.

98. Spinowitz AL, Rumsfield J: Stability-time profile of trichloroacetic acid at various concentrations and storage, *J Dermatol Surg Oncol* 15:9, Sept 1989.
99. Spira M, Dahl C, Freeman R, et al: Chemosurgery—a histological study, *Plast Reconstr Surg* 45(3):247-253, 1970.
100. Spira M, Gerow F, Hardy SB: Complications of chemical face peeling, *Plast Reconstr Surg* 54(4):397-403, 1974.
101. Stagnone JJ: Superficial peeling, *J Dermatol Surg Oncol* 15(9):924-929, Sept 1989.
102. Stagnone JJ, Gregory J: A second look at chemabrasion, *J Dermatol Surg Oncol* 8(8):701-705, 1982.
103. Stagnone GJ, Orgel MG, Stagnone JJ: Cardiovascular effects of topical 50% trichloroacetic acid and Baker's phenol solution, *J Dermatol Surg Oncol* 13:999-1002, 1987.
104. Stegman SJ: A study of dermabrasion and chemical peels in an animal model, *J Dermatol Surg Oncol* 6:490-497, 1980.
105. Stegman S: A comparative histologic study of the effects of three peeling agents and dermabrasion on normal and sundamaged skin, *Aesth Plast Surg* 6:123-135, 1982.
106. Stegman SJ: Letter to the editor, *J Dermatol Surg Oncol* 12:5, May 1986.
107. Stegman SJ: Medium-depth chemical peeling: digging beneath the surface, *J Dermatol Surg Oncol* 12(12):1245-1246, 1986.
108. Stegman SJ, Tromovitch TA: *Cosmetic dermatologic surgery*, St Louis, 1984, Mosby–Year Book.
109. Stegman SJ, Tromovitch TA, Glogau RC: *Cosmetic dermatologic surgery*, ed 2, St Louis, 1990, Mosby–Year Book.
110. Stough DB: The chemical face peel, presented at the 16th annual meeting of the North American Clinical Dermatology Society, 18:239-240, 1976.
111. Stough DB, Irwin WG: Chemical peel for facial wrinkles, *Am Family Physician* 10(6):106-108, 1974.
112. Stuzin J, Baker TJ, Gordon HL: Chemical peel: a change in the routine, *Ann Plast Surg* 23:166, 1989.
113. Swinehart JM: Test spots in dermabrasion and chemical peeling, *J Dermatol Surg Oncol* 16(6):557-563, June 1990.
114. Truppman ES, Ellenby JD: Major electrocardiographic changes during chemical face peeling, *Plast Reconstr Surg* 63(1):44-48, 1979.
115. Urkov J: Surface defects of skin: treatment by controlled exfoliation, *Ill Med J*, pp 75-81, 1946.
116. Van Scott EJ, Yu RJ: Hyperkeratinization, corneocyte cohesion and alpha-hydroxy acids, *J Am Acad Dermatol* 11:867-879, 1984.
117. Warner MA, Harper JV: Cardiac dysrhythmias associated with chemical peeling with phenol, *Anesthesiology* 62(3):316-367, 1985.
118. Wexler MR, Halon DA, Teitelbaum A, et al: The prevention of cardiac arrhythmias produced in an animal model by the topical application of a phenol preparation in common use for face peeling, *Plast Reconstr Surg* 73(4):595-598, 1984.
119. Wolfe SA: Chemical face peeling following therapeutic irradiation, *Plast Reconstr Surg* 69(5):859-862, 1982.
120. Wolfert FG, Dalton WE, Hoopes JE: Chemical peel with trichloroacetic acid, *Br J Plast Surg* 25:333-334, 1972.
121. Woodley DT, et al: Treatment of photoaged skin with topical tretinoin increases epidermal-dermal anchoring fibrils, a preliminary report, *JAMA* 263(22): 3057-3059, June 1990.

Index

A

Acetaminophen, 127
  with codeine, 127
Acid treatment, history of, 31
Acne scarring, 71
  treatment of, history of, 31
Acneiform dermatitis, 218
  after chemical rejuvenation, 175
Acyclovir, 127, 173, 174, 218
Aftercare
  for first 5 days, 126-127
  for first 48 hours, 120-135
Aggressive facial rejuvenation, complications of, 152-154
Alpha streptococci, 126
Alpha-hydroxy acids as peeling agents, 67-70, 219
Anesthesia, 96-99, 213
  field block, 97
  need for, 86
  technique for, 98
Anesthesiologist, 96-99, 213
Antihistamines for itching, 176
Antiinflammatory agents, 215
Aquanil lotion, 175
Arrhythmias, cardiac, 138-139, 214
Aspirin, 127
  for itching and burning, 176
Atrophy of skin complicating chemical rejuvenation, 139

B

Bactoban, 120, 123
Baker, Thomas J., 32-33
  discussion with, 210-219
Baker formula phenol peeling solution, 103-104
  and dermabrasion, skin treated with, compared to sun-damaged skin, 58-59
Baker-Gordon phenol solution, 103-104
Bames, H.O., 16-18
Betamethasone for scarring, 141, 144
Bleach cream for hyperpigmentation, 158
Blepharoplasty and face lift combined with chemical peel, 79
Break time between chemical applications, 105, 106, 108
Bupivacaine hydrochloride for anesthesia, 97, 213
Burning after chemical rejuvenation, 176

C

Carbolic acid; *see* Phenol
Carbon dioxide/trichloroacetic acid combination as peeling agent, 66
Cardiac arrhythmias, 138-139, 214
Cetaphil lotion, 175
Cheeks, chemical application to, 108
Chemabrasion; *see* Chemical rejuvenation
Chemexfoliation, TCA, 62-64
Chemical application, 101-109, 204
Chemical face lifting; *see* Chemical rejuvenation
Chemical peel
  blepharoplasty and face lift combined with, 79
  histology of, 51-59
Chemical rejuvenation
  aftercare for next 4 days after, 126-127
  aggressive, complications of, 152-154

225

Chemical rejuvenation—cont'd
  appearance 1 week after, 128-129
  appearance 24 hours after, 121
  chemical application in, 101-109, 204
  clinical correlations of, 54-55
  combined with surgery, 136-137
  complications of, 136-179
  contraindications to, 80
  culture of exudate 48 hours after, 126
  excellent candidate for, 48
  facial cosmetic surgery combined with, 51
  facts about, 90
  follow-up after, 207
  growth in use of, 42
  histology of, 51-59
  historical investigations on, 53-54
  historical review of, 1-39
  ideal candidate for, 43-47, 50, 71, 72
  indications for, 71-95
  information about, 86-90
  long-term skin care after, 130-135
  marking of face before, 100, 101
  mask removal after, 205
  in men, 194-201
  of neck and chest, 186-192, 214-215
  occlusive dressings applied during, 204
  order of treatment in, 104-105
  overview of, 41-51
  patient selection for, 71-95, 212-213
  "perfect" candidate for, 49
  physiology of, 41
  poor candidates for, 71, 74
  postoperative facial skin care and cosmetic tips, 132-135
  postpeel management, 215
  preoperative preparation for, 100-101, 203
  procedure for, 100-119
  results of, 208-209
  retaping of wrinkled areas after, 206
  skin care after, 128
  step-by-step technique for, 202-209
Chemosurgery; see Skin peeling
Chest and neck peels, 186-192
Cleocin, 175
Cleopatra VII, 3-4
Cloxacillin for toxic shock, 174
Collagen disease, peeling patient with, 212
Color disparity with male skin peeling, 200-201
Complications, 136-179
Conjunctiva, application of peel solution onto, 105-106
Consent to treatment, 93-94
  consultation and, 81-95
Consultation
  and informed consent, 81-95

Consultation—cont'd
  preoperative, 92
Continuous Coverage, 217
Cooley, Arnold J., 10-12
Cordran tape, 142
Cornea, application of peel solution onto, 105-106
Corticosteroids
  for itching, 176
  for scarring, 141
Cosmetic surgery, facial, combined with chemical rejuvenation, 51
Cosmetics, use of
  after chemical rejuvenation, 132-135
  historical review of, 2-7
Crisco, 215
Croton oil added to phenol, 62, 210, 211
Crusting after chemical rejuvenation, 126, 127
Culture of exudate after peel, 126, 217
Cysts, inclusion; see Milia

D

Dark circles under eyes, peeling for, 212
Dark nevi, emergence of, after chemical rejuvenation, 176, 177
"Deep peel," face immediately after mask removal after, 123
Degreasing of skin before surgery, 100-101, 102
Demarcation, line of; see Line of demarcation
Depigmentation after chemical rejuvenation, 216-217
Dermabrasion
  and Baker's formula, skin treated with, compared to sun-damaged skin, 58-59
  history of, 28-29
"Dermal scar," 53
Dermatitis, acneiform, after chemical rejuvenation, 175, 218
Diabetes, patient with, 211
Diazepam, 213
Dioscorides, Pedanius, 4, 7
Diphtheroids, 126
Diprolene; see Betamethasone
Dressing
  occlusive, application of, 114-119
  removal of, and aftercare for first 48 hours, 120-135

E

Eczema, peeling patient with, 212
EES, 175
Egypt, ancient, skin rejuvenation in, 2-3

Eller, Joseph J., 18-19
Enterobacter species, 126
Epidermis, sun-damaged, 51, 54
Eruptions, herpetic, after chemical rejuvenation, 173-174, 217-218
Erymax solution or gel, 175
Erythema, prolonged, 215, 218
Erythromycin, 127
Exodermology; *see* Chemical rejuvenation
Exudate, culture of, after peel, 126, 217
Eyelid, lower, peeling technique for, 106
Eyes, dark circles under, peeling for, 212

F

Face
  chemical rejuvenation of, historical review of, 1-39
  cosmetic surgery of, combined with chemical rejuvenation, 51, 136-137
Face block, local anesthesia, 97
  sites for, 99
Face lift and blepharoplasty combined with chemical peel, 79
Face lifting
  chemical; *see* Chemical rejuvenation
  in history, 31
Face peel, phenol, history of, 8-33; *see also* Chemical rejuvenation
Facial rejuvenation; *see* Chemical rejuvenation
Facial rejuvenation patient questionnaire, 75
Female hormones, 217
Fentanyl, 213
"Fibrosis," 53
Field block anesthesia, 97
"Flushing" after chemical skin peeling, 45
Forehead, chemical application to, 104-105
Forehead hairline, carrying chemical application to, 104, 105
Fox, Tillbury, 12
"Frost," 103

G

Galen, 4, 5
General anesthesia, operating room for, 98
Gordon, Howard L., 32-33
Granular skin after chemical rejuvenation, 155-157, 216
Greece, ancient, skin rejuvenation in, 3

H

Hairline, chemical application beyond, 104, 105
Heart
  arrhythmias of, 138-139, 214

Heart—cont'd
  monitoring of, during chemical rejuvenation, 97, 100
Hebra, Ferdinand, 9-10
Herpes simplex after chemical rejuvenation, 173
Herpetic eruptions after chemical rejuvenation, 173-174, 217-218
Hirsutism after chemical rejuvenation, 179, 218
Histology of chemical peels, 51-59
Hi-Tape, 119
Hormones, female, 217
Hydrocortisone in bleach cream, 158
Hydrocortisone ointment, 128, 130
Hydroquinone in bleach cream, 158
Hyperpigmentation
  postinflammatory, 160-162
  postpeel, 76, 158
  reversal of, 217
  treatment for, 163-164
Hypertrophic scarring after chemical rejuvenation, 141-142, 147-148, 150-151, 152-154, 216

I

Inclusion cysts; *see* Milia
Infection
  after chemical rejuvenation, 173-174, 217
  herpetic, 217-218
  pyogenic, after chemical rejuvenation, 174
Informed consent, consultation and, 81-95
Itching after chemical rejuvenation, 128, 176, 215

J

Jessner's solution as peeling agent, 64-76
  on neck and chest, 186
Jessner's/trichloroacetic acid combination as peeling agent, 65

K

Karp, Florentine L., 23-28
Klebsiella species, 126
Klingman bleach cream, 157, 158, 160
Kromayer, Ernst, 29

L

Lacticare HC, 155
Letessier's modification of Unna's paste as peeling agent, 67
Line of demarcation, 100, 101, 158-168, 217
  difference in, 165

228 INDEX

Line of demarcation—cont'd
　inconcealable, 166
　minimizing, 167-168
　obvious, 166
　placement of, 165
Local anesthesia face block, 97
　sites for, 99
Lower eyelid peeling technique, 106

M

MacKee, George Miller, 14, 15, 21-26
Marcaine; see Bupivacaine hydrochloride
Marking of face before surgery, 100, 101
Mask removal, 122, 205
　appearance immediately after, 123
　drying skin after, 120, 124
　supplies and equipment for, 121
Medrol Dose Pak, 128
Men, facial peeling in, 194-201, 212
Meperidine, 213
Methadone, 127
Middle Ages, cosmetic use in, 6-7
Milia after chemical rejuvenation, 130, 178, 218
Minocin, 175
Monitoring, heart, during chemical rejuvenation, 97, 100
Montgomery, Douglass W., 14-16
Mouth, retaping around, 120, 124

N

Narcotics, premedication with, 96-97
Neck, swelling of, 125
Neck and chest peels, 186-192, 214-215
Nevi, dark, emergence of, after chemical rejuvenation, 176, 177
Nonsteroidal antiinflammatory agents, 127, 128
　for itching and burning, 176
Nose area, chemical application to, 105

O

Occlusion, tape, 118, 119, 214
Occlusive dressing
　application of, 114-119, 204
　removal of, 120
Omniderm, 214
Operating room, 98
Orbital area, chemical application to, 105-106

P

Patch testing, 77-79, 213
Peeling
　perioral, 109
　skin; see Chemical rejuvenation

Peeling—cont'd
　spot, and retaping, 120
Peeling agents, 60-70
Peeling solution, phenol, Baker formula, 103-104
Peeling technique, lower eyelid, 106
Penicillin for toxic shock, 174
Perioral peeling, 109
Persistent erythema, 218
Persistent redness after chemical rejuvenation, 169, 170, 172
Petrolatum over surgical area, 119, 216
Phenol
　and cardiac arrhythmias, 138-139
　croton oil added to, 62
　dilution of, 61
　discovery of, 2
　as peeling agent, 60-62
　septisol added to, 62
　toxicity of, 61-62, 105
Phenol face peel, history of, 8-33
Phenol peeling solution
　Baker formula, 103-104
　Baker-Gordon, 103-104
Phenol-induced changes in skin, historical studies of, 53-54
Photoaging, skin signs of, 51
Photographic record, 81-83
Piffard, Henry G., 12
Pigmentation
　change in, after chemical rejuvenation, 158-168
　irregular, after chemical rejuvenation, 159
　problems with, after chemical rejuvenation, 130
Pliny the Elder, 4-5
Polano, M.K., 18
Polysporin ointment, 126
Postinflammatory hyperpigmentation, 160-162
Postpeel hyperpigmentation, 76
Postpeel take-home kit, 127
Preoperative consultation, 93-94
Preoperative consultation report, 91
Preoperative instructions, 95
Pretreatment use of retinoic acid, 81
Pruritus after chemical rejuvenation, 174
Pseudomonas aeruginosa, 126
Purpose soap, 175
Pyogenic infections after chemical rejuvenation, 174

Q

Questions answered, 88-89

R

Radiation, previous, peeling of patient after, 211-212
Rayer, Pierre, 8-9
Redness, persistent, after chemical rejuvenation, 169, 170, 172
Rejuvenation, chemical; *see* Chemical rejuvenation
Rejuvenation work sheet, 110-113
Repeeling, 180-185, 214
Resorcin as peeling agent, 67
Retaping
   of deeply wrinkled areas, 206
   spot peeling and, 120
Retin-A as pretreatment, 218
Retinoic acid
   in bleach cream, 158
   pretreatment use of, 81
Rome, classical, skin rejuvenation in, 3-5
Runge, Friedlich Ferdinand, 8

S

Saalfeld, Edmund, 13-14
Salonpas, 118, 119, 120
Sanding of face, history of, 31
Scarring
   acne, 71
      treatment of, history of, 31
   after chemical rejuvenation, 139-154, 216
   unusual, 149
Sedatives, premedication with, 96-97
Septisol added to phenol, 62
Shock, toxic, after chemical rejuvenation, 174-175
Sites for local anesthesia face block, 99
Skin
   atrophy of, complicating chemical rejuvenation, 139
   drying, after mask removal, 120, 124
   granular, after chemical rejuvenation, 155-157, 216
   long-term care of, after chemical rejuvenation, 130-135
   normal and sun-damaged, comparison of, 56-57
   phenol-induced changes in, historical studies of, 53-54
   sun-damaged, skin treated with phenol Baker's formula and dermabrasion and, comparison of, 58-59
Skip areas, 106, 107
Soap added to phenol, 211
Spot peels, 214-215
   and retaping, 120
Staphylococcus, 126

Steroids for scarring, 141-142
"Stratum papillare," 53
Streptococci, alpha, 126
Sun exposure after chemical rejuvenation, 158, 160
Sun-damaged skin, 51, 54
   normal and, comparison of, 56-57
   skin treated with phenol Baker's formula and dermabrasion and, comparison of, 58-59
Sundowner 15, 217
Sunscreen, 217
Surgery, cosmetic, facial, combined with chemical rejuvenation, 51, 136-137

T

Tape, reapplication of, 124
Tape dressings, removal of, 120
Tape occlusion, 118, 119
TCA; *see* Trichloroacetic acid
Telangiectasia after chemical rejuvenation, 169, 171
Temaril for itching, 128, 215
Texture change after chemical rejuvenation, 155-158, 216
Toxic shock syndrome after chemical rejuvenation, 174
Treatment, consent to, 93-94
Triamcinolone
   in bleach cream, 158
   for scarring, 142
Trichloroacetic acid
   as peeling agent, 62-64
   pretreatment with, 101-102, 103
   various combinations of, for skin peeling, 62
Trichloroacetic acid/carbon dioxide combination as peeling agent, 66
Trichloroacetic acid/Jessner's combination as peeling agent, 65
TS solution or gel, 175

U

Unna's paste, Letessier's modification of, as peeling agent, 67
Urkov, Joseph C., 19-21

V

Valium; *see* Diazepam
Versed, 213

W

Willam, Robert, 8
Winter, L., 21
Wolff, Shirley, 18-19
Work sheet, rejuvenation, 110-113

Wrinkling
  persistent, repeeling for, 181-183
  premature, ideal candidate for chemical skin peeling to remove, 50
  retaping for, 206

Wrinkling—cont'd
  treatment of, history of, 30

Z

Zovirax; *see* Acyclovir